THE LOW BACK and PELVIS

Clinical Applications

A.L. LOGAN SERIES IN CHIROPRACTIC TECHNIQUE

The Knee: Clinical Applications
The Foot and Ankle: Clinical Applications
The Low Back and Pelvis: Clinical Applications

THE LOW BACK and PELVIS
Clinical Applications

A.L. Logan Series in Chiropractic Technique

Chris J. Hutcheson

With a contribution by
Joseph W. Howe

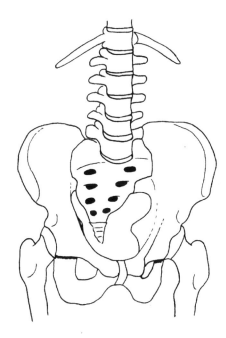

Chris J. Hutcheson, DC
Private Practice
Auburn, California

and

Joseph W. Howe, DC, DACBR, FICC
Professor of Radiology
Los Angeles College of Chiropractic
Private Practice of Radiology
Los Angeles and Sylmar, California

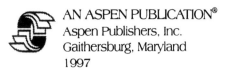

AN ASPEN PUBLICATION®
Aspen Publishers, Inc.
Gaithersburg, Maryland
1997

Library of Congress Cataloging-in-Publication Data

Hutcheson, Chris J.
The low back and pelvis: clinical applications/Chris J. Hutcheson; with a contribution by Joseph W. Howe.
p.   cm.—(A.L. Logan series in chiropractic technique)
Includes bibliographical references and index.
ISBN 0-8342-0689-7
1. Spine—Diseases—Chiropractic treatment. 2. Pelvis—Diseases—Chiropractic treatment.
I. Howe, Joseph W. II. Title. III. Series.
[DNLM: 1. Spinal Diseases—therapy. 2. Lumbosacral Region. 3. Chiropractic—methods. WE 725 H973L 1996]
RZ265.S64H88 1996
617.5'606—dc20
DNLM/DLC
for Library of Congress
96-26305
CIP

Orders: (800) 638-8437
Customer Service: (800) 234-1660

About Aspen Publishers • For more than 35 years, Aspen has been a leading professional publisher in a variety of disciplines. Aspen's vast information resources are available in both print and electronic formats. We are committed to providing the highest quality information available in the most appropriate format for our customers. Visit Aspen's Internet site for more information resources, directories, articles, and a searchable version of Aspen's full catalog, including the most recent publications:
http://www.aspenpub.com
Aspen Publishers, Inc. • The hallmark of quality in publishing
Member of the worldwide Wolters Kluwer group

The authors have made every effort to ensure the accuracy of the information herein, particularly with regard to technique and procedure. However, appropriate information sources should be consulted, especially for new or unfamiliar procedures. It is the responsibility of every practitioner to evaluate the appropriateness of a particular opinion in the context of actual clinical situations and with due consideration to new developments. Authors, editors, and the publisher cannot be held responsible for any typographical or other errors found in this book.

Editorial Resources: Ruth Bloom
Library of Congress Catalog Card Number: 96-26305
ISBN: 0-8342-0689-7

Printed in the United States of America

1 2 3 4 5

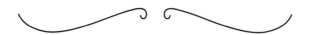

Anyone who has been to school can remember at least one teacher whose influence inspired him to learn more fully, to appreciate the subject being taught, and perhaps to realize a life's work. I have been fortunate enough to have had several such teachers. In high school, my biology teacher moved me into the sciences, and a humanities teacher instilled in me the desire to think and reason. While studying chiropractic, I found Dr. A.L. Logan. I first met him when he voluntarily did clinical rounds at the Los Angeles College of Chiropractic (LACC).

Roy Logan had a capacity to understand how the human body works, and a curiosity about it that kept him constantly searching and researching for ways to help heal it. The profession is full of personalities teaching a variety of techniques, some insisting theirs is the only way, but it has few true professors who can cull the various teachings, and present to the student a clear and concise way to approach a patient, without personality and ego getting in the way. Roy had these abilities, and, fortunately for us, he had a desire to teach others. He never missed an opportunity.

He saw the need in our profession for a way to link the rote clinical sciences and the various ways of executing an adjustment. He gave us an answer to the commonly asked question of when and where to adjust. He was constantly pushing the profession to realize the importance of effective clinical application of chiropractic principles at a time when there seemed to be more emphasis on fitting into the health care industry by wearing a white coat and using big words.

Around the world, students of Dr. Logan use his methods of diagnosis and treatment every day and are reminded of his wonderful contributions to the profession. He lectured repeatedly before several state associations, and taught an eight month post-graduate course at LACC for eight years. He was Chairman of the Technique Department at the Anglo-European College of Chiropractic for five years.

In spite of his many contributions, Roy's work remains unfinished. He passed away in April of 1993, after fighting a terminal illness. He was working hard on his textbooks up to the end, hoping to transfer as much of his knowledge and wisdom to paper as he could.

Dr. Logan has a number of students dedicated to continuing his work and seeing it evolve in the way he envisioned. There is no "A.L. Logan Technique," but rather a compilation of various teachings, combined with a unique understanding of the interdependencies of the human structure. We hope to do his work justice and see more students of chiropractic become as effective as possible in the treatment of human disorders.

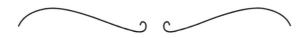

Table of Contents

Series Preface

"... The application of principles ... involves higher mental processes than their memorizing; every student should be given a thorough drill in clinical analysis in which he should be made to see the relationship which exists between the fundamental facts and their clinical application."

Francis M. Pottenger, MD

The education that a modern chiropractor undergoes includes the clinical sciences and the manipulative arts. A graduate doctor of chiropractic has a thorough grasp of the diagnostic and clinical skills and is trained in basic manipulative techniques. With this knowledge, the practicing doctor begins to gain the experience that makes the application of this knowledge successful. A successful doctor is one who continues to learn beyond what is minimally required, for he or she is constantly renewed and stimulated.

Dr. A.L. Logan was a successful chiropractor, a doctor that, like D.D. Palmer, continued to expand his understanding of the human body in health and disease. He studied the works of many of the chiropractic profession's leading educators. He researched and developed his own theories which he applied in his practice, and like most chiropractors, developed a successful, diversified approach to diagnosing and treating his patients. Dr. Logan recognized the need for a practical way to blend basic and advanced manipulative techniques with clinical skills.

From this recognition came over 20 years of teaching. It was his hope that his ideas would generate continued dialogue and interest in expanding the clinical application of chiropractic principles.

Dr. Logan did clinical rounds at the Los Angeles College of Chiropractic, since the early seventies. He lectured often for various state associations, and taught at the Anglo-European College of Chiropractic. During this time Dr. Logan continued to learn and grow as a clinician and teacher. His decision to write a series of texts on the clinical application of chiropractic principles came out of his experience in teaching undergraduate technique at AECC and seeing the difficulty upper division students had in understanding when, where, and why they should adjust.

This series of textbooks will be a comprehensive reference on chiropractic clinical applications. Dr. Logan believed this approach should be the basis for an undergraduate course in adjustive and clinical technique. It is, at the same time, a welcome addition to the knowledge of any practitioner.

Pottenger FM. *Symptoms of Visceral Disease*. St. Louis: Mosby; 1953.

Chris Hutcheson, DC
Auburn, California

This is the third in a series of texts conceived by Dr. A.L. Logan. The concept for these works is based on Dr. Logan's experience in teaching graduate and undergraduate clinical technique and offers a better way to approach the instruction of students. This series started with the knee and followed with the foot and ankle, and now moves up into the pelvis and spine. It is necessary to have an understanding of the lower extremities and their influence on the structures above before being able to fully comprehend the clinical aspects of the pelvis, spine, and upper extremities.

Dr. Logan completed the first two texts even though seriously ill. Before his passing, he outlined the ideas for his third book on the lower back and pelvis. I was honored that he asked me to carry on his work by completing this text thereby continuing the work he so lovingly pursued.

I have written this text based on my understanding of his work and the extensive lecture materials he left in my custody. I have attempted to present his work as he would have done. I think Dr. Logan would be satisfied with the outcome.

Dr. Logan's work is important because it is an intelligent digestion of a diverse collection of techniques handed down from the earliest days of the profession. It is an excellent starting point for research into the most effective manipulative techniques—a needed foundation for the scientific verification of chiropractic manipulative therapy. Dr. Logan's work is a great contribution to the chiropractic profession.

This series is designed to be a working manual of clinical aspects in the diagnosis and treatment of musculoskeletal conditions. It is no easy task to teach manipulative procedures from a text. The illustrations are simple on purpose. Dr. Logan felt that simple line drawings can more accurately focus the emphasis intended. More sophisticated photographic illustrations may present too much confusing information. These texts are our attempt to explain in words and drawings a dynamic process.

—*Chris Hutcheson*

Acknowledgments

This book could not have been written without the aid and support of many people. I would like to thank, especially, the following:

My wife, Rebecca, for her encouragement and advice.

Judy A. Logan, DC for her courageous, tireless support of Dr. Logan in his efforts to complete as much of this series as he could, and for her encouragement in my assuming Dr. Logan's work.

Paula Regina Rodrigues de Fritas Hillenbrand for her many hours of modeling for photographs, and her husband Stephen Hillenbrand for his expertise in photography. Their efforts made the illustrations possible.

Richard Wilcox, DC, Maui, Hawaii, for providing me with videotapes of one of Dr. Logan's last seminars. It proved invaluable in verifying much of Dr. Logan's later work.

Joseph Howe, DC, DABCR for contributing his time and knowledge of radiology to this text.

Herbert I. Magee, Jr., DC and Merill Cook, DC for the use of their extensive libraries for research.

Nehmat G. Saab, MA, MLS, Director, Learning Resource Center, Los Angeles College of Chiropractic, for her aid in researching the literature for Dr. Logan and myself.

The anatomy of the lower back and pelvis encompasses much more than the five lumbar vertebrae, the innominates, and related soft tissues. It cannot really be separated from the influence of the surrounding structures. In understanding the intricacies of the lumbar/pelvic mechanism, it is necessary to understand the influence of the lower extremities as well as the upper body.

The most important anatomy to consider in diagnosing and treating disorders of the lower back and pelvis must include the hip joints, the dorsolumbar junction, and the twelfth ribs. For the purpose of this text, the anatomy will not necessarily be detailed or complete, but will focus on certain important considerations and that which is pertinent to a clinical evaluation and treatment of lower back and pelvic disorders.

BONEY STRUCTURES

The Pelvis

The pelvis is a basin-like structure that holds the pelvic organs and supports the abdominal organs. It provides a stable base for a moveable spinal column and rests upon the lower limbs, balancing over the hip joints (Fig. 1–1).

It comprises four bones: the sacrum, the two innominates, and the coccyx. There are also four joints: the two sacroiliac joints, the pubic symphysis, and the sacrococcygeal joint.

Each innominate bone is actually three bones (the ilium, ischium, and pubis) that, by adulthood, have become fused at the acetabulum, the cup-shaped receptacle for the head of the femur. A lateral view of an innominate (Fig. 1–2) could re-

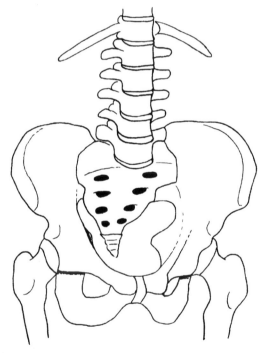

Fig. 1–1 Boney structures of the low back and pelvis.

mind one (with a little imagination) of a two-bladed marine propeller. The acetabulum is the hub of the prop. The wide blades of the ilia form the sides of the pelvic bowl. The lower blade is a ring formed by the rami of the pubis and ischium and is bent inward. Viewed medially, the articular surfaces of the sacrum and pubis can be seen (Fig. 1–3).

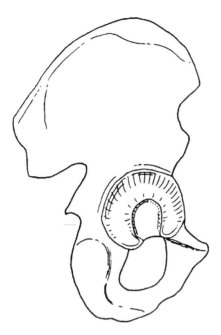

Fig. 1–2 Innominate bone, lateral view.

The sacrum is the end result of the developmental fusion of five segments of the spinal column. Viewed face-on (Fig. 1–4), it looks triangular with the base at the top that forms a platform for the moveable spinal column. The apex points inferiorly and articulates with the coccyx, or tailbone. A lateral view shows the large surface for the sacroiliac articulation and the apex that angles forward (Fig. 1–4).

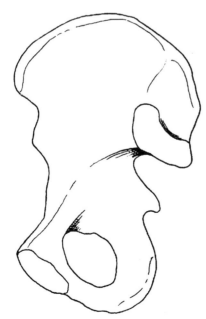

Fig. 1–3 Innominate bone, medial view.

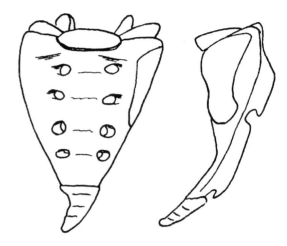

Fig. 1–4 Sacrum, oblique and lateral views.

The coccyx is usually formed by four rudimentary spinal segments, tapering to a "mere nodule" as described in *Gray's Anatomy*.[1] It is a bumpy little bone providing attachment surfaces for muscles and ligaments that support the pelvic floor.

The sacrum is wedged between the pelvic bones, forming two complex articulations, the sacroiliac joints. According to *Gray's Anatomy*,[1] the ear-shaped joint is a blend of a rigid synchondrosis and a freely moveable joint that gradually develops a synovial space as persons age. Kapandji[2] emphasizes the "wide structural variations" that can be seen in the shape and symmetry of the sacroiliac joints. Opinions on the anatomy and function of the sacroiliac joints vary greatly. In chiropractic, the anatomy and function of these joints are considered of key importance.

The sacrum is wedged, caught, and suspended on irregular outcroppings between the innominates and bound internally by patchy areas of fibrocartilage. A complex array of ligaments attach the sacrum to the pelvic bones. The posterior sacroiliac ligament (Fig. 1–5) is composed of several layers of fibers running in different directions. The most central portion of the posterior ligament has been labeled the short axial ligament by Kapandji.[2] It is considered by some to be the axis of sacroiliac movement.

The sacrotuberous ligament (Fig. 1–5c) is a broad structure arising from the posterior inferior iliac spine, sacrum, and coccyx. It twists upon itself and attaches to the ischial tuberosity. The iliolumbar ligament (Fig. 1–6a) stabilizes the L5 and sometimes L4 vertebrae, running from the transverse process and blending with the anterior sacroiliac ligament. The anterior sacroiliac ligament (Fig. 1–6b) is composed of two bands running obliquely across the anterior aspect of the joint. The sacrospinous ligament (Fig. 1–6c), a triangular group of fibers, runs from the lateral border of the sacrum and coccyx to an apical attachment at the spine of the ischial tuberosity.

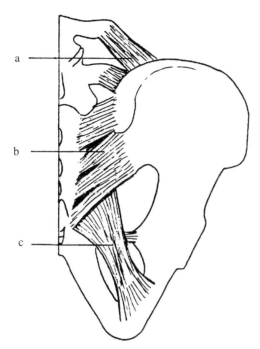

interosseous ligament with a central cleft. The symphysis is bound by ligaments in all planes. The anterior aspect has ligaments that are contiguous with the aponeurosis of abdominal and adductor muscles (Fig. 1–7).

The sacrococcygeal articulation is also a cartilaginous joint united by a disk-like interosseous ligament. It also has an array of ligaments supporting the articulation anteriorly, posteriorly, and laterally (Fig. 1–8).

In examining the pelvis, important palpation landmarks to note are:

1. anterior superior iliac spine
2. iliac crest
3. pubic symphysis
4. posterior superior iliac spine

Fig. 1–5 Posterior sacroiliac ligaments. a. iliolumbar ligament, b. posterior sacroiliac ligament, c. sacrotuberous ligament.

The pubic symphysis is the anterior connection between the pubic bones, completing the rim of the pelvic bowl. It is a cartilaginous joint, a symphysis, which is a slightly moveable joint. Like the intervertebral joint, it has a disk, a fibrocartilage

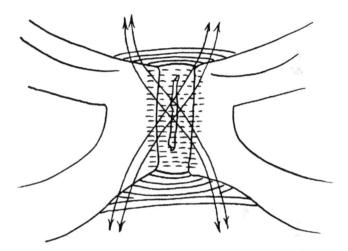

Fig. 1–7 Pubic symphysis: arrows depict fibers blending with abdominal and adductor muscles.

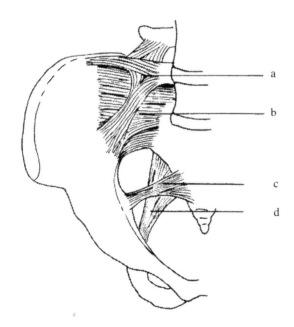

Fig. 1–6 Anterior sacroiliac ligaments. a. iliolumbar ligament, b. anterior sacroiliac ligament, c. sacrospinous ligament, d. sacrotuberous ligament.

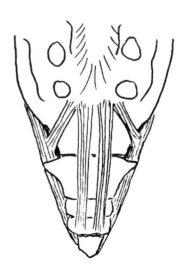

Fig. 1–8 Sacrococcygeal articulation and ligaments.

5. ischial tuberosities
6. sacroiliac joints
7. coccyx
8. lateral sacrum

The Hip Joints

The hip joints are enarthrodial or ball-and-socket joints. The acetabulum, the socket in the innominate, receives the head of the femur, the ball. Hip joints provide a solid foundation for the pelvis to balance upon and have an extensive range of motion.

The femur (Fig. 1–9) is the longest, strongest bone in the body. At its proximal end, the neck bends medially at an almost right angle and terminates in a cartilage coated ball, the head. The neck gradually decreases its angle, becoming more of a right angle as persons grow from infancy to adulthood.[1]

The acetabulum (Fig. 1–9) has a semilunar shape to its articular surface. Within that is a depression, the acetabular notch, filled by a fat pad and covered by a synovial membrane.

The greater trochanter (Fig. 1–9) is a large prominence projecting laterally from the base of the femoral neck. It is the most lateral boney prominence of the hip and provides a large surface area for the attachment of muscles. The lesser trochanter is inferior and medial to the greater trochanter, on the opposite side of the femoral shaft. It is situated at the inner junction of the neck and shaft of the femur.

The ligaments of the hip allow a vast range of motion while keeping the ball firmly in its socket. At the same time, the ligaments support the pelvis, checking posterior rotation of the pelvis on the hips. Internally, a most prominent, but unimportant, ligament, the ligamentum teres (Fig. 1–9), arises from a depression in the head of the femur, the fovea capitis. The ligamentum teres spreads out forming three bands that attach to the acetabular notch and blends with the transverse ligament. The ligamentum teres is considered to be rudimentary and, although strong, appears to have little significance in the stability of the joint. The most tension placed on this ligament is during adduction of the hip.

The acetabular labrum is a fibrocartilaginous rim that extends and deepens the rim of the socket. It is continuous with the transverse ligament that bridges the bottom of the acetabular notch and forms a foramen for nutrient arteries.

The articular capsule is stronger and thicker proximally and anteriorly, but thinner distally and posteriorly. Circular fibers, the zona orbicularis, form a collar, which is stronger posteriorly and distally, around the neck of the femur. The longitudinal fibers are more prominent proximally and anteriorly and blend with accessory ligaments.

The articular capsule is reinforced by external ligaments that wrap clockwise from posterior to anterior around the hip joint. The ischiofemoral, iliofemoral, and pubofemoral ligaments (Fig. 1–10) are tense in the erect position, becoming tighter with further extension. In flexion, they are increasingly relaxed. This "screw-home" mechanism pulls the head of the femur tight into the acetabulum and prevents excessive posterior rotation of the pelvis.

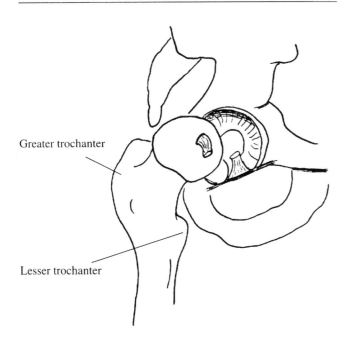

Greater trochanter

Lesser trochanter

Fig. 1–9 Femoral head and acetabulum: ligamentum teres (severed).

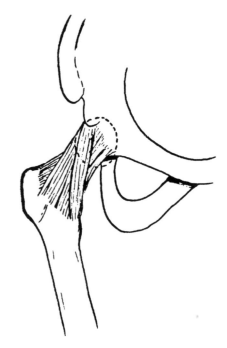

Fig. 1–10 Ligaments of the hip joint (dotted area—iliopectineal bursa).

Between the iliofemoral and pubofemoral ligaments, the articular capsule is thinner. The iliopectineal bursa overlies this area, cushioning the iliopsoas muscle (Fig. 1–10). There is often a communication between the capsule and bursa.

Palpation of the hip is difficult as it is deep under layers of muscle and connective tissue. In evaluating the low back, pelvis, and hips, the greater trochanter is an important area to palpate. It is the attachment point for a number of important muscles and can provide information about the function of the hips; for instance, comparing tension bilaterally can reveal the state of muscle tone, and palpation of muscle insertions can provide information on the muscles of the hip.

The Lumbar Spine

The lumbar spine, as a functional unit, includes the five lumbar vertebrae, the twelfth thoracic vertebra and the twelfth ribs. T12 is a transitional vertebra with characteristics of both the thoracic and lumbar vertebrae. The transition begins with T11 as the body, pedicles, and processes become larger and heavier.

The lumbar spine, viewed anteriorly, is straight and relatively symmetrical (Fig. 1–11). From T12 to L5, one can see that the vertebrae and transverse processes become wider. T12 has divided loyalties and a pivotal role in the mechanical function of the spine. The twelfth ribs, like the eleventh, are floating ribs, having no costotransverse articulation. These ribs are short, incline caudally, and are subject to much variation in size and shape.

From a lateral perspective (Fig. 1–11), the lumbar spine is curved anteriorly. The lumbar lordosis is a complementary curve to the thoracic kyphosis and cervical lordosis. These curves are a necessary component in giving humans the ability to stand erect and walk in balance with minimal effort. Ramamurti,[3] among others, considers the lumbar lordosis to underlie the human predisposition to low back pain.

Farfan[4] describes the anatomical factors that encourage the lumbar lordosis. He points out that the bodies of the lumbar vertebrae are wedged, higher anteriorly, and decrease posteriorly. The disks show similar wedging. This wedging shapes the lumbar curve. Other factors that influence the lordosis are the degree of pelvic tilt and the sacral base angle.

Cailliet[5] describes the spine as an "aggregate of articulated, superimposed segments each of which is a *functional unit*." He divides the unit into an anterior portion: two vertebral bodies and the disk in-between. Its role is that of weight-bearing and shock absorption. The posterior portion consists of two vertebral arches, paired facetal joints, and spinous and transverse processes (Fig. 1–12).

The posterior portion, the motor/neural unit, provides protection for the delicate neural structures and levers for the attachment muscles. The facetal joints give guidance to the movement of the vertebrae as well as bearing some of the weight of the body.

The lumbar vertebrae (Fig. 1–13) are distinguished by several anatomical factors. The pedicles are set higher, forming a deep vertebral notch. The spinous processes are broad, flat, and rectangular. The body is wider than it is deep and taller anteriorly than it is posteriorly. The transverse processes are set ventral to the articular processes instead of dorsally as in the thoracic spine. They are considered to be rib vestiges. There are three tubercles related to the transverse process. The

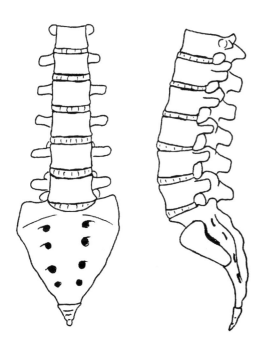

Fig. 1–11 Anterior and lateral views of lumbar spine and sacrum.

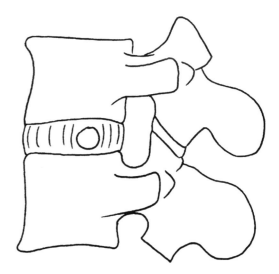

Fig. 1–12 Vertebral functional unit.

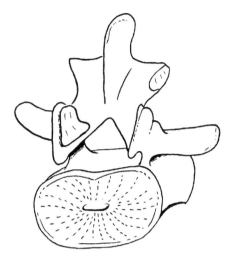

Fig. 1–13 Typical lumbar vertebra.

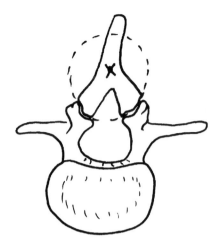

Fig. 1–14 Lumbar axis of rotation.

inferior one, considered to be homologous with the actual transverse process, is called the accessory process. The superior one, the mamillary process, is prominent and connected with the superior articular process. In palpating the lumbar spine, it is the mamillary process, and not the transverse process, that is used to palpate for function. The transverse process is too deep to palpate accurately.

Under general observation, the lumbar facetal joint appears to have both a vertical and sagittal plane of articulation. This would give the lumbar spine control of flexion and extension. The thoracic spine has facetal articular planes that encourage lateral flexion, but in the cervical spine rotation dominates.

Farfan[4] describes the facetal articulations as having a more complex shape, with different roles attributed to the upper (T12 to L3) and lower (L4 to S1) segments. The upper segments have dual facetal joint planes. The posterior two-thirds of the joint has a plane parallel to the longitudinal axis of the spine. The anterior third bends at almost 90° to face posteriorly. Farfan[4] concludes that this design restricts forward displacement of the vertebrae in flexion. Kapandji[2] attributes to this shape a guide for limited rotational movement. The central axis for the rotation is at the base of the spinous process (Fig. 1–14).

The L4–5 and L5–S1 facets have a more rounded shape in the transverse plane. They also face in a more oblique direction mediolaterally and superoinferiorly. Farfan[4] suggests that the movement at the facetal joint is not a gliding action, but a more complex "ball-and-socket" one.

Cailliet[5] mentions, in describing the posterior part of the functional unit, that it is non–weight-bearing. Barge[6] has concluded from his research that lower lumbar facets do bear weight. He refers to this as the "tripod theory." Weight is divided between the posterior aspect of the vertebral body and the articular processes (Fig. 1–15.)

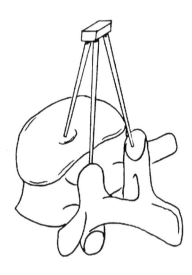

Fig. 1–15 Tripod weight-bearing concept.

The intervertebral disk is the most prominent structure of attachment seen in the spine. The anterior intervertebral joint is classified as a symphysis. It is composed of two end plates and the disk. The disks make up approximately 25% of the height of the spinal column. A healthy disk is hydrophylic, drawing water in like a sponge when the load is off. Consequently, the spine can gain and loose height in 24 hours, corresponding to periods of weight and non–weight-bearing. The structure of the disk is designed to absorb shock, allow for limited movement, and provide a strong attachment between vertebrae. The multiple contributions from each disk make the spine amazingly versatile in its range of motion.

The disk is a fluid-filled container. The wall of the container, the annulus fibrosis (Fig. 1–16), is a thick laminate of

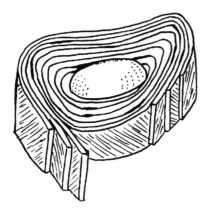

Fig. 1–16 Schematic of a disk.

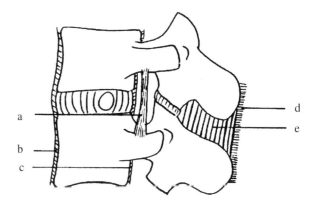

Fig. 1–17 Ligaments of the functional unit. a. intertransverse, b. anterior longitudinal (ALL), c. posterior longitudinal (PLL), d. supraspinous, and e. interspinous.

concentrically arranged fibers at varying oblique angles. Kapandji[2] describes the layers as being vertical at the periphery, becoming more oblique and almost horizontal at the center. The annulus is attached above and below to the end plates. This complex arrangement is what gives the vertebrae the capacity to flex, extend, bend laterally, rotate, and shear with strong limits and stability.

Cailliet[5] describes the disk as having all the characteristics of a hydraulic system. The nucleus pulposis (Fig. 1–16) is a gelatinous substance, mostly water, that is tightly bound by the annulus. The fluid can accept compressive forces and distribute them evenly, keeping the vertebral bodies separated. The movement of one vertebra upon the other is possible due to the ability of the fluid to shift in its semielastic container.

The elastic properties of the disk are the result of annular elasticity. In a young, healthy disk, the fibers are predominantly elastic, and the nucleus is hydrophilic. As aging and injury or both occur, the annular fibers are replaced by more fibrous, less elastic ones, and the colloidal hydrophilic properties of the nucleus decrease. The disk becomes less of a shock absorber.

The disk also gradually loses its vascular supply, and by the third decade, it is dependent upon diffusion, imbition, and movement for its nutrient and waste exchange. This reduces the disk's ability to regenerate or heal effectively.

The spinal column is bound anteriorly by the anterior longitudinal ligament (ALL; Fig. 1–17). It runs from the occiput to the sacrum and is attached to the disks as well as the vertebral bodies. It acts as a reinforcement for the disk in its control of forward shear and also checks hyperextension.

The posterior longitudinal ligament (PLL; Fig. 1–17) courses from the occiput to the sacrum on the posterior aspect of the vertebral bodies. It is adherent to the disks and the superior and inferior margins of the vertebral bodies. A paravertebral venous plexus is housed under the PLL in the midportion of the vertebral body. The PLL has a lesser role in checking flexion than the ALL has in checking extension, as it is closer to the center of rotation. Cailliet[5] notes that the PLL begins to taper as it descends into the lumbar spine and is half as wide when it reaches the sacrum. He attributes the frequency of disk ruptures to this tapering at a point where maximum movement and stresses are produced.

The vertebral arches are connected by segmental ligaments, the lamina, by the ligamentum flavum, a thick ligament that meets its opposite in the midline and completely encloses the vertebral canal. In the lumbar spine, this ligament joins with the capsular ligament anterolaterally and deepens the superior articular process. It tends to hypertrophy and can create stenosis, a narrowing of the vertebral canal.

The apophyseal or facetal joints are diarthrodial joints with a synovial membrane and a surrounding capsule. Farfan[4] dismissed the notion that the facetal capsules are loose. He contends that they are no more lax than the interphalangeal joint capsules.

The interspinous ligament (Fig. 1–17) provides a strong bond between the spinous processes, but the tips of the processes are interconnected by the supraspinous ligament. The supraspinous ligament is contiguous with the lumbodorsal fascia and, according to Farfan,[4] may not be attached to the L4, L5, or S1 segments, leaving a gap from S2 to L3 and a "check" ligament with thin attachments. The intertransverse ligaments are well developed in the lumbar spine and interconnect the transverse processes.

The lumbodorsal fascia (Fig. 1–18) envelops the erector spinae muscles and contributes to the ligamentous support of the lumbar spine. It has attachments to the spinous and transverse processes, the iliac crest, and sacrum. It is also contiguous with abdominal muscles and the latissimus dorsi. It acts as a check ligament against excessive flexion and can absorb some of the shear stresses of flexion or extension by the forces exerted by muscle contractions in a tight compartment adjacent to the spine.

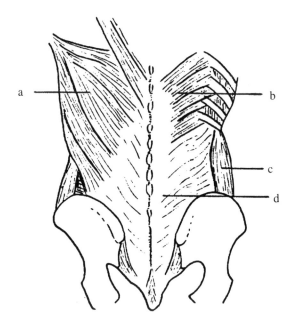

Fig. 1–18 a. latissimus dorsi, b. serratus posterior inferior, c. posterior abdominals, d. lumbodorsal fascia.

The iliolumbar ligaments (Fig. 1–6) are important stabilizers of the L4 and L5 segments. Kapandji[2] describes the iliolumbar ligaments as running inferolaterally from the transverse processes of L4 and L5 to the iliac crest, with an inferior slip down to and then blending into the anterior sacroiliac ligaments. These ligaments check flexion, extension, and, most importantly, lateral flexion.

Anomalous Anatomy

At first glance, our anatomy seems symmetrical. It is a wonder that in the development of a human being from a single cell that it is nearly perfect every time. Upon closer scrutiny, however, we often see little "flaws" in the symmetry of the body. Most of these are insignificant, and we have an amazing ability to adapt and compensate so that these anomalies go unnoticed. It is interesting that an individual with one anomaly will often have more. A patient with a bifid spinous process at S1 may also have a transitional vertebra or facetal asymmetry.

Boney anomalies that are commonly seen in practice and can interfere with normal biomechanical function or alter the approach to treatment include long or short transverse processes, asymmetries in the sacroiliac joints, asymmetries of the facetal joints, transitional vertebrae, and leg length insufficiency. Exaggerated differences in the length of the transverse processes can alter the leverage produced on a particular vertebra and cause aberrant movement or stresses.

The sacroiliac articulations are irregularly shaped and often different in their configuration from right to left. When assessing radiographs of the low back and pelvis, note any significant differences that might require some innovation in manipulation or might explain a patient's symptoms. For instance, one side may have a notched configuration, but the opposite side may be straight. The straight-sided joint would have a tendency to shift superoinferiorly (Fig. 1–19).

Anomalous facetal joints are common in the lumbar spine. Variations from the normal plane of articulation to a more sagittal, coronal, or horizontal one can occur (Fig. 1–20). These variations can be bilateral or unilateral. Unilateral asymmetries (Fig. 1–21) can be verified by radiograph and in some cases by accurate palpation.

Transitional vertebrae usually involve the L5 and S1 segments. A blurring of the difference between a separate vertebra and a fully fused portion of the sacrum has numerous variations. The most clinically significant varieties are those with pseudoarticulations that cause aberrant motion (Fig. 1–22). Palpation can hint at these anomalies, but a radiograph is necessary to determine the exact degree of anomaly, direction of articular planes, and how best to adjust the segment.

Spondylolisthesis (Fig. 1–23) is not an uncommon finding. Most often found at the L5–S1 level, it has several causes. A bilateral defect in the pars due to a failure of ossification centers to fuse has been the accepted explanation. It has become more accepted to think of these anomalies as actual stress fractures rather than congenital defects when they are present at an early age. Other anomalous factors that cause a forward slippage of the vertebrae are elongated pedicles or pars with no break. Degenerative changes in the connective tissues surrounding the segment can also allow a slippage. Spondylolisthesis appears to have a hereditary tendency, and early degenerative changes are likely.

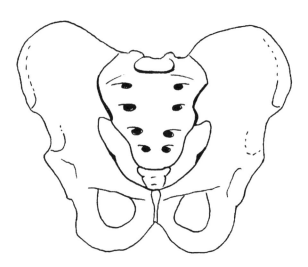

Fig. 1–19 Sacroiliac asymmetry.

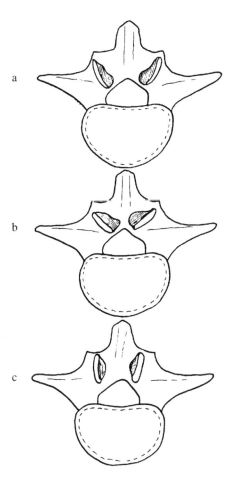

Fig. 1–20 Facetal arrangement. a. normal, b. coronal, c. sagittal.

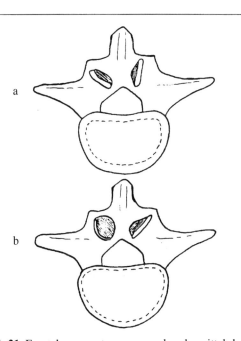

Fig. 1–21 Facetal asymmetry. a. normal and sagittal, b. horizontal and normal.

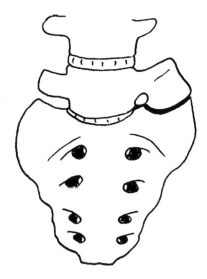

Fig. 1–22 Sacralization with pseudoarticulation.

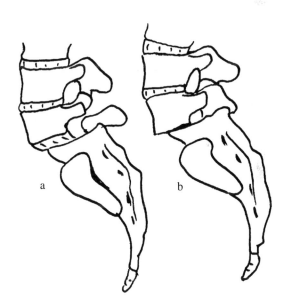

Fig. 1–23 Spondylolisthesis. a. spondylolytic, b. degenerative.

Leg length insufficiency (LLI) is an important factor in the function of the lower back and should be ascertained in an evaluation. There has been much discussion about the effects of an anatomically short leg and, consequently, great controversy as to its importance. A short leg will cause an unleveling of the pelvis and a series of compensatory mechanisms. In evaluating a patient, it is necessary to differentiate between an actual LLI and a functional LLI.

MUSCLES

To fully appreciate the relationship between joint and muscle, it is imperative to thoroughly understand the anatomy and function of the muscles.

Muscles of the Hip and Pelvis

The Gluteal Region

The buttock is composed of successively deeper layers of muscles. The most superficial, the gluteus maximus, is of key importance. It is a large, coarsely fibered muscle, particularly oversized in humans, when compared to other quadrupeds. The gluteus maximus (Fig. 1–24) plays a key role in the erect stance. It originates from the posterior superior ilium (including the crest for a short distance above the superior iliac spine), the lower posterior surface of the sacrum, and side of the coccyx. It also attaches to the aponeurosis of the sacrospinalis muscles, the sacrotuberous ligament and the gluteal aponeurosis, which covers the muscle.

The fibers run inferolaterally to a dual insertion. The larger proximal and superficial distal fibers become thick and tendinous and blend into the iliotibial band of the fascia lata. The deeper distal fibers insert into the femur below the greater trochanter. The actions of the gluteus maximus include extension and lateral rotation of the thigh, stabilization of the knee through the fascia lata, and posterior rotation of the ilia.

The gluteus medius (Fig. 1–25) originates over a broad area of the ilium, including most of the crest, thinning out to just the crest anteriorly. It also arises from the overlying gluteal aponeurosis. Its fibers converge into a tendon that inserts on the lateral aspect of the greater trochanter with a bursa under it to cushion the trochanter. The posteriorly originating fibers attach anteriorly, and the anterior fibers insert posteriorly. This twisting of the muscle gives it a multiple function. The main action is abduction of the thigh. The posterior fibers assist in lateral rotation and extension, and the anterior fibers aid medial rotation and flexion. This muscle is important in walking, as it holds the pelvis level during the swing phase of the opposite side. The gluteus medius has the ability to mimic sciatic neuritis when inflamed, according to Dr. Robert Klein, a rheumatologist at the Sansum Medical Clinic in Santa Barbara, California.

The gluteus minimus (Fig. 1–26) is deep to the medius, attaching broadly across the inner aspect of the ilium. The fibers converge in a tendinous attachment to the anterior surface of the greater trochanter. Its action is first, medial rotation, then abduction. It can assist in flexion as well.

The piriformis (Fig. 1–27) runs almost parallel to the posterior border of the gluteus medius. It is flat and pyramidal in shape, the base originating from the anterior sacrum at the level of the second, third, and fourth foramen and the area adjacent to the greater sciatic foramen. It also has attachments originating from the anterior surface of the sacrotuberous ligament. The muscle exits through the greater sciatic foramen, and at its apex, forms a rounded tendon that inserts into the superior border of the greater trochanter. Its main action is lateral rotation and abduction of the thigh. It can also assist in extension. The piriformis is known for spasms. Its close proximity to the sciatic nerve as it exits the sciatic notch makes it likely to irritate the nerve causing sciatica. In a significant

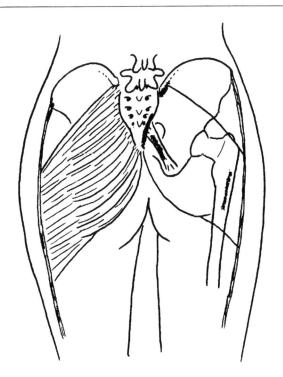

Fig. 1–24 Gluteus maximus.

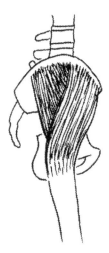

Fig. 1–25 Gluteus medius.

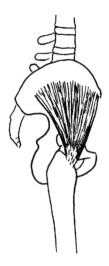

Fig. 1–26 Gluteus minimus.

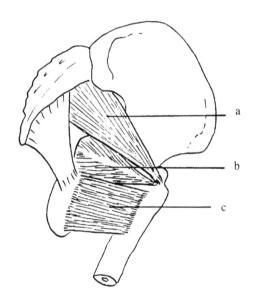

Fig. 1–27 Lateral rotatores. a. piriformis, b. gemelli, c. quadratus femoris.

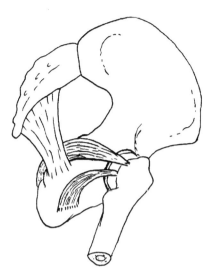

Fig. 1–28 Obturator internus and externus.

quadratus femoris (Fig. 1–27) is the lowest in the group arrangement, just above the adductor group. The obturator externus (Fig. 1–28) makes up the anterior wall of the pelvis.

The tensor fascia lata (TFL; Fig. 1–29) originates along the outer border of the anterior iliac crest and spine. It blends into the fascia lata over the greater trochanter in the thick iliotibial track. The gluteus maximus also inserts into the track at this level. The tensor muscle participates in flexion of the thigh and has a small contribution to medial rotation. It is also responsible for tensing the fascia lata, which helps stabilize the knee.

The rectus femoris (Fig. 1–30), the most superficial of the quadriceps femoris group, crosses two articulations. It originates on the anterior inferior iliac spine and joins with the other muscles of the quad group to insert on the anterior aspect of the tibia. It plays a role in flexing the thigh as well as extending the knee. In the erect position, it assists in influencing the ilia anteriorly.

The sartorius and gracilis (Figs. 1–30 and 1–31) have a common insertion on the medial aspect of the proximal tibia. The sartorius is the longest muscle in the body, originating from the anterior superior iliac spine. It runs obliquely across the thigh to its insertion. It flexes and medially rotates the thigh and also flexes the leg. With the leg flexed, it can assist in medial rotation of the tibia. The sartorius plays a role in iliac stability. A weakness of the sartorius can be a factor in a posterior rotation of the ilia. If the sartorius were in a state of hypertonicity, it could pull the ilia anteriorly.

The gracilis (Fig. 1–31) arises from the pubic symphysis and arch joining the sartorius to insert on the tibia. It is the most superficial muscle on the medial aspect of the thigh. It is an adductor of the thigh, flexor of the leg and assists in medial rotation of the tibia with the leg flexed.

number of people, the sciatic nerve passes through the piriformis. This location can make it even more vulnerable to irritation. The piriformis will become hypertonic, compensating for a weak gluteus minimus.

The other lateral rotatores of the thigh are arranged around the obturator foramen. They include the obturator internus (Fig. 1–28), interesting for its internal pelvic origin, right angle turn, and pulley-like action as it rides over the groove above the ischial tuberosity. The obturator internus is flanked by the gemelli (Fig. 1–27), two muscles that run above and below the internus to attach into the greater trochanter. The

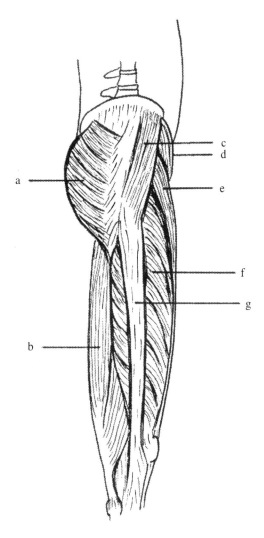

Fig. 1–29 Lateral view, pelvic and thigh muscles. a. gluteus maximus, b. biceps femoris, c. tensor fascia lata (TFL), d. sartorius, e. rectus femoris, f. vastus lateralis, g. iliotibial tract.

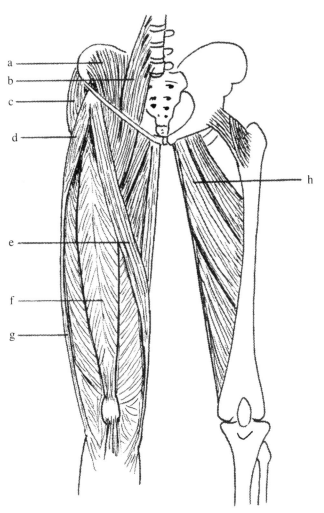

Fig. 1–30 Anterior view, pelvic and thigh muscles. a. iliacus, b. psoas, c. gluteus medius, d. tensor fascia lata (TFL), e. sartorius, f. rectus femoris, g. iliotibial tract, h. adductor group.

The pubic ischial rami provides strong attachment for the adductor group, which adduct and medially rotate the thigh. The group is made up of the pectineus, and the adductors, longus brevis and magnus (Fig. 1–30).

The hamstrings are an important muscle group to consider when evaluating the actions of the hip and pelvis. They cross two joints, the hip and knee, doubling the actions, flexing the knee and extending the thigh. In the erect position, they help (slightly) to check anterior rotation of the pelvis, more so when the pelvis and back are flexed. The hamstrings together provide lateral stability. The biceps femoris (Figs. 1–29 and 1–31) is the lateral string. Its short head originates on the femur, the long head from the ischial tuberosity. Both heads insert on the head of the fibula and lateral tibial condyle. Besides extending the thigh and flexing the leg, the biceps can laterally

rotate the tibia when the knee is flexed and can assist in lateral rotation of the thigh when it is extended. The biceps has an influence on the fibula. If hypertonic, it can pull the fibula superiorly or, if weak, allow it to shift inferior under the influence of the opposing muscles in the calf.[7]

The medial hamstring (Fig. 1–31) is composed of two muscles. The semitendinosus runs more laterally and the semimembranosus more medially. They originate from the ischial tuberosity. The tendons join the sartorius and gracilis to insert on the anteromedial tibia. The medial hamstrings can medially rotate the tibia with the knee in flexion. The hamstrings are often found to be shortened especially in patients who tend to be sedentary in their jobs and at home.

Two muscles in the perineum, the transversus perinei and coccygeus, are involved in pelvic problems. The transversus perinei (Fig. 1–32) originate on the medial ischial tuberosity and join at a central tendinous point anterior to the anus. Their

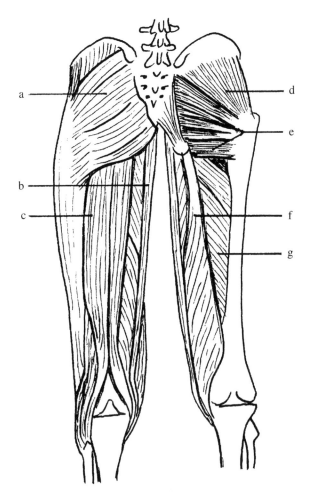

Fig. 1-31 Posterior view, pelvic and thigh muscles. a. gluteus maximus, b. gracilis, c. hamstrings, d. gluteus medius, e. lateral rotators, f. semimembranosus, g. adductors.

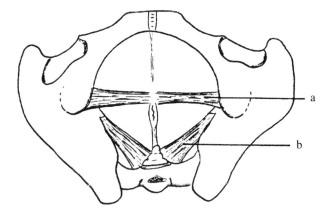

Fig. 1-32 Inferior view of pelvic basin. a. transversus peroneus, b. coccygeus.

orly. The fibers on and close to the sacrum run in an anterior oblique direction. Keep in mind that the different sections of the muscle can have different effects on the function of the ilia and sacrum. The basic function of the iliacus is flexion of the thigh. It is also a principal anterior rotator of the ilia, and the more lateral fibers may oppose lateral flare of the ilia. The fibers with a sacral origin can influence the base of the sacrum anteriorly.

Muscles of the Lumbar Spine

The psoas (Fig. 1-33) is a major player in the normal and abnormal function of the lower back. Kapandji[2] describes the psoas as being composed of two sheets, one originating from

simultaneous contraction fixes the perineum drawing the ischia medially. Dysfunction of these muscles can cause iliac flare or medial ischium distortions. The coccygeus (Fig. 1-32) is a triangular, flat, fibrous muscle. Its apex origin is from the spine of the ischium and the sacrospinous ligament. The insertion is on the last sacral and all the coccygeal segments. They draw the coccyx anteriorly and can be a principal player in coccygeal problems.

The iliacus (Fig. 1-33) is often found to be involved in low back and pelvic problems. It has a broad origin, taking up most of the inner surface of the ilium. The origin extends from the anterior iliac spines, around the iliac fossa, and onto the anterior sacral base. It also has attachments to the anterior sacroiliac and the iliolumbar ligaments. The fibers converge with the psoas tendon, inserting into the lesser trochanter of the femur.

The muscle fibers of the iliacus run in varying directions depending on their point of origin. The fibers closer to the anterior spines run inferomedially. The middle fibers run inferi-

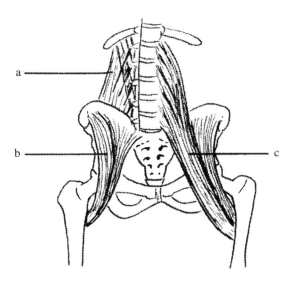

Fig. 1-33 Anterior view: deep muscles. a. quadratus lumborum, b. iliacus, c. psoas.

the transverse processes of the five lumbar vertebrae. The second sheet is more anterior, originating from adjacent bodies and disks from T12 to L5. The muscle descends obliquely and is reflected over the pelvic brim, under the inguinal ligament. The iliacus joins with the psoas to insert on the lesser trochanter. It has a variety of actions: (1) flexing the thigh, (2) flexing and lateral bending the lumbar spine, and (3) influencing the lumbar lordosis and pelvic tilt. Depending on the position of the hip, it can medially or laterally rotate the femur.

The psoas minor (often absent) arises from the sides of the vertebral bodies from T12 and L1. It has a long tendon that inserts on the pubic bone at the iliopectineal eminence. It flexes the lumbar spine and posteriorly rotates the pelvis.

The quadratus lumborum (Q-L; Figs. 1–33 and 1–34) is another important, but often ignored, muscle in lower back dysfunction. It is a thin, roughly rectangular shaped muscle running between the iliac crest and the last rib, with slips to the transverse processes of the lumbars. Closer observation shows the muscle to have three layers. The most posterior layer is made up of fibers running directly from the last rib to the iliac crest. The middle layer has fibers running from the last rib to the transverse processes of all five lumbars. The anterior layer runs from the transverse processes of the first four lumbars to the iliac crest. The most often described function is related to the depression of the last ribs and lateral flexion of the lumbar spine. This muscle also has important functions in the stabilization of the lumbar spine and pelvis. In his research, Dr. Logan[7] found the Q-L to have a significant role in chronic low back instabilities.

The muscle group, sacrospinalis or erector spinae (Fig. 1–34), makes up the more superficial of what Gray considers the deep muscles of the spine.[1] The muscle group arises from a broad, thick tendon attaching to the middle crest of the sacrum and the spinous processes from L5 to T11. The group also has attachments to the lateral crest of the sacrum and inner posterior iliac crest, blending with the sacroiliac and sacrotuberous ligaments and origins of the gluteus maximus. The lumbo-dorsal fascia covers the group in the lumbar and thoracic region. The sacrospinalis muscles start out thin and mostly tendinous, becoming thick and fleshy in the lumbar region. The muscle group is divided into three distinct groups, gradually thinning out again as they continue upward.

The erector spinae lies in the groove adjacent to the vertebral column. Its function is to extend and laterally bend the vertebral column. The medial division, the spinalis thoracis, originates from the spinous processes of the last two thoracic and first two lumbar vertebrae. Running superiorly, it attaches by as many as eight slips into the upper thoracic spinous processes. The longissimus thoracis is the largest division. At its origin, it is blended with the spinalis and iliocostalis groups with some fibers attaching to the lumbar accessory and transverse processes. This division inserts into the tips of the tho-

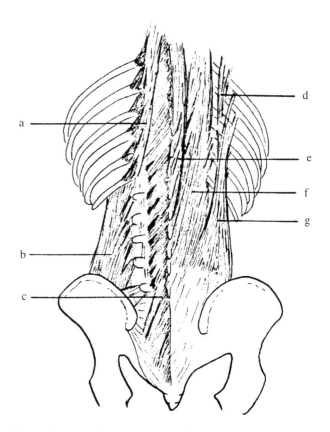

Fig. 1–34 Posterior view erector spinae muscles. a. semispinalis dorsi, b. quadratus lumborum, c. multifidus, d. iliocostalis dorsi, e. spinalis dorsi, f. longissimus thorasis, g. iliocostalis lumborum.

racic transverse processes and into the last nine or ten ribs. The iliocostalis lumborum is the most lateral group. Its fibers originate from the iliac crest and insert into the angles of the last six or seven ribs.

The deeper layers of the spinal muscles can be lumped together as the paravertebral muscles. They all have vertebral origins and insertions, and are short, running between one to five segments. They can be further differentiated by their attachments and basic function. The paravertebrals include the multifidus (Fig. 1–34), interspinales, intertransversarii, and the rotatores. They extend and rotate the vertebral column in general and move individual vertebrae, or several at a time, upon each other.

The abdominal muscles are the anterior muscles of the lumbar spine. The rectus abdominus (Fig. 1–35) is the anterior-most, running vertically on either side of the midline. It originates by wide bands from the fifth, sixth, and seventh ribs, at the anterior arches and costal cartilages. The bands become narrower as they descend to be attached to the pubic crest and symphysis by a string tendon. The recti are attached at the midline by the linea alba, a portion of the abdominal aponeurosis.

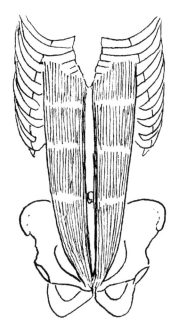

Fig. 1–35 Rectus abdominus muscle.

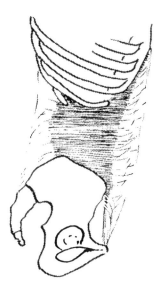

Fig. 1–36 Transversus abdominus muscle.

The transversus abdominus (Fig. 1–36) is the deepest layer, originating at the tips of the lumbar transverse process (TPs), the cartilages of the last six ribs, the iliac crest, and the lateral inguinal ligament. The fibers run horizontally to the anterior, blending into the aponeurosis of the rectus sheath, joining its opposite. The transversi make up the inner abdominal wall surrounding the viscera.

The obliquus internus (Fig. 1–37) is the layer anterior to the transversus. Its fibers fan out from its attachments along the iliac crest and the inguinal ligament, running superomedially. The inferior fibers, which attach to the inguinal ligament, run horizontally and inferiorly, to attach to the pubic crest and symphysis. The superior fibers run obliquely superomedially to attach into the tips of the last two ribs. The middle fibers run from the iliac crest, blending into an aponeurosis that contributes to the linea alba and attaches to the tenth costal cartilage and xiphoid process.

The obliquus externus (Fig. 1–38) makes up the outermost layer of the abdominal wall. The fibers run obliquely superoinferiorly and lateromedially, originating from the lower eight ribs. The lower segments run almost directly inferior to insert on the anterior half of the iliac crest. The upper segments run obliquely inferomedially to blend with a broad aponeurosis becoming the linea alba at the midline.

When considering the abdominal muscles as a whole, one can see that they support the viscera, that they are involved in flexion and rotation of the trunk, and that they support the pelvis anteriorly, pulling it superiorly. The posterior fibers of the obliques, attaching into the posterior aspect of the iliac crest, can produce posterior rotation or allow anterior rotation of the ilia.

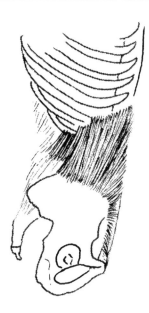

Fig. 1–37 Obliquus internus muscle.

The serratus posterior inferior (Fig. 1–39) can influence the upper lumbar spine. It arises from the spinous processes of the last two thoracic and first three lumbar vertebrae. It runs upward obliquely and laterally to insert on the inferior borders of the last four ribs. Its main action is to draw the lower ribs out and down in opposition to the diaphragm.

The latissimus dorsi (Fig. 1–39) has attachments into the lumbodorsal fascia, which gives it attachments also to the spinous processes of the lower thoracic, lumbar, and sacral segments as well as the iliac crest. It is conceivable that the

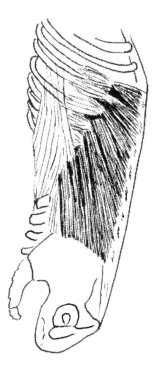

Fig. 1–38 Obliquus externus muscle.

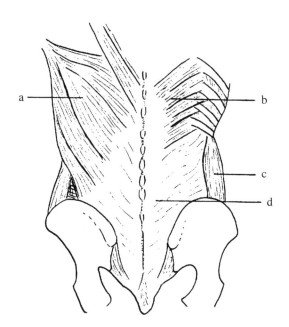

Fig. 1–39 a. latissimus dorsi, b. serratus posterior inferior, c. posterior abdominals, d. lumbodorsal fascia.

latissimus dorsi can influence function in the low back and pelvis.

The diaphragm has attachments to the lumbar spine. Its tendinous cura and lumbocostal arches attach into the lumbar vertebrae. The cura and the origins to the psoas interdigitate and can be affected by each other.

VASCULAR ANATOMY

A detailed study of the vascular system is not relevant to the purpose of this text; however, there are several clinical vascular considerations that need evaluating when examining the lower back and pelvis. Pathology of the aorta is a very important contraindication to forceful manipulation. The aorta, the main artery descending through the abdomen, lies along the anterior lumbar spine. Before bifurcating at L4, it gives off numerous visceral and parietal branches. The bifurcation forms the two common iliac arteries, which divide into the internal and external iliac arteries (Fig. 1–40). Occlusive and in-

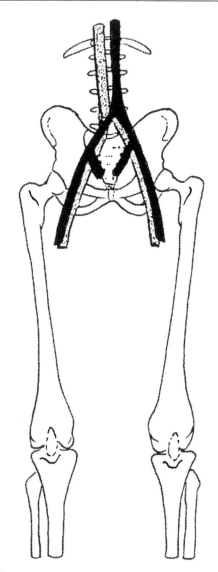

Fig. 1–40 Aorta, external and internal iliac arteries, and venous return.

flammatory diseases and aneurysm of the vessels can be important considerations in determining a course of manipulative therapy.

The internal iliac, or hypogastric artery, supplies the pelvic walls, viscera, and reproductive organs. It also supplies the buttock and medial thigh. The external iliac artery descends along the medial border of the psoas and under the inguinal ligament at which point it is named the femoral artery.

The femoral triangle (Fig. 1–41) is an anatomical landmark important in examining the circulatory system. The area bordered by the inguinal ligament, adductor longus, and sartorius allows palpation of the femoral vein, artery, and nerve.

NEUROANATOMY

The examination of the lower back and pelvis includes an evaluation of the nervous system. This text will focus on the clinical aspects of neurology, rather than a detailed discussion of neuroanatomy.

The spinal nerve (Fig. 1–42) originates from the spinal cord via two roots, the ventral or motor root and the larger dorsal or sensory root. The dorsal root contains the spinal ganglion, which is usually situated in the intervertebral foramen, beyond the dural sheath. The two roots join immediately beyond the ganglion.

The roots of the lumbar, sacral, and coccygeal segments are long, descending from the end of the cord, in the cauda equina. The cord ends at the L1–L2 level. Because the roots in the

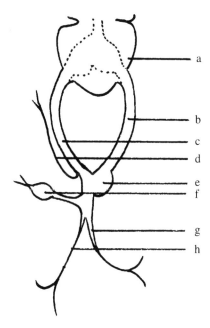

Fig. 1–42 Spinal nerve. a. spinal cord, b. dorsal root, c. ventral root, d. meningeal branch, e. dorsal root ganglion, f. sympathetic trunk ganglion, g. posterior primary division, h. anterior primary division.

lower lumbar and below originate higher up anatomically, it has been found that manipulating the spine at the origin of the roots, as well as where they exit, may be effective. For instance, a weakness in the quadratus lumborum innervated by T12 and L1 nerves often responds to adjusting of the T9–10–11 segments.

The spinal nerve splits into dorsal and ventral primary divisions. The dorsal division is generally smaller. In the lumbosacral spine, medial and lateral branches supply the deep paravertebral and sacrospinales muscles, with cutaneous branches supplying the buttock area. The ventral primary divisions will distribute nerves to the rest of the body. In the thoracic region, the ventral primaries remain segmental and in the cervical and lumbosacral areas, they form plexuses.

The pelvis and lower extremity are innervated by nerves from four plexuses: the lumbar, sacral, pudendal, and coccygeal. These plexuses are formed from the ventral primary divisions of the five lumbar, five sacral, the coccygeal, and a contribution from the twelfth thoracic spinal nerves.

The lumbar plexus (Fig. 1–43) is formed by the twelfth thoracic, first three, and most of the fourth lumbar divisions. The plexus lies against the posterior abdominal wall against the psoas, often intertwined in the fasciculi of the muscle. Its terminal branches are as follows:

1. iliohypogastric	T12, L1
2. ilioinguinal	L1
3. genitofemoral	L1–2

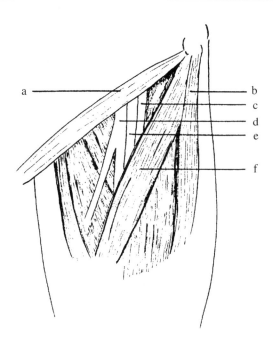

Fig. 1–41 Femoral triangle. a. inguinal ligament, b. TFL, c. femoral vein, d. femoral artery, e. femoral nerve, f. sartorius.

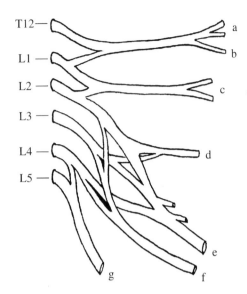

Fig. 1–43 Lumbar plexus. a. iliohypogastric nerves (T12, L1), b. ilioinguinal nerve (L1), c. genitofemoral nerves (L1, 2), d. lateral femoral cutaneous nerve (L2, 3), e. femoral nerve (L2, 3, 4), f. obturator nerve (L2, 3, 4), g. lumbosacral trunk.

4. lateral femoral cutaneous	L2–3
5. obturator	L2–3–4
6. femoral	L2–3–4
7. lumbosacral trunk	(to the sacral plexus)

The first three nerves innervate the tissues of the lower abdominal wall, including the muscles and skin of the buttock, proximal thigh, and groin. The lateral femoral cutaneous supplies the skin of the anterolateral thigh to the knee. The obturator nerve is the motor nerve for the adductors and gracilis, with an articular branch to the knee. The femoral nerve supplies sensory nerves to the anteromedial thigh and, via the saphenous branch, the medial leg and foot. Motor branches supply the sartorius, pectineus, and quadriceps group. Branches to the psoas leave the plexus at or near the beginning of the femoral nerve.

The sacral plexus (Fig. 1–44) is a combination of a portion of the fourth, all of the fifth lumbar, and first three sacral nerves. It lies against the piriformis on the posterior wall of the pelvis. The sacral plexus converges on the greater sciatic foramen. The bulk of the combined fibers make up the sciatic nerve. The sacral plexus has the following branches:

1. to the quadratus femoris and gemellus inferior	L4–5, S1
2. to the obturator internus and gemellus superior	L5, S1–2
3. to the piriformis (not shown in Fig. 1–44)	S1–2
4. superior gluteal	L4–5, S1
5. inferior gluteal	L5, S1–2

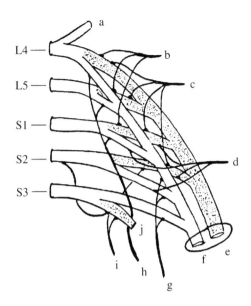

Fig. 1–44 Sacral Plexus. a. to lumbar plexus, b. superior gluteal nerve (L4–5, S1), c. inferior gluteal nerve (L4, S1, 2), d. posterior femoral cutaneous (S1, 2, 3), e. common peroneal nerve, f. tibial nerve, g. to obturator internus and gemellus superior (L5, S1, 2), h. to quadratus femoris and gemellus inferior (L4, 5, S1), i. inferior medial cluneal nerve (S2, 3), j. to pudendal plexus.

6. posterior femoral cutaneous	S1–2–3
7. perforating cutaneous	S2–3
8. sciatic (Fig. 1–44 e, f)	L4–5, S1–2–3
9. to pudendal plexus	S2–3–4
10. inferior medial cluneal	S2–S3

The first three branches are 3self-explanatory as to their function. The superior and inferior gluteal nerves innervate the gluteal muscles. The posterior femoral cutaneous nerve supplies the skin of the posterior thigh, leg, and perineum. The perforating cutaneous nerve supplies the skin over the medial and lower gluteus maximus.

The sciatic nerve is subdivided into the tibial and common peroneal, which travel together from the piriformis to the distal third of the posterior thigh before splitting up. The sciatic nerve supplies the skin of the foot and most of the leg, all the joints of the lower extremity, the posterior thigh muscles, and all the muscles of the leg and foot. The tibial portion of the sciatic nerve continues down the back of the leg, splitting into the medial and lateral plantar nerves as it rounds the medial malleolus on its way to the underside of the foot. The common peroneal nerve crosses the popliteal fossa, winds around the neck of the fibula, splitting into the superficial and deep peroneal nerves.

The pudendal and coccygeal plexuses (Fig. 1–45) have branches from the lower four sacral and the coccygeal nerves. They supply the perineal structures.

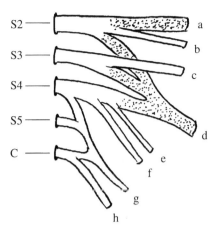

Fig. 1–45 Pudendal and coccygeal plexuses. a. b. c. to sacral plexus, d. pudendal nerve (S2, 3, 4), e. f. to levatorani, coccygeus, sphincter ani externus, g. h. anococcygeal nerves.

VISCERAL ANATOMY

The abdominal and pelvic viscera are contained and supported by the various pelvic structures and musculature. Every patient should have a visceral palpation examination. This will broaden examiners' diagnostic skills and increase their confidence in their ability to recognize abnormalities. When using the organic reflex techniques, knowing where the organs or reflex points are located can make the difference between the success and failure of treatment.

The organs are affected by the condition of the pelvic structures as well as the tone and function of the muscles. The psoas shelf supports the kidneys, ileocecal valve, appendix, ureters, and renal veins. The psoas can affect these structures if it is dysfunctional. The abdominal muscles hold the viscera in place. A weak, sagging abdomen can cause ptosis and alter the function of the organs. An anterior tilt to the pelvis can encourage ptosis and may affect the uterus adversely.

FUNCTIONAL ANATOMY

To fully appreciate the validity of diversified technique, it is necessary to develop a complete mental moving picture of the functional anatomy of the human body. Functional anatomy is a combination of biomechanics, kinesiology, and anatomy.

Not only the range of motion of individual articulations, but the combined actions of many joints must be understood. Muscles often have additional roles beyond their main actions. They can function in synchronization bilaterally and affect the body one way or operate unilaterally in various combinations that can complicate the clinical picture beyond the basics. It is easy to overlook important biomechanical considerations when examining a patient; therefore, it is important to understand the body's functional anatomy.

Range of Motion

The sacrum, as described earlier, is suspended between the ilia. Gillet[8] describes it as "floating" in the pelvic ring, passive in its movements, following along with the movements of the ilia and lumbars. Nutation of the sacrum is the rotational tilting of the sacrum over the horizontal axis at the axial ligament. The sacrum can rotate around a vertical axis and tilt obliquely (Fig. 1–46). It should be noted that the sacrum has no direct muscle attachments, except for a small segment of the iliacus and is in essence a passive player in the movements of the pelvis.

The ilia can rotate posteroanteriorly on the sacrum. The posterior superior iliac spines become closer to or further from the midline as the plane of rotation is tangential to the sagittal plane. The ilia can flare, the ischial tuberosities converging medially (Fig. 1–47), and they can shift inferiorly. The pubis can shift either inferiorly or superiorly. The hip joints have a wide range of motion, including flexion, extension, abduction, adduction, circumduction, and rotation.

The vertebrae have three basic movements upon each other: anterior to posterior (A-to-P; flexion/extension), lateral flexion, and rotation. The lumbar spine has a total flexion of approximately 40° and an extension of 30°. Most of the movement occurs at the L4 and L5 segments. Kapandji[2] notes that lateral bending is about 30°. All movements are greater early in life and diminish with age. Kapandji also considers the shape of the lumbar facetal articulations and the resistance to shearing of the disk restrictive to rotation and cites studies that give the total rotational movement of the lumbars as 10° in either direction. Interestingly, in these studies it was found

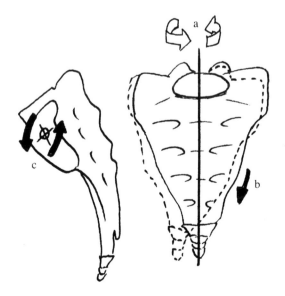

Fig. 1–46 Sacral movements. a. rotation around a vertical axis, b. oblique or inferior, c. nutation.

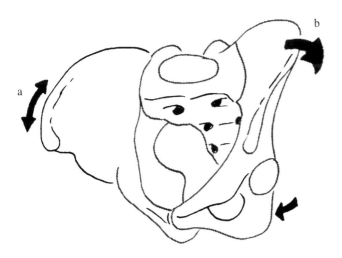

Fig. 1–47 Movements of the ilia. a. A-to-P rotation, b. flare.

that the thoracic spine has four times the rotational ability of the lumbar spine, in spite of the rib cage.

Gillet[9] describes lumbar flexion and extension as having less forward and backward gliding than the dorsal or cervical spine. He also describes the combination of flexion/rotation involved in lateral bending and states that the Lovett principle is only truly present in the lower dorsal and lumbar spine. According to the Lovett principle, the rotation of the vertebrae in lateral flexion is normal or positive if the body rotates toward the convexity and the spinous toward the concavity (Fig. 1–48).

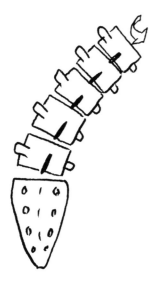

Fig. 1–48 Lumbar lateral flexion with rotational component.

Lordosis and Pelvic Tilt

The pelvis is balanced over the hip joints. The A-to-P tilt of the pelvis affects the lumbar lordosis (Fig. 1–49). The interplay of the muscles above and below has a vital role in this balancing act that also includes a sacroiliac component. The A-to-P rotation of the ilia on the sacrum adds a slight degree to pelvic tilt, without affecting the lordosis. Kendall[9] describes the neutral pelvic position as having the anterior superior iliac spine (ASIS) and the pubic symphysis in the same vertical plane. Kapandji[2] refers to the interspinous line between the anterior and posterior iliac spines as level in a neutral pelvis. Both methods are good indicators.

When the pelvis tilts anteriorly, the lumbar curvature is increased and the hip joints are flexed. In a posterior tilt, the curve is decreased and the hip joints are extended. Excessive posterior tilt is checked by the iliofemoral ligaments, which become taut.

In the erect stance, the abdominals, gluteus maximus, and hamstrings influence the pelvis posteriorly (Fig. 1–50). The abdominals can be thought of as the anterior muscles of the lower spine. The rectus and the oblique fibers help support the pelvis, pulling upward on the pubis while the posterior fibers pull posteriorly on the iliac crests, reducing the lordosis as well as the pelvic tilt. The abdominal oblique and transverse fibers, especially the more posterior fibers, are often involved in low back and pelvic conditions and are often overlooked in evaluation and treatment.

The gluteus maximus works with the abdominals to pull the pelvis posteriorly in the erect stance. With the legs planted, the gluteus maximus, with its attachments to the femur, iliac crest, and sacrum, keeps the pelvis from tilting too far anteriorly. The hamstrings provide further pull on the ischia, keeping them from riding superiorly. The gluteus maximus is often

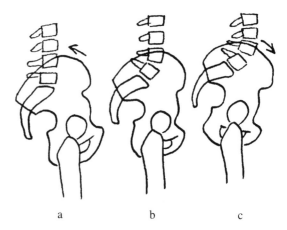

Fig. 1–49 Pelvic tilt and lordotic curve changes. a. posterior, decreased curve, b. neutral, c. anterior, increased curve.

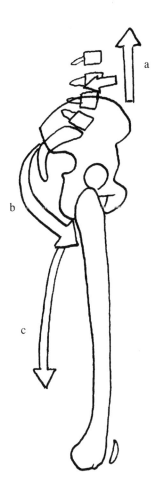

Fig. 1–50 Muscles that influence the pelvis posteriorly. a. abdominals, b. gluteus maximus, c. hamstrings.

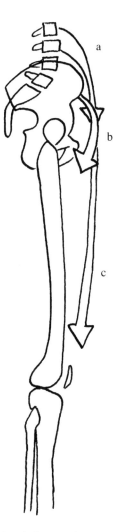

Fig. 1–51 Muscles that influence the pelvis anteriorly. a. psoas, b. iliacus, c. sartorius, TFL, rectus femoris.

found to be weak or have weak portions. The hamstrings are often too short and often contractured.

The psoas, iliacus, and, to a lesser extent, the sartorius' TFL and rectus femoris influence the pelvis anteriorly (Fig. 1–51). The psoas influences the lumbar spine into lordosis. Bogduk[10] feels that the design of the psoas adds a compressive force to the lumbar spine increasing the lordotic tendency. The iliacus pulls the ilia anteriorly. It is principally the middle fibers of the iliac fossa that are responsible. The more anterior fibers near the ASIS pull the iliac crest more inward.

With their attachments to the anterior and inferior iliac spines, the sartorius and rectus femoris pull from their respective knee insertions encouraging the pelvis to tilt anteriorly.

In the erect stance, the pelvis is balanced by a concert of synergistic and antagonistic actions by the above described muscles. Kendall[9] believes the erector spinae contributes to lordosis when they are chronically contracted. The erectors are not as significant in affecting the tilt of the pelvis as the previously mentioned muscles; however, if contracted, they

are responsible for increasing the lumbar curvature without involving the pelvis. Kapandji[2] notes that, with the sacrum fixed, the erectors are powerful extensors acting on the lumbosacral and thoracolumbar joints. This extension will increase the lordosis. They may also be contracted secondary to a chronic lordotic lumbar syndrome (see Chapter 6 on Conditions and Treatment.)

Transverse Pelvic Stability

In the optimal erect stance, the pelvis is level horizontally across the iliac crests and at the posterior superior iliac spines. The dynamic actions translated through the hips and pelvis in all phases of movement are the counterpart of the stability that the pelvis provides in supporting the body.

The important muscles in lateral stability include the adductors, abductors, hamstrings, oblique abdominals, quadratus lumborum, psoas, and the iliacus and transversus perinei (Fig. 1–52).

In the erect position, the gluteus medius is the major lateral stabilizer. It is a very important muscle in walking and running. Its function is that of a hip abductor, but from another perspective it can be viewed as a lateral flexor of the pelvis on the hip. With a major weakness of the medius, the pelvis will drop on the opposite side when the contralateral leg is lifted (a positive Trendelenberg sign; Fig. 1–53). The medius is often found to be weak enough to cause adaptive problems without showing a positive Trendelenberg sign. The gluteus minimus

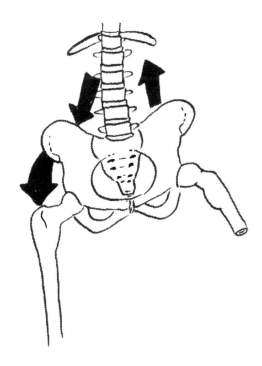

Fig. 1–53 Action of gluteus medius and Q-L in Trendelenberg's test. Q-L supports lumbar spine on right and lifts pelvis on left.

and the TFL play a significant role in supporting the medius.

The oblique abdominals can lift the pelvis. The ipsilateral internal oblique and the contralateral external oblique work together to lift the iliac crest (Fig. 1–52). For instance, in lifting the left leg, the right gluteus medius, minimus and external oblique, and the left internal oblique abdominals are acting in concert to keep the left side of the pelvis from dropping.

At the same time the quadratus lumborum is working bilaterally, the left will be lifting the ilium, and the right will be stabilizing the lumbar spine, keeping it from bending to the left (Fig. 1–53). The psoas on the right will also be holding the lumbars.

If the weight remains on the right leg and the pelvis is anterior or posterior of neutral, there is a recruitment of additional abductors. In neutral, the medius is the main muscle. With the pelvis in a posterior tilt, the TFL and minimus can be called into action. As the pelvis tilts anteriorly, the maximus, then the piriformis, obturator externus, and quadratus femoris will successively come into play keeping the pelvis level.

The hamstrings act as stabilizers in the erect posture and assist in moving the pelvis from side to side. Standing with both feet on the ground, transverse stability is accomplished by the synergistic/antagonistic check and balance of all these muscles.

The transverse perinei muscles will approximate the ischial tuberosities (Fig. 1–54). They act as a check to prevent the

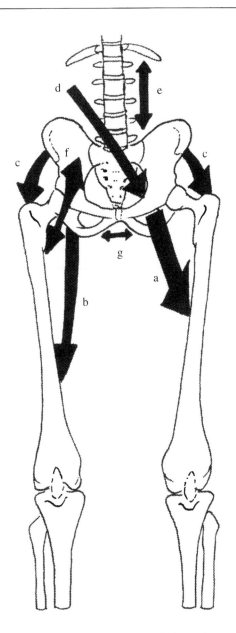

Fig. 1–52 Lateral stability. a. adductors, b. hamstrings, c. abductors, d. oblique abdominals, e. Q-L, f. iliopsoas, g. transversus perinei.

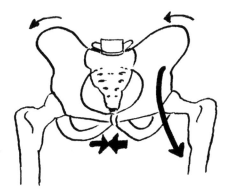

Fig. 1–54 Transversus perinei pull ischia medially causing iliac flare, anterior fibers of the iliacus pull ilia medially reducing flare.

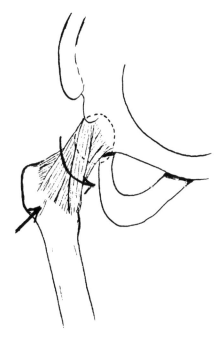

Fig. 1–55 "Screw-home" design of the hip capsule.

tuberosities from spreading too far apart. Lateral flexion or flare of the ilia on the sacrum is produced by the transverse perinei pulling the tuberosities medially (Fig. 1–54). The anterior fibers of the iliacus counter this by pulling the iliac crests medially, which spreads the tuberosities and encourages a medial flexion of the ilia on the sacrum. The internal oblique abdominals lend support, pulling inward on the iliac crests. With these muscles acting in concert, the pelvis remains relatively balanced and stable. The transversus perinei need to be strong to oppose the pull of the adductors. They contract first before the adductors can begin to work.

Gillet[8] describes the mechanisms of lateral and medial flexion of the ilia involved in sitting and standing. He describes the ilia as flaring, the ischia coming together upon standing. When persons sit, the ischia spread out to provide a wider base for distribution of weight. The synergistic actions of the transversus perinei and anterior iliacus fibers are major stabilizers in this action.

Hip Actions

The hip joint is held together by fibrous extensions of the acetabulum, the labrum, and zona orbicularis. The acetabulum is not a deep enough socket alone. Its articular surfaces are firmly coapted by atmospheric pressure. The head of the femur is very difficult to remove from the socket without allowing air into the joint space.

While erect, the weight of the body also keeps the femoral head in place. The ligaments of the joint capsule wrap around the joint from posterior to anterior and become taut in extension, checking further extension and, conversely, posterior rotation of the pelvis. The femoral head is "screwed" into the acetabulum by this ligamentous configuration (Fig. 1–55). It is interesting to note that the anterior hip joint has heavy ligaments and less musculature, but the posterior aspect has the

opposite. The hip is much more stable in extension than any other position.

The muscles that are in line with the femoral neck work to hold the femur in place. The piriformis, obturator externus, and the gluteus medius are noted by Kapandji[11] to be the main muscles of hip apposition (Fig. 1–56). He notes that the longitudinal muscles, like the adductors, can be a strong force to

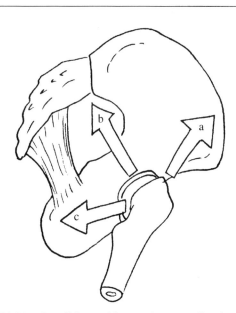

Fig. 1–56 Muscles of hip aposition. a. gluteus medius, b. piriformis, c. obturator externus.

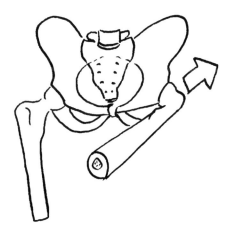

Fig. 1–57 Hip in adduction and flexion—weakest position for dislocation.

dislocate the hip. The hip is weakest in adduction with flexion (Fig. 1–57). Hip dysplasia or a shallow acetabulum can facilitate dislocation as the roof of the socket can be angled more superiorly.

The extensor muscles of the hip are primarily the gluteus maximus and the hamstrings, assisted by the fibers of the gluteus medius and minimus and the adductors (mostly the magnus; Fig. 1-58) Kapandji[11] divides the extensors into two groups. The gluteus maximus along with the medius and minimus extend and abduct. The hamstrings and adductor magnus extend and adduct. Pure extension requires a balance between these two sets of synergists and antagonists. The hamstrings cross two joints, the hip and knee. The more extended the knee, the more efficient their extensor action at the hip.

Hip flexion is primarily the responsibility of the iliopsoas. Assisting the iliopsoas are the sartorius, TFL, rectus femoris, pectineus, adductor longus, and gracilis (Fig. 1–59). When these muscles act in concert, one sees pure flexion. The individual flexors are also capable of abduction, adduction, and medial and lateral rotation. The rectus femoris is a biarticular muscle, flexing the hip and extending the knee. The more the knee is flexed, the more efficient the rectus is at hip flexion.

A combination of flexion-abduction-medial rotation is accomplished with the aid of the anterior fibers of the gluteus medius and minimus. Flexion-adduction-lateral rotation is produced with the iliopsoas, pectineus, and the adductor longus predominating. In flexion-adduction-medial rotation, the adductors and TFL predominate.[11]

The main abductor of the hip is the gluteus medius (Fig. 1-60). It is situated nearly perpendicular to its lever arm. The minimus is essentially an abductor, and the TFL is a strong abductor in the erect stance. The most superior fibers of the maximus assist in abduction, and the piriformis, a main lateral rotator, kicks in with the hip flexed (Fig. 1–61).

The principal adductors are the adductor group, the largest being the magnus. It lies posterior to the adductors longus and brevis and has some extension capability, but the longus and brevis can assist only in flexion. Other important muscles assisting in adduction are the hamstrings, gluteus maximus,

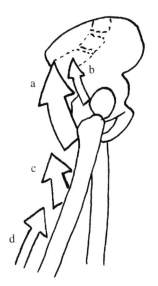

Fig. 1–58 Muscles of hip extension. a. gluteus maximus, b. gluteus medius and minimus, c. adductor magnus, d. hamstrings.

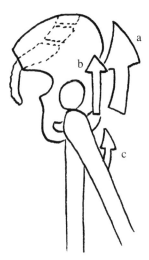

Fig. 1–59 Muscles of hip flexion. a. iliopsoas, b. sartorius, TFL, rectus femoris, c. adductor longus, gracilis, pectineus.

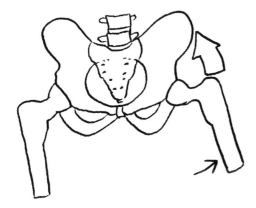

Fig. 1–60 Gluteus medius—main hip abductor.

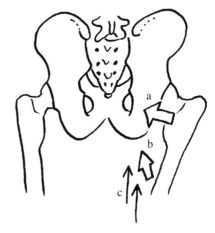

Fig. 1–62 Muscles of adduction. a. quadratus femoris, pectineus, obturators, b. adductor group and gluteus maximus, c. hamstrings, gracilis.

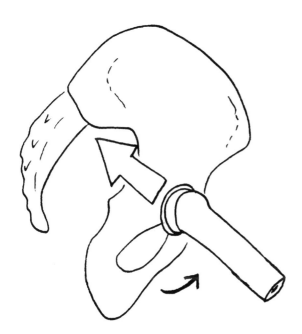

Fig. 1–61 With hip flexed, piriformis acts as an abductor.

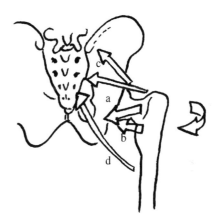

Fig. 1–63 Lateral rotatores. a. piriformis, obturators, gemelli, b. pectineus, quadratus femoris, c. gluteus medius, maximus, d. adductors.

quadratus femoris, pectineus, both obturators, and the gracilis (Fig. 1–62).

Lateral rotation is accomplished by numerous powerful muscles (Fig. 1–63). The piriformis, the obturators, and gemelli are the principal rotatores and are assisted by the quadratus femoris, pectineus, fibers of the gluteus maximus, medius, and adductor magnus. The obturator externus has some flexor influence and is a more powerful lateral rotator with the hip in flexion. The piriformis does more abduction with the hip in flexion.

Medial rotation is accomplished with less force and fewer muscles, the TFL and anterior fibers of the gluteus medius and most of the minimus (Fig. 1–64). When the hip is in extreme medial rotation, the obturator externus and the pectineus become medial rotatores. This is an example of what Kapandji[11] calls inversion of muscular action. It is easy to see that the main function of a muscle can become altered, demonstrating secondary functions, or even be reversed depending on the position of the joint. Another example is the previously mentioned secondary abduction function of the piriformis in hip flexion (Fig. 1–61). With extreme flexion, the piriformis becomes capable of medial rotation and extension.

Lumbar Mechanics

The lumbar spine sits on the sacral base, taking off at a forward tilt. The lordotic curve is maintained and influenced by

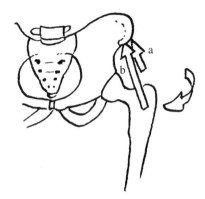

Fig. 1–64 Medial rotatores. a. TFL, b. gluteus medius and minimus anterior fibers.

the pelvic tilt, the wedge of the L5–S1 functional unit, the sacral base angle, and the action of the related muscles.

The paravertebral muscles, all the deep muscles covering one to several segments, are responsible for extending, rotating, and laterally bending individual or groups of segments. Clinically, they are considered in a general context when examining and treating a back condition. They will often be found to be hypertonic and inflamed in areas of dysfunction.

The last two vertebrae are rather tightly bound to the ilia by the iliolumbar ligaments and therefore have a limited range of motion compared to L3 and above. Kapandji[2] gives L3 a significant role in the erect posture. It is at the apex of the lordosis and is generally parallel to the horizontal plane. L3 has a beefier arch, anchoring the ascending spinalis fibers and the descending iliolumbar fibers from the lats. It is itself anchored and pulled inferiorly by erector spinae fibers from the sacrum and ilium (Fig. 1–65).

T12 is considered to be the point of inflexibility between the lumbar and thoracic spine. It acts as a swivel and is bypassed by some of the vertebral muscles attaching above and below it.[2]

When considering the lumbar spine clinically, there are several important muscles that need to be fully understood for a clinician to be successful in treating the low back and pelvis. The iliacus, psoas, gluteus maximus, and quadratus lumborum are most often involved in one combination or another in low back and pelvic dysfunctions.

In the erect stance, the lumbar spine and pelvis are supported by the synergistic/antagonistic actions of the surrounding muscles. Anteriorly, the abdominals are powerful flexors of the trunk. They also work in the opposite direction to lift the pelvis, which can reduce the lordosis (Fig. 1–66). This is an act of flexion as well with a reversal of stabilization and affected points.

The psoas muscles, principally hip flexors, act to compress the lumbars and tend to increase the lordosis, especially the

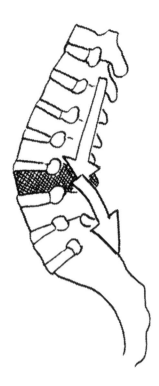

Fig. 1–65 L3: anchor for lower fibers of erector spinae and ascending fibers of spinalis and descending latissimus dorsi.

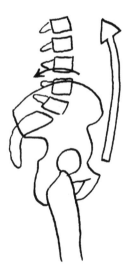

Fig. 1–66 Abdominals' effect on posterior pelvic rotation.

upper lumbar fibers (Fig. 1–67). L4 and L5 are more flexed by the psoas. When the pelvis and lumbar spine are in full flexion, as in bending over, before the body can begin to arise, L5 is further flexed by its psoas slip. This holds L5 in flexion, which facilitates the extension of the rest of the lumbar spine

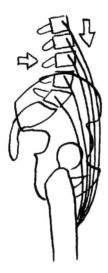

Fig. 1–67 Psoas effect on compression of lumbars, increasing lordosis.

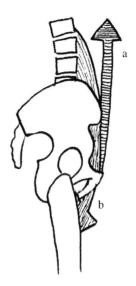

Fig. 1–69 Antagonistic action of a. abdominals and b. psoas in erect posture.

and pelvis by increasing leverage (Fig. 1–68). The L5 psoas slip is often found to be dysfunctional, either hypo- or hypertonic. Bending and lifting injuries commonly involve the psoas, especially the L5 slip.

There is a relationship between the psoas and the abdominals. They work together in an act such as a sit-up. The abdominals initiate the act, and the psoas kicks in at the halfway point. They antagonize each other in the standing position, the abdominals lifting or influencing the pelvis posteriorly, while the compressive influence of the psoas increases the lordosis, and by flexing the hips, influences the pelvis, tilting it anteriorly (Fig. 1–69).

Posteriorly, the erector spinae and the deep paravertebrals are important extensors. The gluteus maximus keeps the pelvis in check, facilitating extension by pulling the pelvis posteriorly (Fig. 1–70). The maximus is considered the most powerful muscle in the body, yet it is often found to be weak.

The Q-L is a much more important muscle than originally thought. The Q-L runs between the iliac crest and the last rib, with two of its three layers giving slips to the first four lumbar (not the fifth) transverse processes. These slips run in a lateral and slightly anterior direction (Fig. 1–71). In the erect stance,

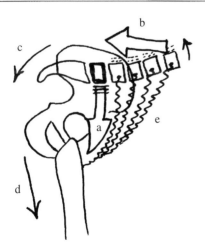

Fig. 1–68 Initial stage of arising from a bent position. a. L5 psoas slip contracts hard—keeping L5 flexed, b. erector spinae contracts, c. gluteus maximus contracts, d. hamstrings contract, e. relaxed upper psoas fibers.

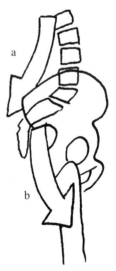

Fig. 1–70 Erect posture—extension of spine and pelvis by a. erector spinae and b. gluteus maximus.

the Q-L helps the lumbars to resist the forward pull of the psoas (Fig. 1–71). The individual slips from the transverse processes can influence the movement and position of the first four lumbars. These slips play a part in lumbar dysfunction and subluxation. The Q-L slip from the fourth lumbar is an important check on anterior rotation of the ilium if the lumbar spine is fixed by its support muscles.

The Q-L's principal function is described as lateral flexion of the spine. In tandem, they resist the anterior pull on the lumbars. They work with the abdominals, psoas, and paravertebrals to rotate the spine and trunk.

One can see by this multitude of seemingly conflicting functions that a muscle can operate in a variety of directions depending on the demands of the moment and the position of its origin or insertion. The Q-L is often found to have significant weakness, often unilateral, which can have a significant impact on spinal and pelvic stability.

Static and Dynamic Posture

In evaluating the biomechanical function of a patient, the unilateral function of the various muscles must be considered. To further complicate things, each muscle is actually a collection of smaller muscle bundles that can be considered as separate muscles. One must consider that portions of a muscle may be dysfunctional. It is possible to have part of a muscle hypertonic, part hypotonic, and part functioning normally, and the muscle may test normal!

Most lower back and pelvic problems involve the muscles in various combinations of hyper- and hypotonic states. In looking at the mechanics of the area, the examiner must consider the muscular interactions and determine which muscle or muscles are malfunctioning and if the involvement is bilateral, unilateral, oblique (diagonal), or internal.

When investigating a patient's complaints, the kinesiology of the area should lead the examiner to look at the muscles that produce the perceived imbalance, those that allow it, and those that provide secondary support. Careful scrutiny will reveal the muscles most likely to be involved. They could be above, below, next to, diagonally across, or obliquely above or below. Determining whether the whole or only a portion of a muscle is involved will help pinpoint the problem, which may even be caused by one of the more obscure muscles. If not discovered, any muscle dysfunction will prevent a complete recovery.

Posture is maintained by the coordinated effort of these muscles. The coordination is provided by the proprioceptive nervous system. The patients' basic posture will reveal much about their condition and how their body is adapting to stresses and dysfunction. We must visualize patients biomechanically and mentally compare the image to our understanding of ideal function. A key to successful treatment, which in chiropractic involves the reduction of subluxations, is the correction of any kinesiopathology.

Ideal Posture

We often refer to normal posture, but rarely is the normal specimen found except in text books. Even Kendall[9] admits

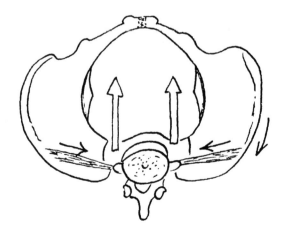

Fig. 1–71 Anterolateral pull of Q-L fibers influences ilia posterior and resists anterior pull of psoas (large arrows).

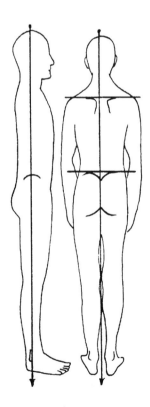

Fig. 1–72 Ideal (plumb line) posture.

that they had never seen a subject that fit all their criteria for perfect posture.

As chiropractors, we guide our patients toward maximum health. A smooth-functioning, balanced musculoskeletal system is fundamental to the successful reduction of subluxations and their effects on the nervous system. Kendall[9] describes ideal posture as it would be seen upon examination. Figure 1–72 demonstrates the ideal plumb line posture and should become a mental standard in patient evaluations.

When a Homo sapien stands erect, he or she is using minimal muscle power and the proprioceptive nervous system to keep the balancing act together. If we compare the Homo sapiens to other primates, we see that we have had to adapt to the erect position. We have had to curve the spine in the sagittal plane. The lower back sits on a base that tilts forward. The lumbar spine has to curve back and then goes into a kyphotic curve as it ascends to the neck where it curves anteriorly again, all necessary to balance the body.

The lumbar lordosis is adaptive, and there are muscular adaptations as well that are necessary to support the upright position. According to Michele[12] in his book *Iliopsoas*, the elongation of the iliopsoas is a primary adaptation to the upright stance. He contends that it is often incomplete and that the failure of the muscle to fully elongate is a primary factor in low back and pelvic problems. Dr. Logan stressed the importance of the iliacus and psoas. However, in his studies, he concluded that the two muscles cannot be considered as one. He even stressed the idea of viewing the psoas as five distinct muscles, one for each lumbar segment. It is important to recognize that portions of the muscle can be hypertonic and others hypotonic.

The psoas and iliacus can be out of balance, which will alter the relationship between the lumbar lordosis and pelvic tilt. If the psoas were hypertonic and the iliacus normal or hypotonic, the lordosis would be increased with the pelvis neutral or tilted posteriorly (Fig. 1–73). If both are hypertonic, swayback can result (Fig. 1–74) with an increased lordosis and anterior pelvic tilt, especially if the abdominals and gluteus maximus are not able to compensate. If the psoas and the iliacus were hypotonic (Fig. 1–75), a clinical picture of a flat back could be seen with a decreased lordosis and posterior pelvic tilt. If the psoas is weak and the iliacus hypertonic (Fig. 1–76), there could be a decreased or normal lordosis and anterior pelvic tilt, exaggerated by weak abdominals.

The neutral, ideal standing posture has the feet placed evenly apart under the hip joints and the pelvis level in the sagittal and coronal planes. The knees are in slight flexion (not hyperextended and locked). The head is over the shoulders, which are, in turn, over the rib cage. The use of the plumb line is helpful, but it should become easy to spot imbalances once the ideal mechanical image is ingrained. If the pelvis is deviated from the ideal neutral position, the distortion in the lower back will transfer upward into the thoracic and cervical spine,

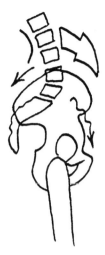

Fig. 1–73 Psoas hypertonic, iliacus weak—increased lordosis with pelvis neutral or posterior.

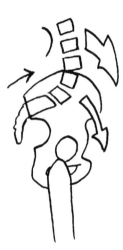

Fig. 1–74 Psoas and iliacus hypertonic—increased lordosis, anterior pelvis.

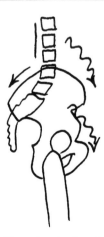

Fig. 1–75 Psoas and iliacus hypotonic—decreased lordosis, pelvis neutral or posterior.

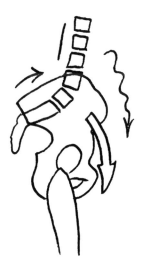

Fig. 1–76 Psoas hypotonic, iliacus hypertonic—decreased lordosis, anterior pelvis.

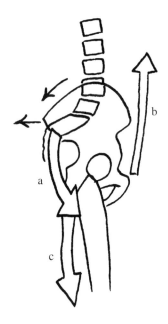

Fig. 1–77 Muscles that produce a posterior shift. a. gluteus maximus, b. abdominals, c. hamstrings.

either exaggerating or reducing the normal curvatures accordingly.

As mentioned earlier, muscles fall into one of three categories when analyzed for specific biomechanical function: (1) those that allow an action, (2) those that produce an action, and (3) those that support an action. When a muscle allows an action to occur, it is relaxing or contracting eccentrically (lengthening the muscle) against the opposing load. The concentric contraction of a muscle (causing the muscle to shorten) is a producer of an action. The support muscles are the synergists assisting in stabilizing the skeletal system around the area of action. The support muscles would be in a sustained contraction during the action.

Looking at the A-to-P balancing mechanism, the muscles that produce a posterior shift of body weight are those that produce a posterior tilting of the pelvis, primarily the gluteus maximus, abdominals, and, to a lesser degree, the hamstrings (Fig. 1–77). The muscles that allow this posterior shift are the psoas, iliacus, and the sartorius and rectus femoris. They must relax and let the producers take over.

Anterior shifting is a reversal of the above with the producers being the psoas, iliacus, and other synergists (Fig. 1–78). Those that allow it are the gluteus maximus, abdominals, and synergists. Recall that the fourth segment of the quadratus lumborum has a significant role in the A-to-P stability of the ilium. Its line of pull from the transverse process of L4 to the iliac crest gives it the ability to support the ilia when the lumbar spine is fixed. Therefore, it can be significantly involved in the production of posterior rotation of the ilia or allow anterior rotation.

The balancing act of the pelvis in the erect stance is accomplished by the interplay of these pelvic muscles in the A-to-P plane and by the lateral stabilizers in the transverse plane. As

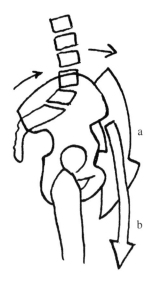

Fig. 1–78 Muscles that produce an anterior shift. a. psoas, iliacus, b. TFL, rectus femoris, sartorius.

the pelvis is influenced posteriorly by the weight of the body, it is checked by the psoas, iliacus, and, ultimately, the iliofemoral ligaments. The abdominals hold the pelvis up, and the erector spinae supports the spine by extending it. The gluteus maximus pulls back on the pelvis countered by the iliacus and psoas. There are other muscles in the lower extremities that also play important roles in maintaining the erect stance (see texts on *The Knee* and *The Foot and Ankle* by Dr. Logan).

Postural Faults

Postural faults are frequently seen in lower back patients. The most common is the lordotic lumbar syndrome (LLS). This is due to an exaggeration of the lumbar lordosis and anterior rotation of the ilia, shifting the body weight forward (Fig. 1–79). It is produced by hypertonic, tight psoas and iliacus, weak, stretched gluteus maximus, and weak or nonfunctioning abdominals (Fig. 1–80). There may or may not be significant changes in the upper spinal curvatures. Such changes would include an increased thoracic kyphosis and anterior displacement of the head and neck.

A flat-back fault is the opposite of the LLS with a posterior rotation of the pelvis with the gluteus maximus being hypertonic and the psoas weak (Fig. 1–81). This is seen less often clinically.

Unleveling of the pelvis in the transverse plane is another common fault often seen with leg length insufficiency (LLI), either anatomical or functional. Opposing or unilateral rotations of the ilia and corresponding muscular adaptations occur in an attempt to correct the unleveling.

Posture in Motion

In diagnosing the mechanical cause of a low back condition, knowing what is occurring during specific actions that precipitate symptoms is vital to a successful treatment outcome. For

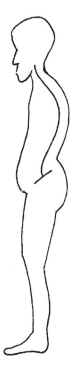

Fig. 1–80 Chronic LLS.

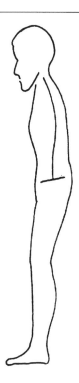

Fig. 1–81 Flat-back posture.

example, a patient with an acute low back episode will often arise with weight borne on one leg to reduce stress on the injured area (see Chapter 2 on Examination).

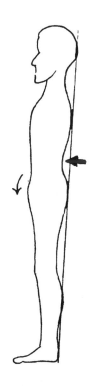

Fig. 1–79 Lordotic lumbar syndrome (LLS).

Standing on One Foot

When the weight in the standing position is placed on one foot, the low back and pelvis must adapt in order to remain level and support the upper body. The pelvis will tend to drop on the non–weight-bearing side, and the lumbar spine will curve away from the supported side. The thoracic spine will compensate by curving back, and the neck could tend in the direction of the lumbars. In a healthy body, this is minimized. The support muscles will go to work to see that balance is maintained.

The gluteus medius is a key muscle in this position. The medius on the weight-bearing side, assisted by other abductor muscles, will be working to keep the pelvis as level as possible (Fig. 1-82). A significant weakness of the medius will be seen as a positive Trendelenberg test with a significant drop of the pelvis on the unsupported side. The Q-L will be active on both sides (Fig. 1–82). On the weight-bearing side, the Q-L and psoas will be retaining the lumbar spine, reducing its tendency to curve convexly toward the unsupported side. On the resting side, the Q-L will be lifting the pelvis superiorly, aided by the oblique abdominals. Clinically, any lack of balance or weakness observed when evaluating this function should lead the examiner to investigate these muscles and correct any dysfunction.

Arising

The act of arising from a seated position involves many muscles acting in concert. Some will be active, contracting concentrically (CC), producing the action; others will be eccentrically contracting (EC), allowing the action; and others will be supportive (S). The act of arising can be broken down into four stages: (1) forward movement of the trunk, (2) initiation of elevation of the buttocks from the seat, (3) midway to erect, and (4) final movement to erect. Exhibit 1–1 describes the various functions of the most significant muscles in the stages of arising.

In reviewing Exhibit 1–1, the bold concentric contractions (CC) captions in the second stage indicate that the Q-L, gluteus maximus, and the quadriceps femoris are contracting hard and are the most important muscles in the act of standing up.

Arising on One Foot

The act of standing up with the weight on the right foot emphasizes a unilateral change in the efforts of the Q-L and gluteus maximus and activates harder contractions from other muscles (see Exhibit 1–2).

Exhibit 1–2 shows that the Q-L must contract harder on the left side to lift the unsupported side while the gluteus maximus works much harder on the weight-bearing side as does the quadriceps femoris. Both Exhibits 1–1 and 1–2 demonstrate the great importance of the Q-L and gluteus maximus—two muscles that should be considered early in the investigation of lower back disorders.

Bending and Lifting

The lumbar-pelvic rhythm is the coordinated movement of the lumbar spine and the pelvis necessary for a smooth movement into full flexion, as in bending over, and a return to the upright position. Cailliet[5] describes the rhythm as a precise ratio of lumbar flexion and anterior pelvic rotation over the hip

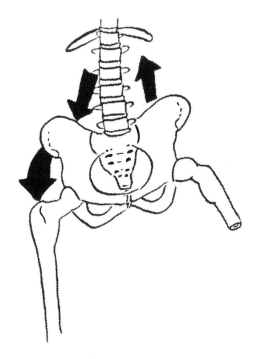

Fig. 1–82 Gluteus medius and Q-L function standing on one foot.

Exhibit 1–1 Muscle Function in Stages of Arising

Muscle	Stage 1	2	3	4
erector spinae	EC	S	CC	CC
psoas	CC	S	EC/S	EC/S
iliacus	CC	EC	EC	EC
abdominals	CC	—	—	—
quadratus lumborum	EC	**CC**	CC	CC/S
gluteus maximus	—	**CC**	CC	CC
transverse peroneal	CC	S	S	—
piriformis	CC/S	CC	CC	—
gluteus medius	S	S	S	—
quadraceps femoris	—	**CC**	CC	CC
hamstrings	S	EC	EC	—
adductors	S	S	S	—
gastrocnemeus	EC	EC	EC	—

Exhibit 1–2 Muscle Function in Stages of Arising on One Foot

Muscles	Stage							
	1L	*R*	*2L*	*R*	*3L*	*R*	*4L*	*R*
erector spinae	EC	EC	S	CC	CC	CC	CC	CC
abdominals	CC	CC	S	CC	CC	S	EC	EC
quadratus lumborum	**CC**	CC	**CC**	CC	**CC**	CC	**CC**	S
psoas	CC	CC	S	S	EC	EC	EC	EC
gluteus maximus	—	—	CC	**CC**	CC	**CC**	CC	**CC**
transverse peroneus	—	—	CC	CC	S	S	S	S
piriformis	—	—	S	CC	S	CC	S	CC
gluteus medius	—	—	CC	CC	S	CC	S	CC
quadriceps femoris	—	—	CC	**CC**	S	**CC**	S	**CC**
hamstrings	—	—	EC	EC	EC	EC	EC	EC

joints. The lumbar spine flexes maximally by the time the trunk is inclined 45°. The pelvis, which has been tipping anteriorly, continues to tilt to complete the process. The reverse action is exactly the opposite. If this is a normal rhythm, the pelvic tilt is responsible for probably 70% of the overall action.

Kapandji[2] describes the muscular action in bending over as beginning with the paravertebrals and erectors contracting hard. As the trunk is lowered, there must be an eccentric contraction of the erectors gradually allowing the body to flex. The gluteus maximus is next in the sequence contracting hard, then eccentrically lowering the pelvis. The hamstrings are the last to kick in, lowering the pelvis the rest of the way. Cailliet[5] mentions the mechanical advantage of flexing the knees which contracts the quadriceps femoris tightening the iliotibial tract giving the gluteus a better purchase. This is an advantage in lifting, taking the stress off the spine.

The act of arising is essentially the opposite, the hamstrings then the gluteals contract concentrically, tilting the pelvis posteriorly. Dr. Logan found that the psoas slip from L5 will contract hard to hold L5 in flexion as the rest of the psoas is relaxing and the erectors and paravertebrals are extending the spine above. This appears to provide better leverage for extension.

Reclining and Active Straight Leg Raising

In the supine position, with the legs extended, the tension of the psoas muscles will accentuate the curvature of the lumbar spine leaving a gap between the spine and the table. If the psoas muscles are hypertonic, the gap can be significant. This position can be uncomfortable at best. By flexing the legs, allowing the pelvis to rotate posteriorly, the tension can be reduced flattening the spine and bringing it closer to the surface of the table.

In the supine position, an active straight leg raise (SLR) provides another look at muscular integration in the low back and pelvis. If the right leg is actively raised, the first thing that has to happen is a stabilization of the pelvis and lower back.

The left side of the lower back must be supported more aggressively to offset the weight change on the right as the leg is lifted. The left Q-L, iliocostalis lumborum, and serratus posterior inferior contract. The abdominals contract to support the pelvis preventing it from tilting anteriorly. The muscles that produce the lift are the psoas, iliacus, sartorius, rectus femoris, and TFL. If examiners place their fingers on the lumbar spinous processes while the right leg is rising, the vertebrae will be felt to rotate to the left away from the active leg raise. This is a sign that the support muscles are in play, pulling against the spine and countering the weight of the rising leg. The maximum degree of rise may be restricted by shortened hamstrings.

CONCLUSION

The static and functional anatomy of the human body is of paramount importance in the diagnosis and treatment of musculoskeletal conditions. A thorough understanding of the way muscles attach and operate the various articulations will enable practitioners to be competent in analyzing their patients and innovative in their approach to treatment.

As has been demonstrated, most muscles have actions beyond their main function. Synergistic actions, antagonistic actions, and support actions can be performed by the same muscle in different situations. Reciprocal inhibition, the neurological phenomenon where the contraction of one muscle is coupled with the inhibition of its antagonist, can occur in an A/P plane, a superior/inferior plane, or a diagonal plane, either horizontally or vertically.

Several of the most common structural dysfunctions have also been demonstrated. The vast majority of low back complaints will be found to have one to several of these common dysfunctions. However, there is no limit to the variety of possibilities that could occur. With a keen knowledge of structure and function, there are no limits on the abilities of the practitioner.

REFERENCES

1. Gray H. *Anatomy of the Human Body.* (29th Am ed). Philadelphia, Pa: Lea & Febiger; 1973.
2. Kapandji A. *The Physiology of the Joints. The Trunk and Vertebral Column.* New York, NY: Churchill Livingstone; 1974.
3. Ramamurti. *Orthopedics in Primary Care.* Baltimore, Md: Williams & Wilkins; 1982.
4. Farfan HF. *Mechanical Disorders of the Low Back.* Philadelphia, Pa: Lea & Febiger; 1973.
5. Cailliet R. *Low Back Pain Syndrome* (3rd ed.) Philadelphia, Pa: Davis; 1981.
6. Barge F. *Tortipelvis.* Davenport, Iowa: Bawdin; 1986.
7. Logan AL. *The Knee: Clinical Aspects.* Gaithersburg, Md: Aspen; 1994.
8. Gillet H. *Belgian Chiropractic Research Notes 1985.* Huntington Beach, Calif: Motion Palpation Institute; 1985.
9. Kendall H. *Posture and Pain.* Malabar, Fla: Robert E. Krieger; 1985.
10. Bogduk N. Anatomy and biomechanics of psoas major. *Clin Biomech.* 1992;7:109–119.
11. Kapandji A. *The Physiology of the Joints. Lower Limb.* New York, NY: Churchill Livingstone; 1974:2.
12. Michele A. *Iliopsoas.* Springfield, Ill: Charles C Thomas; 1962.

Many symptoms in the upper body stem from problems in the lower back, pelvis, or lower extremities. Therefore, no chiropractic examination is complete without determining the condition of the lower torso. With a clear understanding of the functional anatomy of the area of complaint and its relation to the body as a whole, it becomes easier for the clinician to objectify the musculoskeletal findings and develop a treatment plan.

OBSERVATION

The exam should begin with the examiner's observation of the patient. Does the patient appear to be in pain? Facial expression can give important clues. How does the patient position himself? Is she able to sit? Does he sit level or off to one side? How easily does he arise? Does she arise with weight balanced equally on both feet, or with most of the weight on one foot?

Is there an antalgic lean to the side, or is there an exaggerated flexion posture? Does she need assistance or hold on to things for support? With what difficulty does she lie upon the exam table? Is he able to extend the legs, or is one or both kept bent?

HISTORY

In taking a history, it is important to really watch and listen to the patient. There can be many subtle signals of dysfunction that will be evident if the physician is paying close attention. Patients often try to minimize significant factors about their health or attempt to disguise the facts to make them look bet-

ter. The use of pain drawings and pain-rating scales can help in assessing the patient's perception of his or her condition and how much emotional overlay exists.

How and when did the condition begin? Is it a traumatic injury or does it appear to have no causal incident? Is it an acute, subacute, or chronic condition? Was the onset sudden or gradual? Getting patients to relate as accurately as possible the factors surrounding their complaint can result in important clues about the nature of the injury giving direction to the examination.

If the patient was bending over to lift a box, did the pain start on the way down or on the way up? The answer to that question will lead the examiner to the muscles likely to be involved. For instance, pain starting on the way down would more likely involve the gluteus maximus, but pain at the initiation of the lift would involve the fifth segment of the psoas. Recall that the gluteus will be eccentrically contracting while a person is bending down, but upon arising the fifth segment of the psoas will contract hard in order to stabilize L5 while the rest of the spine is extending.

Knowing how long the patient has had the condition will indicate the stage of the condition. If it is a recent injury (less than 8 hours), inflammation will be minimal. If the condition is over 12 hours old, swelling will be advanced and, therefore, an important factor in the initial treatment. A chronic condition will have tissue changes and adaptive habits that will complicate treatment and recovery.

The patient's past history provides clues for better understanding of the current complaint. Previous episodes should be discussed. Were they severe, worse, or mild in comparison? Are there any residuals from past injuries? Any surgeries? Serious illnesses and family history should be explored. The patient's lifestyle is important. Diet, exercise habits, and stress levels should be assessed. Always ask about sleeping habits. Many people are in the habit of sleeping on their stomachs. This will often cause neck, low back, hip, and knee problems.

If the patient cannot relate a specific incident or activity that precipitated his or her complaint, inquire about activities over the last six to eight weeks. It is often found that an event occurring that far back could precipitate a current episode of back pain. An out-of-shape 45-year-old man who goes downhill skiing without any attempt to get into shape will (six weeks later) have an onset of excruciating low back pain while bending over for a pencil on the floor. Picking up the pencil gets the blame. This action is not really the cause, but the last straw in a back that has tried to compensate for damage done earlier.

EXAMINATION

The format of an initial examination may be altered by the severity of the patient's symptoms. A patient with a hot low back may not endure a detailed history or systematic evaluation. There will be no way to proceed except to assess the patient for the most effective way to relieve pain as quickly as possible. Obviously, once the patient is more comfortable, the exam can be completed.

Standing Exam

The examination of a low back complaint should start with the patient in the standing position, proceed to a seated exam, and then on to a supine, and finally to a prone assessment. There will be significant variations in posture and structural findings between these positions that are indicative of the underlying pathology.

First, ask the patient to stand without saying that you are observing posture. Not knowing what you are observing, the patient will assume a position of comfort. This is a good way to see how the patient carries him- or herself. Look at the position of the feet. Are the legs far apart, or close together (they should be under the hips)? Are the feet rotated out beyond the accepted 5° to 10°, or is one rotated out farther than the other? Unilateral toeing-out (Fig. 2–1) is a common finding in anatomical leg length insufficiency (LLI) and hip problems. The patient with such a habit will resist the anatomically correct position, feeling uncomfortable. This resistance is an indication that the patient has compensated for the abnormality. Standing in a corrected position will likely reveal the true distortion. To continue the exam without correcting the foot placement would be a mistake. This also applies to radiograph positioning in the weight-bearing position.

If possible, the patient should stand in the corrected position for at least one minute. It takes that long for the muscles to

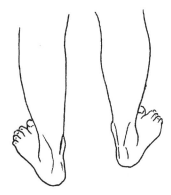

Fig. 2–1 Observe for unilateral toeing-out. Note the right foot shows greater lateral rotation of hip and leg.

readjust to the normal stance. Any movement should be noted as the patient attempts to adapt to the stance.

Ask the patient to describe where he or she feels weight is distributed on the soles of the feet. Patients should be instructed to not look down, but remain still and think about how the feet are sensing weight distribution. In a normal situation, patients should not be able to discern any area with a greater sensation of weight-bearing. Weight that is forward on the balls of the feet could be a sign of anterior tilting of the pelvis, often due to hypertonic psoas and a weak gluteus maximus or both. If this forward weight is unilateral, it could be due to an anterior rotation of that particular ilia with associated muscle dysfunction. If the weight is backward on the heels, the opposite is a likely finding, i.e., a posterior pelvic tilt with the gluteus maximus hypertonic and the psoas weak.

If weight is felt on the outside of the feet, look for a weakness in the peroneus tertius and extensor digitorum longus that allows inversion of the foot. If weight is felt on the medial aspect of the foot, it could be the anterior tibialis contributing to pronation.

Antalgic Posture

Note any antalgic lean. The patient may be leaning to either side or have a flexed stance with a flat back, one knee bent, or a combination of flexion and lateral bending. Note the degree, and compare the direction of lean and the location of pain. For instance, a presentation of left lateral lean with radiating pain into the right leg may indicate a discopathy with nerve root compression on the right caused by a lateral disk protrusion. However, if the radicular symptoms are on the left, the cause may likely be a central protrusion.

With the patient standing in as close a compliance with the desired posture, start at the feet. Instruct the patient not to move and to avoid turning to answer questions. This keeps the patient from shifting out of the "normal posture" or disguising faults. The logical approach to examining any structure is to start with the base. Any imbalance will produce a reaction of the structures above, enabling the body to compensate and re-main standing. Keep in mind the patient's foot position and note any excessive outward deviation, especially if unilateral. Postural faults ranging from a tilted head or pelvis to unlevel shoulders or spinal distortions may be either contributing to or caused by a lower extremity problem.

Pronation of the Calcaneus

Look for signs of pronation and determine if the calcaneus is involved. There will be an obvious deviation of the Achilles tendon (Fig. 2–2). Pronation involving the calcaneus reduces the distance from the tibia to the floor and will produce a func-tional shortening of that leg causing consequences above. If the pronation is in the forefoot only, there will be no effect on the leg length. Unilateral pronation without trauma usually in-dicates poor body mechanics and should lead to further inves-tigation. Pronation may itself be adaptive, the result of a later-ally rotated femur, anatomical leg length insufficiency, or a valgus knee deformity.

Knee Fold Height

Compare knee fold height (Fig. 2–3). With both feet the same, a low knee fold may indicate a possible anatomically short tibia.

Flexion-Extension of the Knee

Compare the knees for any flexion-extension imbalance (Fig. 2–4). Are the knees hyperextended? Unilateral flexion could indicate an anatomically long leg, a way to adapt to pain or an adaptation to pelvic distortion. A unilateral hyperexten-sion could indicate damaged ligaments, a weak popliteus, or pelvic distortion.

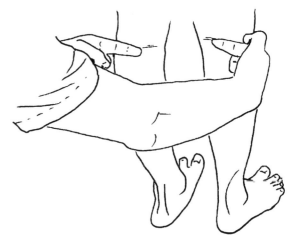

Fig. 2–3 Comparing knee fold heights.

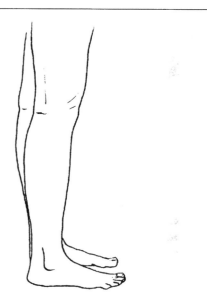

Fig. 2–4 Unilateral flexion-extension imbalance.

Gluteal Folds

Compare the gluteal folds (Fig. 2–5). Any unleveling or unilateral exaggeration suggests an unlevel pelvis or unilateral rotation.

Iliac Crests and Posterior Superior Iliac Spines (PSIS)

Bring the index fingers down on the iliac crests to determine the level of the pelvis (Fig. 2–6). Palpation should compare the levels at three points along the crest. The posterior, middle, and anterior crest should be compared to obtain a complete idea of the nature of the imbalance. Is it an inferiority or a rotation of the ilia, or a combination? Hook the thumbs under the posterior superior iliac spines and compare levels. Uneven levels indicate a rotation of one or the other or both ilia in

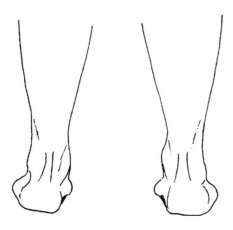

Fig. 2–2 Left Achilles tendon shows medial curve suggestive of pronation.

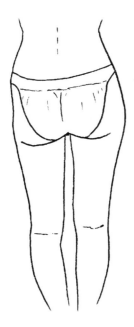

Fig. 2–5 Compare gluteal folds.

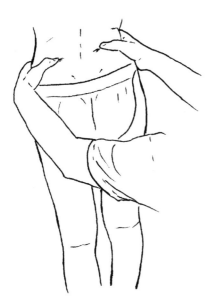

Fig. 2–6 Palpation of iliac crests and PSIS.

different directions. At this point, motion palpation of the sacroiliac joints can be performed. Passive motion palpation of the pelvis can provide more information and is done later with the patient in the supine exam.

Spine and Upper Torso

Note any obvious abnormalities in the spinal curvatures, either a loss or increase in the anterior to posterior (A-to-P)

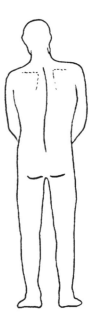

Fig. 2–7 Note any unleveling of shoulders and scapulae.

curves or any sign of scoliosis. Note the position of the scapulae and if they are level (Fig. 2–7). Note any head tilt. Note the degree of tension in the paravertebrals and if there are any differences from side to side.

Pelvic Tilt

From the side, assess the pelvic tilt and whether the spinal curvatures are normal, decreased, or exaggerated. Is the abdomen protruding? Note the position of the shoulders and the head, which is often set forward (Fig. 2–8).

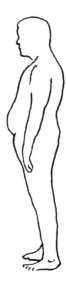

Fig. 2–8 Anterior pelvic tilt with weak abdominals and anterior head displacement.

Valgus/Varus Deformity

From the front, note if there is any valgus or varus deviation of the knee, which can contribute to a functional leg length insufficiency (Fig. 2–9). Further evaluation of the knee should be done with the patient in the supine exam. Often subluxation or fixation in the knee can also affect leg length.[1]

Range of Motion (ROM)

Determining the range of motion (ROM) in the lumbar spine gives clues to the mechanical compensations a patient will make to achieve movement. An accurate measurement is also important in the clinical setting to compare findings during the course of treatment, to satisfy the need to keep accurate records, and to justify findings and treatment in a medical/legal setting.

ROM	Normal (in degrees)
Flexion	90
Extension	30
Lateral Bending	20
Rotation	30

Numerous methods of measurement and differences of opinion about the degree of movement considered normal exist. Recently, the use of inclinometers has made the accurate determination of ROM easier with better reproducibility. However, range of motion can be determined by observation alone if the examiner has much experience. Deficiencies in movement are easy to spot. It is important to document the range and be able to compare it with future tests to determine a patient's progress. The best comparison is with the patient's ability to achieve a full (normal for them) ROM without pain, visible deficiency, compensation, or perceived limitations.

It should be remembered that no two people will have the same degree of mobility; what is normal for one would be hypermobility or hypomobility for another. One simple, but accurate, assessment of flexion is to measure the distance from the fingers to the floor if the patient cannot touch the floor. This is an easy way to objectify the patient's progress. If the patient could never touch the floor before, they cannot be expected to do so when they are cured.

Flexion. Ask the patient to bend and attempt to touch the floor, but not to go beyond the point of pain. Note how the patient bends. Is there the appearance of a smooth lumbopelvic rhythm? Do the knees bend significantly? If so, assess the range with the knees straight as well. Watch the spine and pelvis and note any abnormal lateral or rotational movements. Often an examiner can observe a lateral deviation of the lumbars as if the spine is moving around an obstacle as flexion is attempted. When pain is present, note the location of the pain and any radiation.

Extension. Have the patient extend backward to the point of pain and note the location of pain. Note the degree of posterior pelvic tilt. Watch the lordosis and note any exaggerated increase suggestive of hyperextension.

Lateral Bending. Watch for variations in the lateral tilt of the pelvis. Note the way the lumbar spine bends in both directions. Often the degree of movement will be normal and equal, but the spine may bend from different levels, indicating aberrant motion and fixation. Consider that an inequality of side bending may indicate a weak or stretched quadratus lumborum (Q-L) on the excessive side.

Rotation. Keep the pelvis from moving, and note the degree of movement and the location of any pain. The shoulders are the easiest to watch, but it should be kept in mind that rotation of the upper torso involves the thoracic spine and the shoulder girdle.

Evaluating the range of motion of the hips should include active and passive testing. All ranges should be considered. Flexion: the patient should be able to bring the knee almost to the chest (135°). Extension: arising from sitting tests extension. Normal extension beyond neutral is 30°. Abduction: the standing patient spreads the legs as far apart as possible (Fig. 2–10). Normal abduction is 45°. Adduction: crossing one leg over the other should be at least 20°. Internal rotation should be approximately 35°, and external rotation should be about 45°.

Having the patient cross the thighs in the seated position tests flexion and adduction; having the patient place the lateral side of the foot on the opposite knee tests the combined movements of flexion, abduction, and external rotation (Patrick's test). Decreased range of motion can be found with degenerative conditions and muscle contractures.

Sitting and Arising Exam

Important signs and symptoms can be revealed during the act of sitting down and arising from the sitting position. If the

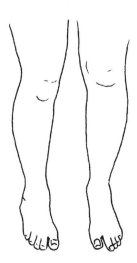

Fig. 2–9 Right knee—valgus deformity.

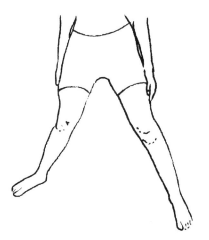

Fig. 2–10 Functional testing for hip abduction.

patient is able, have them sit on the exam table; observe the low back and torso for imbalances. Do the findings in the standing position remain when the patient is sitting, or is there a change? For instance, a patient with an anatomical short leg and a unilateral weakness of the Q-L or both may show a low scapula on one side in the standing posture. But when this patient sits, the low scapula will palpate high. Look at the spinal curves and the pelvis for rotational or level changes.

Have the patient stand; watch for obvious difficulty or unbalanced movements. As the patient lifts the buttock off the table, note whether one side lifts off first and if there is any lateral shifting of the torso. If the patient can rise up straight, but with difficulty, have him or her attempt to rise with the weight on one leg and then the other. If there is a unilateral weakness of the Q-L, it will be more difficult for the patient to arise on the opposite leg. For instance, if the right Q-L is weak, the patient will be able to rise easily on the right foot, but will not be able to rise easily on the left foot. The right Q-L must work harder to raise the right pelvis when the bulk of the weight is on the left.

A patient with a disk abnormality will rise and list to one side or the other and lift one buttock first. Such a patient cannot rise straight because this increases the pressure on the disks. A patient with a facetal strain/sprain will be able to rise easily straight, but will find it painful to rise to one side as there is more stress on the facetal joints. Side of pain and weight-bearing are not directly correlated in this evaluation. The antalgic posture of a patient with a disk problem is affected by the position of the protrusion, medial or lateral (see Chapter 6 on Conditions and Treatment). A facetal injury can cause a variety of compensatory mechanisms.

If a patient cannot rise straight up without pain or difficulty but can rise more easily with the weight on the right leg and less on the left, it is probable that the right Q-L is weak or dysfunctioning. Grasp the right Q-L and assist it to contract while the patient rises (Fig. 2–11). If it is easier or less painful, it is likely the right Q-L is a major factor in the patient's condition.

In patients with sciatic symptoms, support the piriformis during rising and sitting (Fig. 2–12). If the pain is reduced or there is a greater ease in the actions, it is probable that there is a piriformis dysfunction at the root of the problem. In the sitting position with the thigh flexed to 90°, the piriformis is an abductor. As the patient rises, watch for any inward deviation of the knee. This could be a sign of a weakness in the piriformis. Assist the piriformis in its contraction and note any improvement in the ease of rising or decreased pain.

Another area to check is the stability of the ischial tuberosities. In the act of arising, the transversus peronei must contract to pull the tuberosities inward. They spread for a wider base in sitting and come together in the standing position. If an instability is suspected, support the ischial tuberosities pushing them medially as the patient stands (Fig. 2–13). Any reduction in pain or ease of action is a positive indication and should lead to an evaluation of the muscles involved. A severe instability with ligamentous involvement may benefit from a trochanter belt.

Supine Exam

Evaluations in the supine examination include general palpation, passive motion palpation of the spine and pelvis, palpation of the abdomen, orthopaedic and neurologic tests, and a

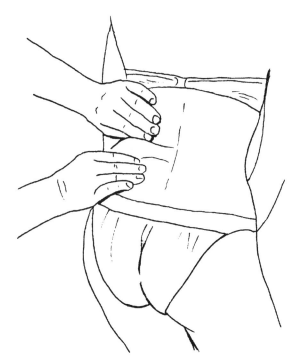

Fig. 2–11 Assisting Q-L as patient attempts to arise.

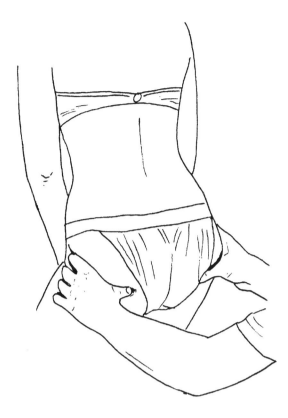

Fig. 2–12 Supporting piriformis bilaterally as patient attempts to arise.

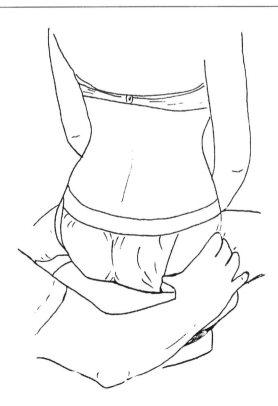

Fig. 2–13 Supporting ischial tuberosities as patient attempts to arise.

kinesiological evaluation of many significant muscles in low back and pelvic function. The supine position is the most ideal for palpation. In evaluating the connective tissue, muscles, and articulations, the examiner should feel for edema, hypertonicity, restricted mobility, and pain.

With the patient as comfortable as possible, grasp both ankles and push firmly several times in a cephalad direction. Push hard enough to make the pelvis rotate posteriorly (Fig. 2–14). This will put a weight-bearing stress on the body and reveal any imbalances or compensatory adaptations. In evaluating for imbalances and subluxations, it must be remembered that the examiner is easily led to subjective opinions about the findings. It is imperative that the examiner make every effort to objectify the findings. Keep in mind that it is easy to form opinions about what to expect and make the findings fit those expectations. Removing as many obstacles to an objective examination as possible is important in such an imprecise arena as the investigation of human ailments. During a postgraduate seminar, Dr. Logan asked the participants in the class to verify the leg length of a subject. He purposely, and with feigned inadvertence, made the class aware of the wrong answer. All but 1 of the 32 participants gave the incorrect answer. They had satisfied themselves that their findings fit what they thought the instructor wanted to hear instead of using what they had been taught.

The first things to consider in the evaluation of the musculoskeletal system are the key landmarks. The anatomical landmarks for evaluating the low back and pelvis are (Fig. 2–15):

1. inferior calcaneus
2. medial malleolus
3. medial femoral condyle
4. anterior superior iliac spines (ASIS)
5. iliac crests

The pubic symphysis and the greater trochanters are often helpful landmarks as well.

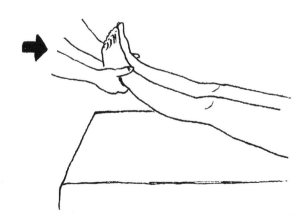

Fig. 2–14 Pushing cephalad to simulate weight-bearing.

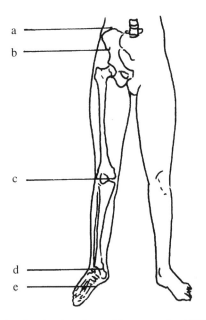

Fig. 2–15 Palpation landmarks. a. iliac crest, b. ASIS, c. medial femoral condyles, d. medial malleolus, e. inferior calcaneus.

Hip Evaluation

The hip joints should be examined for range of motion, areas of pain, edema, and signs of degeneration. With the patient in the supine position, bring the knee and thigh into flexion. Attempt to fully flex the thigh onto the chest and determine the end-feel and ask if any pain is felt. The iliopectineal bursa may be the source of pain with full flexion. Place the patient's foot on the opposite knee and abduct the thigh (Fig. 2–16). Note the degree of movement, end-feel, and any pain. Reduced abduction and a tight end-feel are indicative of contracture of the

pectineus and some of the upper adductors, and possible degenerative changes.

Move the flexed thigh in the opposite direction, into adduction (Fig. 2–17). This action is reduced in degeneration, especially with acetabular rim buildup. Distract the femur with a steady pull and retest the range of motion (Fig. 2–18). This may allow a temporary increase in movement. This can be painful if the iliopectineal bursa is inflamed.

The iliopectineal bursa can be irritated in cases of functional long leg and this irritation can affect the flexor muscles, which could test weak due to pain. Palpate the bursa for pain. Differentiate between bursitis and a pectineus hypertonicity by noting if the ilia is anteriorly rotated and if the iliacus and psoas are hypertonic, both of which can cause the pectineus to shorten and sometimes spasm or undergo contracture in more chronic conditions.

Reduced extension is evident with a degenerated hip, but is also seen with psoas spasm or shortening and with an anatomically short femur (compensatory anterior rotation of the ilia and flexor and lateral rotator muscle hypertonicity; Fig. 2–19).

Edema in the hip can cause the leg to appear longer due to intercapsular swelling. Compress the flexed hip and recheck for a decrease in length that quickly increases again (Fig. 2–20). Pain can be palpated behind the trochanter, superior to

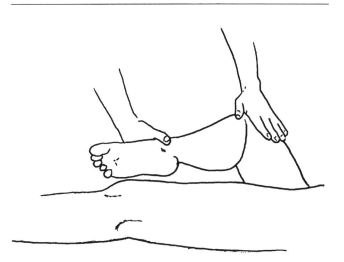

Fig. 2–16 Test for abduction, lateral rotation extension.

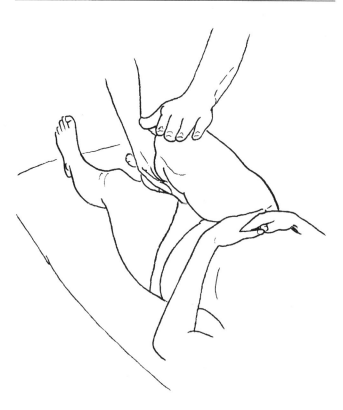

Fig. 2–17 Evaluating hip flexion and adduction.

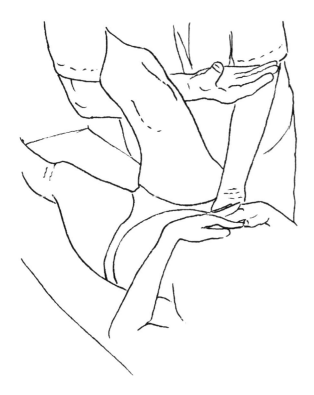

Fig. 2–18 Hip distraction may temporarily improve movement in degenerative conditions.

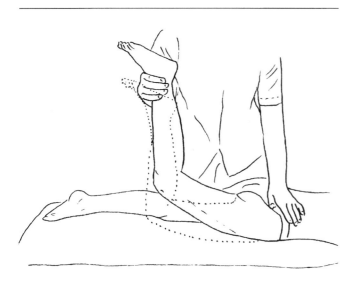

Fig. 2–19 Normal and reduced (dotted outline) hip extension.

the piriformis, and anterolateral to the ischial tuberosity. The patient will often complain of low back pain rather than hip pain. D'Ambrosia[2] describes the pain of hip arthritis as sometimes mimicking sciatica and more often radiating down the anteromedial thigh to the knee. There may be no findings sug-

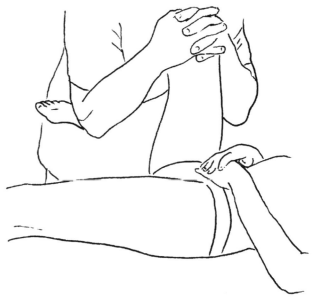

Fig. 2–20 Compress hip checking for edema.

gestive of leg length inequality in the standing position. The hip flexors may test weak.

Leg Length

The evaluation of leg length is a common procedure in chiropractic; however, it is the subject of much controversy and is often misunderstood. The determination of an LLI and whether it is anatomical or functional, is important. Anatomical LLI is found in approximately 10% to 15% of the population, but functional LLI is much more frequently found. Because of its prevalence, the clinical determination of LLI is of major importance in the diagnosis and treatment of low back and pelvic disorders.

The differential diagnosis of anatomical versus functional LLI requires a clear, concise, and consistent method to determine the difference. The biomechanical evidence available does much to explain the causes and means of correction of a functional LLI. Much of the discussion by experts, however, revolves around the numerous methods of measuring the degree of anatomical difference in leg length. Most of the methods are inaccurate and can involve complicated radiological procedures. None of them have been clinically satisfactory thus far.

The intraprofessional discussion of a functional LLI has been limited to the admission that there may be some pelvic distortion that might bear clinical study.[3] The methods developed by Dr. Logan[4] have proved to be accurate in differentiating anatomical from functional LLI and have shown an accuracy in measuring anatomical differences to within 3 mm of the most accepted measurement procedure in limited clinical studies.

Initial determination. After simulating weight-bearing stress, use the thumbs, with equal pressure against the inferior medial malleoli (the proximal tibia). Be sure not to use too much pressure, which could alter the position and distort the findings. By sighting directly over the malleoli, determine if they are even or not (Fig. 2–21). Dorsiflex the feet and check the level of the heels (Fig. 2–22). To confirm the findings at the foot and ankles, use the same thumb technique to press up under the inferior surface of the medial condyle of the femur (Fig. 2–23).

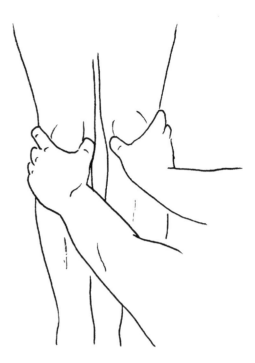

Fig. 2–23 Checking length at medial femoral condyles.

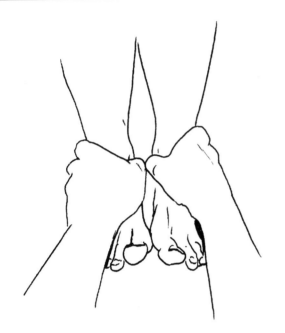

Fig. 2–21 Checking leg length at medial malleoli.

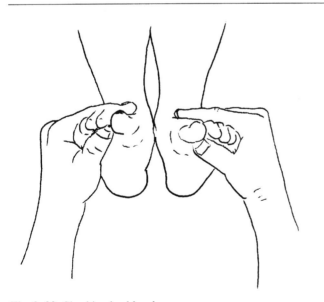

Fig. 2–22 Checking heel levels.

With these above three checks, an initial determination of leg length can be made. If the medial malleoli are uneven but the femur check shows no unevenness, and if the heel check also shows uneven levels, the tibia may be short. If the tibia check shows evenness and the heel check shows unevenness, look for problems in the foot or ankle. A pronation or fixation of the tibiotalar–calcaneus complex may be at fault.[4] Uneven malleoli, confirmed by the heel and the femur check, indicates a possible short femur, or hip and pelvic distortion or both.

Next, check the ASIS levels (Fig. 2–24). Press the thumbs up under both spines with equal pressure and sight down over them. An inferior ASIS is indicative of an anterior rotation of the ilium (an AS ilium), which, by lowering the acetabulum, will increase leg length. A superior ASIS is a sign of a posterior iliac rotation (a PI ilium), raising the acetabulum and shortening the leg.

Bring the hands down on the iliac crests, fingers extended, and the index fingers resting on the crests (Fig. 2–25). Sight down over the area and determine if there is any unleveling. An inferior crest could be a positive sign of an inferior ilium or weak Q-L or both, which could cause an increased leg length sign in the supine patient.

Lateral Rotation of the Femur

Grasp the ankles and lift the legs off the table. Rotate the legs internally and compare the degree of movement (Fig. 2–26). If there is less movement on one side, there may be a lateral rotation fixation of the femur or hypertonicity of the lat-

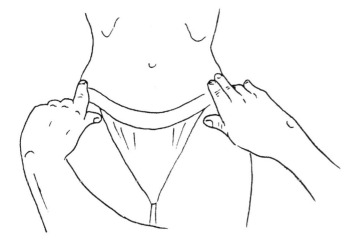

Fig. 2–24 Checking ASIS levels.

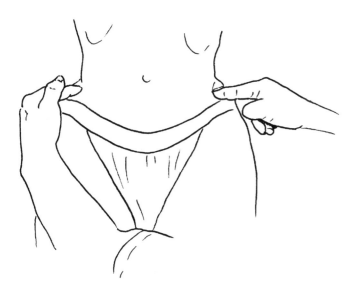

Fig. 2–25 Checking iliac crest levels.

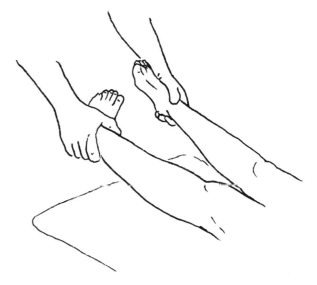

Fig. 2–26 Checking internal rotation of femurs, note decreased rotation on the right.

Differential Diagnosis of Functional and Anatomical LLI

The several causes of functional leg length insufficiency discussed above include an AS or PI rotation of the ilia, an inferior ilia, a lateral rotation of the femur, and knee and foot dysfunctions. These findings can occur alone or in many different combinations. Often an evaluation will reveal several combinations that counteract each other in an effort to compensate and balance out the structure. For instance, a lateral rotation of the femur increasing leg length is compensated by a PI ilium on the same side, which cancels out the long leg (Fig. 2–27). After finding and correcting all imbalances and listings, if there remains a leg length discrepancy, it is highly likely that there is an anatomical LLI.

Lordotic Lumbar Syndrome

Maintaining the weight-bearing stress, examine the lumbar lordosis. A normal lordotic curve will, in the supine position, allow the hands to easily slip in between the spine and table. No gap at all or difficulty in slipping the hands under the back indicate a decrease in the lordosis with a likely weakness of the psoas and iliacus and hypertonicity of the gluteus maximus or both. If there is a significant gap with plenty of room to slip hands under the spine, a lordotic lumbar syndrome (LLS) is likely, with hypertonicity of the psoas and weakness of the gluteus maximus and abdominals. Evaluate the muscles involved in producing and allowing this distortion to occur and treat accordingly (see Chapter 4 on Muscle Testing).

Another sign of LLS in the supine position is the level of the pubic symphysis in relation to the ASIS. In a normal situation

eral rotators. Another sign of lateral rotation fixation is a significant internal position (lateral rotation of the femur) of the leg with maximum flexion of the hip and knee. Normally, if the flexed knee is used to fully flex the hip, the foot should be in alignment with the thigh. If there is a lateral rotation fixation of the hip, or at least hypertonic lateral rotators, the foot will move medially as the hip is fully flexed. Lateral rotation fixation of the femur will increase the length of the leg. It is an incomplete seating of the head of the femur in the acetabulum. Any time the leg length and pelvis findings do not coincide, suspect a laterally rotated femur. This is a common subluxation. The lateral rotators should be checked for hypertonicity and treated accordingly.

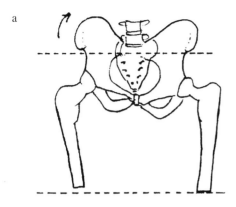

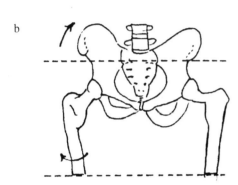

Fig. 2–27 a. PI ilium producing short leg, b. PI ilium and lateral rotation of femur equalizes leg lengths.

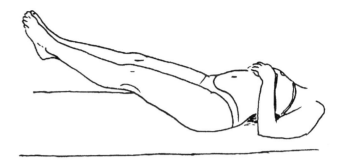

Fig. 2–28 Active bilateral SLR. Note increased lordosis and pubic symphysis lower than ASIS indicative of weak abdominals.

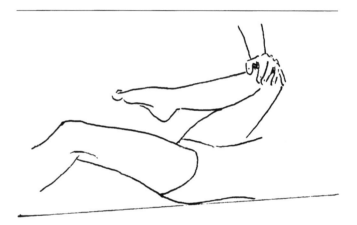

Fig. 2–29 Psoas hypertonicity with Thomas test.

(patient supine, at rest), the symphysis is level with the iliac spines. With an LLS, the symphysis is found to be lower (anterior pelvic tilt). This can become even more evident by having the patient do an active bilateral straight leg raise (SLR; Fig. 2–28). Observe the degree of increased lordosis and anterior pelvic rotation that occurs. If there is significant exaggeration, the abdominals should be evaluated for weakness or underfunctioning.

Iliacus and Psoas Imbalance

The psoas can be checked for hypertonicity by flexing one hip, bringing the knee to the chest, and observing the opposite extended leg (Fig. 2–29). If it is pulled up off the exam table, there is a hypertonicity on that side. Palpation of the iliopsoas insertion for tenderness can confirm irritation. Palpate the iliacus origins along the inner iliac crests and determine the degree of sensitivity. If excessive, it can indicate irritation. A normal lordotic curve in the presence of marked iliacus origin pain and anterior pelvic tilt in the standing position could indicate hypertonic iliacus muscles.

Michele[5] describes the clinical history of psoas myositis. He attributes "psoitis" to chronic failure to elongate during the rapid growth phase. He also mentions the likelihood of mis-

taken diagnosis of appendicitis in cases of right-sided psoas myositis. McBurney's point used in the diagnosis of appendicitis, can be confused, according to Michele, with myositis or fibrositic changes in the iliacus.

Have the patient do an active unilateral straight leg raise. Palpate the lumbar spine and note the movement of the spinous processes. If the psoas muscles are functioning properly, the spinous processes will move away from the side being raised. This indicates that the opposite support muscles, including the psoas, are working properly, supporting the spine against the weight of the rising leg.

Quadratus Lumborum Imbalance

After evaluating the pelvic landmarks, grasp the ankles and ask the patient to completely relax the back and hips. Tug several times, with equal force, in an inferior direction (Fig. 2–30). Tug hard enough to pull the pelvis down almost moving the patient. Recheck the leg length and the iliac crests for any change. If there is a lengthening of one leg and an ipsilateral inferior shift of the iliac crest, there is a likelihood of a unilateral Q-L weakness. Reset the weight-bearing stress and retest to confirm the finding. Excessive anterior movement of the pelvis when distracting the legs is indicative of abdominal weakness.

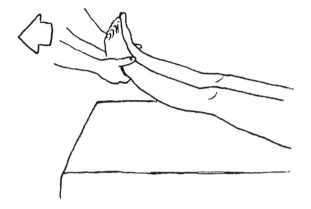

Fig. 2–30 Tug inferiorly for Q-L imbalance.

Hamstring Imbalance

A passive straight leg raise with the patient relaxed will reveal any hypertonicity or contracture of the hamstrings (Fig. 2–31). They are commonly too short. The knee will begin to flex as the leg is raised. In a normal situation, the leg should approach 90° with no significant restriction.

AS and PI Iliac Rotations

One of the most common findings in a chiropractic examination is rotation of the ilia at the sacroiliac joint. As mentioned above, an AS ilium is an anterior rotation of the ilia. The AS designation refers to the position of the PSIS, which moves anterior and superior in the AS distortion. A PI rotation shows a posterior inferior position of the PSIS. In the exami-

nation, the AS and PI ilia are checked by observing the position of the ASIS in the supine position. The ASIS will be inferior with an AS ilium and superior with a PI ilium (Fig. 2–32). The AS ilium will produce a functional long leg, and a PI ilium will produce a short leg. The muscles that allow and produce these rotations need to be evaluated for weakness or hypertonicity. The muscles that produce a PI ilium (gluteus maximus, posterior abdominals, hamstrings—to a minor extent) are the muscles that allow an AS ilium. The muscles that allow a PI (iliacus, transverse abdominals, TFL, rectus femoris, sartorius, gracilis) produce an AS.

Medial Ischium

The medial ischium (MI) and the AS and PI fixation/subluxation complexes are the three most commonly found imbalances in the pelvis. The MI is a flared ilium. The ischial tuberosity will be medially positioned and possibly fixed while the crest is flared out laterally (Fig. 2–33). The muscles involved are the iliacus, posterior oblique and transverse abdominals, and fourth segment of the Q-L, usually found to be weak. The gluteus medius and minimus, tensor fascia lata (TFL), and transverse peroneals are usually hypertonic.

To test for an MI, reach under the patient and grasp the medial aspect of both ischia and pull laterally (Fig. 2–34). With practice, it is easy to differentiate normal play from restricted or excessive movement. In unstable low back patients, a hypermobility is often found at the ischial tuberosities. In this case, the muscle imbalance will be the opposite of the medial ischial fixation. The most important muscles to consider are the transverse peroneal muscles, which are weak and will need to be strengthened (see Chapter 7 on Exercises).

Pubic Symphysis

Pubic symphysis problems are uncommon. They can be seen often in pregnancy with the relaxed ligaments and the stresses on the gravid pelvis. Palpate the pubic symphysis for

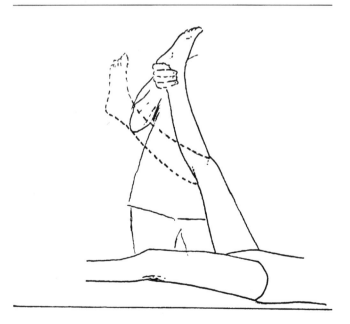

Fig. 2–31 Checking for hamstring contracture, dotted outline shows decreased leg extension.

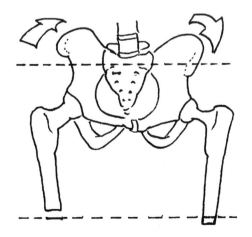

Fig. 2–32 Right PI ilium. Left AS ilium.

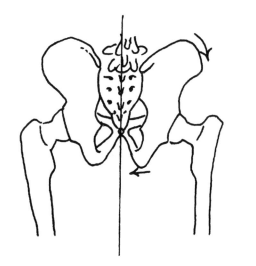

Fig. 2–33 Right medial ischium.

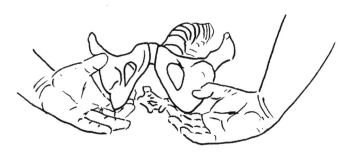

Fig. 2–34 Motion palpation of ischia.

tenderness and alignment. By bringing the thumbs down on the superior aspect of the pubes, it can be determined if they are level. If subluxated, a superior shift can be seen.

Passive Motion Palpation

Passive motion palpation (PMP) is best defined as the motion palpation challenge of an articulation without the influence of weight-bearing. This is not to be confused with motion palpation, developed by Dr. Henri Gillet, and widely used in the chiropractic profession. Passive motion palpation was developed by Dr. Raymond T. Broome and Dr. Alfred Logan while faculty members at the Anglo-European College of Chiropractic. Dr. Broome developed methods for palpating the extremities, especially the feet. Dr. Logan began to develop PMP for spinal and pelvic palpation after using static palpation and motion palpation and finding both to have too many variables that decrease interexaminer reliability.

Static palpation is usually performed with the patient in the prone position, which is convenient for direct observation of

the spine; however, it places abnormal stresses on the vertebrae through pressure on the rib cage and increased lordotic pressure on the lumbar spine as the pelvis rotates anteriorly. Motion palpation is done in the sitting position, which can alter the forces on the spine by reducing the influence of important support muscles that are active in the standing position.

Passive motion palpation is performed in the supine position (Fig. 2–35). This eliminates the prone compression of the rib cage, which tightens the thoracic vertebrae, and anterior pelvic rotation, which increases the lordosis, tightening the lumbars and all the weight-bearing effects of the sitting position. It provides an opportunity to palpate the body in a posture that is as close as possible to the erect posture without weight-bearing stresses.

The patient is in the supine position with the arms at rest and the fingers interlaced over the chest. As described earlier, grasp the ankles and push in a cephalad direction hard enough to rock the pelvis. This puts a weight-bearing stress on the body and sets the usual distortions, dysfunctions, compensations, and adaptations into place. Palpation is accomplished by placing the hands under the patient's body at the levels to be examined. The metacarpophalangeal joints are set against the exam table, acting as a fulcrum, and the finger tips are used to rock and move the individual segments.

The information gained by palpation includes an assessment of the sensitivity of the tissues, the state of muscular tone, the relative position of adjacent articulations, and the degree of joint play. In evaluating the musculoskeletal system for subluxation, fixation, and muscle dysfunction, it is necessary to clearly define the cause of any abnormalities in order to treat the condition with any effectiveness. An age-old chiropractic question is: where, when, and why adjust? PMP is an effective tool for answering this question.

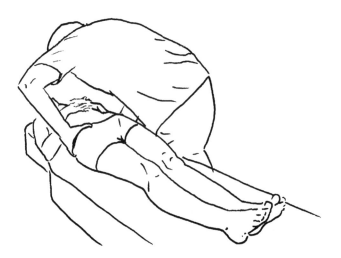

Fig. 2–35 Basic position for palpation of low back and pelvis.

Subluxation/Fixation

The subluxation is the fundamental lesion considered by the chiropractor. It has been defined in many different ways and has been the subject of controversy from a clinical as well as a philosophical standpoint. One definition is that subluxation is any articulation that fails to return to its normal resting place. Biron et al.[6] refers to a subluxation as a slight change in the relative position of contiguous vertebrae. *Dorland's*[7] defines it as an incomplete or partial dislocation.

The International Chiropractic Association defines subluxation as "an alteration of the biomechanical and physiologic dynamics of contiguous spinal structures causing neural disturbances." This excludes extraspinal structures. The American Chiropractic Association defines subluxation as "an aberrant relationship between two adjacent structures that may have functional or pathologic sequelae, causing an alteration in the biomechanical or neurophysiological reflections of these articular structures or both, their proximal structures or other body systems or both that may be directly or indirectly affected by them." This definition is more comprehensive and includes extraspinal structures.

In his teachings, Dr. Logan preferred the term fixation over subluxation and defined it simply as any articulation that fails to move through its entire normal range of motion. Others use both fixation as well as subluxation to define the lesions examiners attempt to diagnose and correct. I consider a subluxation to be a fixation that is pathognomonic for the chiropractic lesion, an aberrant vertebral segment affecting neurological structures. Not all fixations are subluxations, but some may contribute to causing subluxations.

An articulation may be restricted in its movement throughout its normal range of motion by an imbalance of the musculature. The use of static palpation (palpation for position) may determine a malposition; however, it will not differentiate between a fixation and a malposition due to muscle imbalance. An articulation can be in place, but fixed, and PMP would be more likely to detect a problem than static palpation.

If a malposition exists and PMP produces movement through a normal range, no fixation exists and manipulation would be useless. The malposition is produced by muscle dysfunction and should be investigated and treated accordingly. If PMP shows the articulation failing to move normally, a true fixation exists and may be graded as follows:

1. severe $0°$ of movement in the direction tested
2. moderate minimal movement
3. mild   moves yet fails to move through its entire range

The examiner should keep in mind that a fixation may have occurred as a result of muscle imbalance or may have created muscle dysfunction. It is important to consider both possibilities in the evaluation process, and often it is difficult to determine which came first.

PMP for Iliac Fixation

The determination of a fixation is achieved by PMP. To challenge the ilia for an AS fixation, slide the hand from the opposite side under and contact the sacrum just medial to the sacroiliac joint. Use a broad index finger and thumb contact along the iliac crest to be tested. By rocking the ilium in a posteromedial direction and pushing upward with the fingers on the sacrum, the examiner can feel for movement or lack of movement. If the ilium is fixed, it will not move into posterior rotation but is fixed anteriorly (AS; Fig. 2–36).

A PI fixation is tested with the opposite maneuver. Pull medially against the spine of the sacrum while attempting to rotate the iliac crest in an anterolateral direction, feeling for joint play. If none is detected, there is a fixation preventing the anterior rotation of the ilia on the sacrum, a PI fixation (Fig. 2–37).

These fixations may or may not coincide with the static palpation of the anterior superior iliac spines. Often the fixation will not include a malposition. For instance, static palpation may show a posterior rotation of the right ilia (a high ASIS or PI ilia). PMP may show the right ilia to have no fixation. The attempt to pull the iliac crest anterolaterally would show no restriction, which would lead to an investigation of the muscles that allow and produce a PI. PMP of the left ilium could show a lack of movement into posterior rotation, suggesting an AS fixation that would likely need to be adjusted.

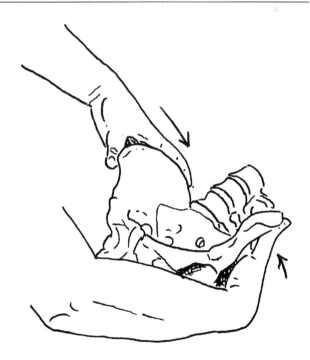

Fig. 2–36 Passive motion palpation for AS ilium fixation.

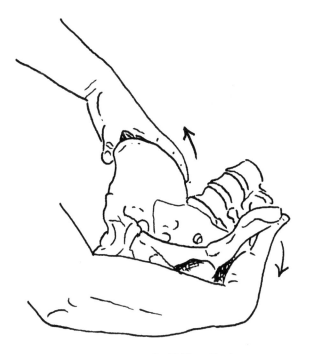

Fig. 2–37 Passive motion palpation for PI ilium fixation.

Testing for AS and PI fixations requires practice and patience. The movements are subtle, and it takes time to develop a feel for what is normal and abnormal. In general, it is common to find more anterior fixations (AS) due to the tendencies of the ilia to rotate anteriorly in the standing position. It is also conceivable to find a neutral position of the ASIS on static palpation and a failure of posterior or anterior movement with PMP, suggesting an AS or PI fixation. In exploring the function of the pelvis, it is possible to find many combinations of fixations and muscle imbalances.

PMP of the Sacroiliac Joints and Lumbar Spine

The supine position increases the accuracy of determining spinal function. As mentioned earlier, it is closer to the standing position without weight-bearing. In the thoracic spine, the rib cage is less likely to distort findings by pressure on the ribs as in the prone posture. The lumbar spine is more relaxed as the pelvis will not tend to rotate anteriorly.

Stand to one side of the patient and slide both hands, from opposite sides, under the patient. Start at the sacroiliac joints and work upward to the thoracic spine. With the knuckles against the table acting as a leverage point, the finger tips press upward on the first sacral segment and on the mamillary processes of the lumbars and transverse processes of the thoracics.

PMP of the Sacroiliac Joints. From a starting place at the sacroiliac (SI) joints, the segments can be moved in all directions and challenged against each other to obtain a clear pic-

ture of intervertebral function. Rock the SI joints and feel for relative position (Fig. 2–38). There should be a perceptible joint play and an equality in the relationship of the lateral sacral body and the posterior superior iliac spine. Common fixations of the SI joints are anterior, posterior, and oblique.

Posterior Sacrum. PMP of the SI joint will show no anterior joint play and the PSIS and sacrum will palpate more evenly (Fig. 2–39).

Anterior Sacrum. PMP is not capable of assessing the movement as it is not possible to influence the sacrum posteriorly. The sacral body will be more anterior in relation to the PSIS (Fig. 2–39). The finding of normal joint play on the opposite side is further clarification. In this case, the first impres-

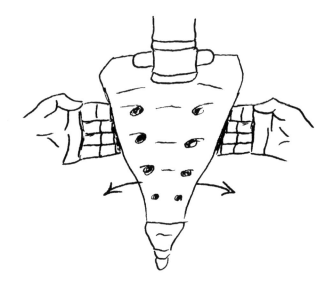

Fig. 2–38 PMP of sacroiliac joints.

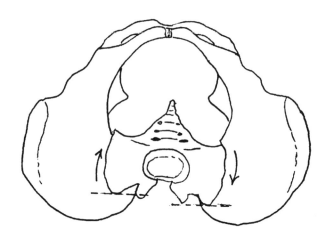

Fig. 2–39 Superior view of sacrum and pelvis, right posterior, left anterior subluxation.

sion would be a possible posterior fixation, but with evidence of normal joint play it is likely to be anteriorly fixed on the opposite side.

PMP of the Lumbosacral Articulations. The lumbosacral joints are subject to anterior, posterior, and oblique fixations. The L5–S1 segments are often subject to anomalies, such as sacralization and facetal asymmetry. With practice, PMP can be an effective tool in detecting these anomalies with an accuracy that makes radiographic confirmation almost secondary. Dr. Joseph Howe has stated that being surprised by what you find on the radiograph means your examination was probably lacking (personal communication to Dr. Alfred Logan, 1989).

Move the hands up to the L5 level and rock it in the same fashion as the SI joints. Feel for position and joint play. Then move one hand down to the S1 segment and press upward on both at the same time and rock one upon the other (Fig. 2–40). Then reverse the position of the contact and repeat (Fig. 2–40). This allows you to play one segment against the other, on both sides, to determine any fixation and the direction of that fixation. L5 can subluxate anteriorly, posteriorly, and inferiorly.

Anterior Fixation L5 on S1. Palpation of an anterior L5 (Fig. 2–41) will feel like a deep depression, giving a more posterior feel on the opposite side. To confirm, the "posterior" side should be rocked anteriorly while stabilizing the S1 segment on the opposite side (Fig. 2–40). If joint play is detected on the "posterior" side, it is likely that no posterior fixation exists, and the opposite side is indeed fixed anteriorly. Palpable pain on the anterior side is often found. The fifth segment of the psoas may be hypertonic on the anterior side.

Posterior Fixation L5 on S1. Palpation of L5 will show a more posterior feel to the side of fixation and an obvious reduction in the joint play when pushing anteriorly (Fig. 2–41). The opposite side will be more normal in its position and show

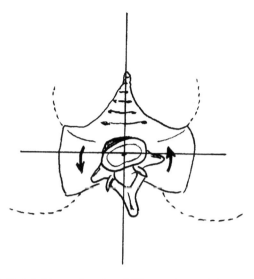

Fig. 2–41 L5–S1 superior view, L5 is anterior on right, posterior on left.

a more normal degree of joint play. The posterior fixation will often be more painful to palpation. The fifth segment of the psoas may be weak or strained.

Oblique or Inferior Fixation of L5 on S1. By taking a stabilizing contact on the S1 segment on one side and pushing the opposite L5 mamillary process superiorly, it is possible to detect any restriction in superior/inferior joint play (Fig. 2–42). This should be done for both sides. It is possible to have an inferior fixation as well as an anterior or posterior fixation on the same side.

Combination Fixations. In many instances, L5 could be fixed bilaterally, anterior on one side, posterior on the other. It could be fixed posterior bilaterally or anterior bilaterally. PMP will indicate the true nature of the fixations. For instance, if L5 is fixed anteriorly on the right and posteriorly on the left, palpation findings would likely show pain bilaterally, with a deep depression on the right and a rigid posterior feel on the left. In

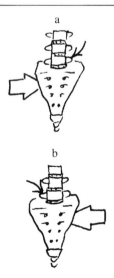

Fig. 2–40 PMP L5–S1. a. stabilize right SI, move L5 on left, b. reverse.

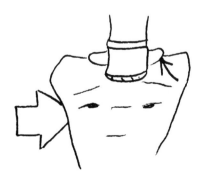

Fig. 2–42 PMP for inferior L5.

correcting these fixations, the posterior fixation could be adjusted and repalpated. If the adjustment is successful, there will be a return of joint play on the left with perhaps a decrease in pain. The deep depression on the right would indicate an anterior fixation that would be adjusted next and repalpated for normal position and play. If there remains any palpable distortion, the fifth segment of the psoas should be checked for imbalance. As one's level of skill in palpation becomes more acute, it is easy to determine these combinations. Obviously, knowing whether a fixation is present, or merely a muscle imbalance, greatly improves one's accuracy in adjusting.

Anomalous L5–S1 Articulations. As one becomes more adept at PMP, the suspicion of anomalous conditions is more easily confirmed. A unilateral sacralized L5 will palpate as rigid and unmoving perhaps more so than a fixation. It will have no anterior/posterior or superior/inferior joint play. If there is a pseudoarticulation, there may be a slight degree of superior/inferior play.

Facetal asymmetry adds a new dimension. A coronal facet will have less anterior/posterior play with superior/inferior play in evidence. A sagittal-facing facet will likely have more of both, sometimes to the degree of hypermobility. In investigating these variations, one may expect to palpate and adjust, then repalpate and continue to correct suspected fixations. A picture will form as to the function of the articulations. Experience and comparison with radiographic findings will enhance one's confidence in assessing these complex fixations.

Spinal Palpation. Continue to palpate the vertebral segments in the same fashion, press upward on each segment, then rock each vertebra to determine basic position. This will reveal if the vertebra is in neutral, or rotated and fixed. Next, move down one level on one side and challenge the vertebra below against the superior one, pressing upward simultaneously on both sides; reverse contacts and challenge again. Then, move the inferior contact to the next vertebra above and challenge in the same fashion on both sides (Fig. 2–43). These challenges will tell if the vertebra is fixed in respect to the segment above or below.

As an example in palpating L4, first press upward on the mamillaries of L4, and feel for a neutral, posterior, or anterior position. Rock it back and forth to determine the degree of joint play. Then move the right contact inferior to the L5 mamillary. Press upward simultaneously feeling for normal joint play between the segments. Then reverse the contacts, L4 on the right and L5 on the left, and repeat the process. Then shift the left contact to L3 and challenge L3–4. Reverse contacts and challenge again. By repeating this process, one can work all the way up to T3 and obtain an accurate assessment of spinal fixations. This seems tedious at first, but familiarity brings speed. In most cases, the significant subluxations stand out. This technique is useful in fine-tuning the specificity of subluxation analysis especially when more general manipulative procedures fail to completely correct the problem.

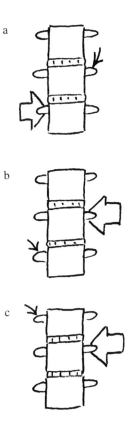

Fig. 2–43 Sequential PMP of vertebral segments. a. stabilize on right, move left, b. reverse, c. move up to next level and repeat.

Muscle Testing

The relative strength of the muscles involved should be tested. Testing should begin with the most important muscles and proceed to the more unlikely muscles. It is not necessary to test all of the muscles in every case. As one's expertise improves, the key muscles will become easier to detect. In the supine position, the psoas, abdominals, quadratus lumborum, TFL, quadriceps femoris, sartorius, gracilis, and the abductors and adductors of the hip can be tested. The gluteus medius and minimus are better tested in the side posture.

Prone Exam

The prone position gives the examiner a look at the back. The condition of the skin and the state of the posterior musculature can be evaluated. Findings from previous sections of the exam can be confirmed.

Leg Length

Take another look at the leg length by hooking the thumbs under the medial malleoli and compare with the supine exam.

Pelvic Rotation

Hook the thumbs under the posterior superior iliac spines and sight down over them. Compare these findings with the supine evaluation. Your findings should be consistent with the findings in other parts of the exam. There are times when you will find that leg length or pelvic rotation or both will reverse when the patient switches from supine to prone.

Dr. Logan's[1,4] research has found that subluxations of the atlas can cause this to happen. I have confirmed his findings in practice. Adjusting the atlas first is likely to either eliminate the findings in the low back or pelvis altogether, or a consistency of findings will establish itself from supine to prone. We have no clear biomechanical explanation for this phenomenon; however, it is an indication of the importance of the atlas in imbalances of the human body.

Another example of this is the finding of an AS ilium with a short leg on the same side. It is not uncommon to find this variation, which makes no sense biomechanically. What seems to happen is that a posterior rotation and fixation of the fifth lumbar can alter the clinical appearance of a pelvic imbalance. This appears to occur far more frequently with a right posterior rotation (spinous left) fixation of L5. With this, the right ilia will palpate AS and the right leg, instead of checking long, checks short. By adjusting L5 before proceeding, the true nature of the pelvic distortion will be revealed. There is no consistency to what shows next. It could palpate as normal, or as an AS with long leg, or PI with a short leg. The phenomenon may be a muscular and proprioceptive reaction influenced primarily by the fifth segment of the psoas.

Oblique Sacrum

Bring the thumbs up on each side of the inferior sacral apex. Sight down over the area and look for any unleveling that would indicate the sacrum has shifted inferiorly on one side (Fig. 2–44). An oblique sacrum is often found with an inferior ilium.

Muscle Tone in the Hip

An assessment of the tone of the gluteus maximus and piriformis can be done by two methods. First, by passively extending the patient's hip by bending the knee to 90° and lifting the relaxed thigh off the table (Fig. 2–45). If the knee "pops" out laterally at the first part of the lift, it is likely that the piriformis is hypertonic. If the knee rides out laterally as the extension is nearing maximum, the gluteus maximus is hypertonic. At the same time, note the degree of passive extension. If it is restricted, it may indicate a shortened psoas or rectus or degenerative changes and is often found with an anatomical short leg due to compensatory rotation of the ilia and femur.

The second method is done by standing at the patient's shoulder, facing footward and contacting the greater trochanters with the fingers. An examiner can detect hypertonicity or weakness in either the gluteus maximus or piriformis by moving the trochanters. By pushing the trochanters anteriorly (medial rotation), the piriformis resistance can be assessed. By pushing in a more inferior direction, the gluteus maximus can be assessed (Fig. 2–46).

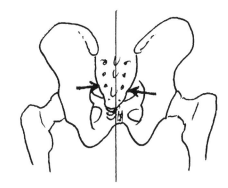

Fig. 2–44 Right inferior or oblique sacrum.

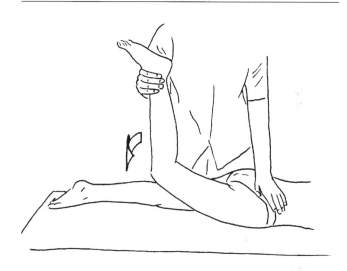

Fig. 2–45 Passive hip extension—lateral flare of knee indicates piriformis or gluteus maximus hypertonicity.

Muscle Testing

With the patient in the prone position, the gluteus maximus, piriformis, and medial rotators of the thigh and the hamstrings can be evaluated.

Differentiating Joint and Muscle Dysfunction

In the course of the examination, by careful observation and palpation techniques, the examiner will be able to differentiate between joint and muscle causes for a patient's complaints.

The sitting and arising exam demonstrated the idea of attempting to rise, determining if there was any pain or difficulty, then supporting various muscles involved in the action.

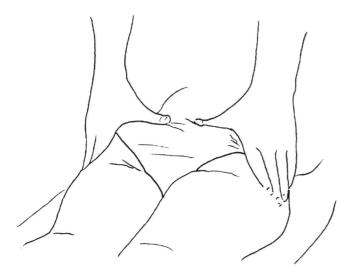

Fig. 2–46 Palpation of greater trochanters for piriformis and gluteus maximus hypertonicity.

Any improvement in the signs and symptoms would indicate muscle dysfunction.

This principle can be applied to other areas and can be used to improvise ways to investigate a variety of suspected imbalances or dysfunctions. For instance, when examination findings reveal a probable unstable pelvis (see Chapter 6 on Conditions and Treatment), palpation of the SI joints produces significant pain. By supporting the ilia in different directions, it may be possible to determine the likely muscle or muscles involved, or whether the condition is inflammatory, and design a more specific treatment plan.

Support the various muscles in the following manner: Stand or sit to one side of the supine patient. Slide the cephalad hand under the patient with the fingers in contact with the SI joint. Use the other hand to put the ilia through various maneuvers. First, push the ischial tuberosity medially, hold, and check for reduced pain at the SI joint. If there is less or no pain, the transversus perinei muscles are likely weak and at fault. Pull the tuberosity laterally, hold, and check for pain. With reduced pain at the SI joint, suspect the transverse abdominals and fourth segment of the Q-L of being at fault. Push the tuberosity anteriorly (posterior rotation of the ilia). With decreased SI pain, suspect the gluteus maximus. With a decrease in SI pain while pushing superiorly on the ischial tuberosity, consider Q-L dysfunction. Pull the iliac crest medially. If pain is lessened at the SI joint, the posterior abdominal fibers and third and fourth segments of the Q-L may be at fault.

If these maneuvers reduce pain, the cause of the pain is muscle dysfunction. If no relief is noted, a joint problem with inflammation, a significant factor, is likely the cause.

In the supine position, the active SLR gives indications as to the patient's ability. Is there pain or limitation? By assisting the support muscles, does the patient find it easier? In this case, the support comes from the opposite Q-L, psoas, and back muscles. Reach under the supine patient, grasp, and hold the muscles as if they were contracted, and have the patient attempt the movement again.

A bilateral active SLR can be impaired by weak abdominals. Press down on the lower abdomen and have the patient repeat the move (Fig. 2–47). In the presence of weak or underfunctioning abdominals, this support by assisting the abdominals makes it significantly easier. This is a common finding in women who have had children. The abdominals cease to function as pregnancy advances. It is common to find that they do not return to normal action even in women who are exercising. The entire abdominal complex must be retrained to function normally.

In PMP of the vertebrae, I have found that the location of pain can aid in the differential diagnosis. After acute inflammation has been reduced, a finding of pain over the lateral aspects of the vertebral motor unit usually suggests a facetal problem including the ligaments and muscles related to that segment. Palpable pain over the spinous, and absent or significantly less laterally over the mamillary process, is a sign of disk involvement. It may be a strain/sprain of the disk, an irritated degenerative condition, or a sign that could indicate protrusion or herniation. Further confirmation is, of course, necessary. The pain with spinous pressure is usually deep and likely to involve the deep innervation of the disk itself and the recurrent sensory nerves.

Orthopaedic Testing

The field of orthopaedic testing is controversial. There are many obscure "tests" usually named for some ancient medical practitioner. As I understand the concept of orthopaedic test-

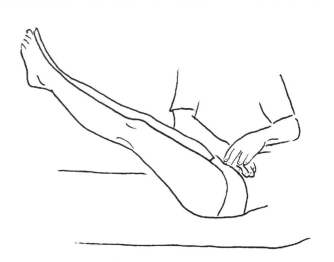

Fig. 2–47 Active bilateral SLR with abdominal support.

ing, it is an attempt to isolate a lesion involving articulations and their supporting structures. Many tests overlap and can be confirmatory, or can contradict and confuse the issue. There are numerous factors that can alter the test findings, including muscle imbalances and subluxation/fixation. It is up to each practitioner to determine which tests best serve his or her own examination procedures, giving one as clear a diagnostic impression as possible. Orthopaedic testing is important in objectifying a patient's complaints, especially in medical/legal reporting.

In understanding orthopaedic testing, it is helpful to understand the biomechanics of the area. Often a thorough palpation and muscle evaluation can give more information. It is recommended that before performing or analyzing orthopaedic tests, the examiner should thoroughly examine and palpate the area. From the concepts presented in Chapter 1 (Anatomy), it should become easier to understand the results of orthopaedic testing, and to establish for oneself the validity of a particular test. During the testing, be sure to observe the patient's reactions. Look for painful reactions that can negate the test, and watch for compensatory reactions that alter the results.

Orthopaedic Tests for the Hip

Trendelenberg's Test. The patient is standing and alternately lifts one foot off the floor. Observe the pelvic level and note any drop of the iliac crest on the side being lifted. Any dropping of the crest is indicative of a weakness of the weight-bearing side abductors, principally the gluteus medius.

Thomas' Test (Fig. 2–48). The patient is supine. Flex the thigh (with knee bent) on the abdomen. Observe the opposite extended leg and note whether the thigh lifts off the table. Also, note any posterior pelvic rotation and feel the lumbar lordosis and note whether it flattens or remains the same during the maneuver. If the extended thigh is lifted by the flexion of the opposite thigh, there is likely a flexion contracture of that (the extended) hip, or at least a hypertonic iliacus or psoas or both. A lack of flattening of the lordosis may also be seen. An increased lordosis may be a compensation for a flexion contracture.

Patrick's Fabrere Test (Fig. 2–49). The patient is supine. The hip is flexed, abducted, externally rotated, and extended. Simply place the ankle of the side being tested on the opposite knee and press down on that knee (the side being tested) abducting the hip. This test is supposedly painful with degenerative hip disease. It may indicate a capsular inflammation. Any restriction in abduction and external rotation demonstrates probable contracture or hypertonicity of the internal rotators and upper adductors, principally the pectineus.

Ober's Test. The patient is lying on his or her side. Grasp the ankle and abduct and extend the leg with the knee flexed to 90°. If the thigh remains abducted with support withdrawn, it suggests a hypertonicity or contracture of the iliotibial band that is related to the muscles attaching into it, the TFL, and the

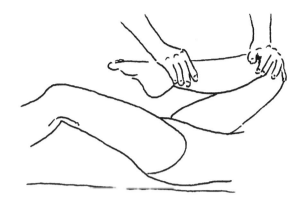

Fig. 2–48 Thomas' test.

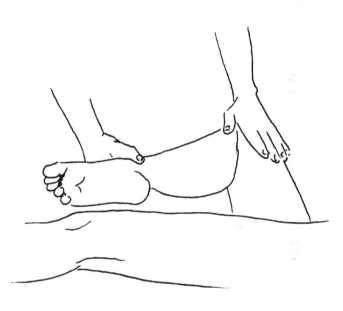

Fig. 2–49 Patrick's Fabrere test.

gluteus maximus. Evans[8] states that Ober's test is positive in cases of transient synovitis of the hip and some cases of lumbosacral disorders.

Orthopaedic Tests for the Sacroiliac Joints

Iliac Compression Test. The patient is side-lying. Apply firm pressure downward over the iliac crest. This stresses the sacroiliac ligaments, especially the posterior ligaments. Resulting increased pain or sensation is indicative of an SI disorder.

Goldthwait's Sign. The patient is supine. Place one hand under the lumbar spine and passively raise the affected leg. If pain is elicited before the lumbars move, suspect the SI, either a sprain or arthritis. If pain comes on after the lumbars move, it is probably a lumbosacral problem. Repeat the test with the unaffected leg. If the pain begins at about the same level, suspect a lumbosacral problem. If the unaffected leg can be raised farther before pain is elicited, the problem is likely with the SI joint.

Yeoman's Test. The patient is prone. Flex the affected leg and extend the thigh while applying a firm downward pressure over the suspected SI joint. If pain is increased in the SI joint, the test is positive. The test puts pressure on the anterior sacro-iliac ligaments.

Orthopaedic Tests for the Lumbar Spine

Kemp's Test. This test can be performed with the patient either sitting or standing. Evans[8] recommends performing the test in both positions. He states that the sitting position increases intradiscal pressure, maximizing stress on the disk. Standing increases weight-bearing stress to the facets. Stabilize the patient with one hand on the iliac crest and with the other on the shoulder. Guide the patient into flexion and around to the right into an obliquely extended position. Repeat to the left side. The test is positive if radicular symptoms are elicited or aggravated and indicate a probable nerve root compression. If low back pain is felt with no radiating symptoms, suspect a facetal lesion.

Minor's Sign. Observe as the patient arises from sitting. The patient supports the weight of the body on the uninvolved side, flexing the knee and hip on the involved side. This is a general finding and can be seen in a variety of low back conditions (see Chapter 1 on Anatomy).

Bechterew's Test. The patient is seated. Attempt to fully extend one leg at a time and then both legs simultaneously. Any resistance or aggravation of radicular pain is indicative of a probable disk lesion. It can also be indicative of inflammation, or subluxation that compromises the nerve root. Often the patient will lean back in an attempt to reduce the stretch on the nerve. Raising both legs increases intradiscal pressure.

Straight Leg Raise (SLR). The patient is supine with the legs extended. The examiner passively raises the affected leg to the point of pain or 90°. Exacerbation of pain is a positive test and may indicate sciatica from lumbar or sacroiliac problems, discopathy, stenosis, or inflammation.

The tension developed by the SLR is sequential. In the first 30° to 35°, there is little or no tension on the nerve roots, and pain generated at this level is likely due to a piriformis syndrome or sacroiliac lesion. Pain elicited between 35° and 70° is likely to be due to a nerve root lesion, such as a disk protrusion, affecting primarily the L5, S1, and S2 levels. Past 65° to 70°, elicited pain will be due to a lumbar joint problem, as the nerve roots are already maximally stretched. The hamstrings are often shortened with contractures. Note how far the leg can be raised before the knee flexes.

Further information can be obtained with an active straight leg raise (ASLR). Ask the patient to attempt to raise the affected leg. Determine the degree and where pain is noted.

Watch for signs of anterior pelvic rotation that suggest weak abdominals. Support the abdominals and note if the patient can raise the leg further or notes less pain or both. If so, attention should be paid to correcting the abdominal weakness. Note whether the opposite Q-L, serratus posterior inferior, and iliocostalis lumborum are contracting to support the leg lift. If dysfunction is suspected, support the muscles by compressing them while the patient attempts to raise the leg. Note any improvement in the patient's ability and decrease in pain. Palpate the lumbar vertebrae for normal rotation away from the side being raised to determine if the psoas is functioning normally.

More information can be ascertained by testing the flexor muscles: the psoas, iliacus, rectus femoris, sartorius, and TFL. Weakness in these muscles can affect the outcome of the SLR and ASLR. In actual practice, the SLR is often inconclusive. Combining the SLR, ASLR, and flexor testing can provide more information with which to form an opinion as to the patient's condition.

Bragard's Sign. If the SLR is positive, drop the leg to just below the point of pain and dorsiflex the foot. If the pain is increased or if there is radiating pain produced along the course of the sciatic nerve, the test is positive and indicates a likely nerve root irritation.

Double Straight Leg Raise. The patient is supine and both legs are raised together. If pain is elicited earlier than during the raising of one leg only, the test is positive and is indicative of lumbosacral joint problems.

Well-Leg Raising. After performing the SRL, the unaffected side is tested with the leg raised and the foot dorsiflexed. If there is pain produced on the symptomatic side, it is probable that a significant herniation has occurred.

Bowstring Sign. Raise the patient's leg above the examiner's shoulder and compress the hamstring muscle and the popliteal fossa. If any radicular or lumbar pain is elicited, suspect a nerve root compression.

Femoral Nerve Traction Test. The patient lies on the unaffected side. The examiner extends the knee and then hyperextends the affected thigh to 15°. At this point, flex the knee. This stretches the femoral nerve. The test is positive if pain is felt radiating down the anterior thigh. Pain in the groin and hip radiating along the anteromedial thigh indicates an L3 nerve root problem, and pain extending to the midtibia indicates L4.[8]

Ely's Sign. The patient is prone. Flex the heel to the buttock and then hyperextend the thigh. This test will elicit resistance or pain or both with a hip problem, psoas contracture, or nerve root irritation.

Neurological Evaluation

The lumbar spine and sacrum distribute nerves to the pelvis and lower extremity. It is necessary to evaluate the integrity of the nervous system to arrive at a complete diagnosis. The nerve supply from this area can be disturbed by numerous conditions including inflammation, muscle spasm, space-occupying lesions, such as disk derangement or tumor, stenosis, and degenerative conditions.

The initial neurological workup should include reflex testing, muscle strength assessment, and sensory evaluation. The texts on neurological testing usually describe the findings for a perfect nerve root disturbance. In the clinical setting, it is usually a muddled picture that develops. In my experience, the more confused the findings (with no clear-cut nerve root lesion discernible), the problem is more likely to be a neurological disturbance due to a strain/sprain injury involving inflammation and muscle spasm. However, a working diagnosis can be quickly discarded if initial treatment fails to improve the condition.

Often, initial treatment directed at reducing inflammation and spasm, may "fine-tune" the signs and symptoms revealing a more obvious nerve root lesion. There are cases of disk herniations at several levels that can present a confusion of signs and symptoms. When the situation warrants, further, more extensive neurological evaluation may be necessary.

Reflexes

The integrity of the reflex arc can provide information about the integrity of the afferent/efferent nerves and their central synaptic connection. The deep tendon reflexes of the lower extremity are the patellar and Achilles reflexes. A decrease or absence of these reflexes may indicate a peripheral nerve lesion or a lesion in the spinal cord or cerebellar disease. Exaggerated reflexes can result when there is a lesion in the upper motor neurons or motor cortex.

As with most all bodily functions, there are a wide variety of responses to stimulating a deep tendon reflex. Some patients will seem to have none at all, yet function normally anyway. Others will flail about with the slightest stimulation with no other evidence of an upper motor neuron lesion. Clinical experience helps to differentiate between a normal and pathological response. The degree of response is compared bilaterally for symmetry. Asymmetrical responses are usually indicative of a problem.

Reflexes are graded clinically as absent, diminished, normal, or exaggerated. Often they are numbered: (1) zero equals absent, (2) plus 1 equals diminished, (3) plus 2 equals normal, (4) plus 3 equals exaggerated but not necessarily pathologic, and (5) plus 4 equals hyperactive and likely pathologic. If the reflexes are difficult to elicit, the Jendrassik maneuver is helpful. Have the patient hook the flexed fingers together and pull as if to separate them. Often a diminished or absent reflex will become normal.

The patellar reflex is usually taken with the patient seated and the legs relaxed and feet clear of the floor. A sharp rap on the patellar tendon just below the patella will demonstrate a knee-jerk response (a quick extension of the leg). The patellar reflex is predominately L4, but includes L2 and L3. The reflex can be tested in the supine position by slightly flexing and supporting the knee.

The Achilles reflex is tested with the patient sitting, but can be obtained with the patient supine or prone. The foot is put into slight dorsiflexion to stretch the tendon, and a sharp rap on the Achilles tendon should elicit a quick plantar flexion response. The Achilles reflex is almost exclusively S1.

Hoppenfeld[9] describes a reflex test for the L5 level, but indicates it to be difficult to elicit. The test is on the posterior tibialis tendon with the foot in slight eversion and dorsiflexion. Strike the tendon on the medial side of the foot just before its insertion into the navicular. The normal response would be plantar flexion with inversion.

The pathological reflexes in the lower limb are usually seen in cases of upper motor neuron lesions. Babinski's sign is most often mentioned. By stroking the bottom of the foot with a pen, as if to tickle, extension of the great toe and a fanning out of the small toes is a positive sign. The normal response would be a flexing of all the toes.

Muscle Strength

When there is a neurological compromise, it will be likely to affect the muscles innervated, weakening them. Testing certain muscles can help in narrowing down a nerve root lesion. Always test bilaterally and compare. It is important to consider the numerous reasons a muscle will test weak besides a nerve root lesion; pain due to injury, spinal subluxation, articular subluxation or dysfunction, lymphatic congestion, and just plain weakness.

The T12 through L1–2–3 levels innervate the iliopsoas. As this is a multileveled innervation, it is not a very accurate muscle test for lesions, and careful assessment of all factors of function should be done. Testing for the iliopsoas is best done in the supine position. Flex to 65° and slightly externally rotate the leg. Contact the patient's thigh just above the knee and ask the patient to resist your effort to extend and slightly abduct the thigh. Test several times to determine the stamina of the muscle (see Chapter 4 on Muscle Testing).

The quadriceps femoris is innervated by L2–3–4 via the femoral nerve. Assessing the strength of knee extension can be achieved in several ways. Noting any difficulty in the sitting patient's ability to fully extend the leg is a sign of extension lag.[9] The last 10° of extension require 50% more muscle power. Testing the muscle can be done in the sitting or supine positions. Ask the patient to resist your attempt to flex the extended leg. In the sitting position, the leg is fully extended. In the supine position, the thigh and knee are flexed to 90°. The patient resists the examiner's attempt to further flex the leg. Test several times to ascertain the stamina of the muscle.

The hip adductors are also L2–3–4 (obturator nerve) innervated. Have the supine patient resist your attempt to abduct the legs from the midline.

The tibialis anterior is mainly innervated by L4 and is a strong indicator of L4 radiculopathy. This muscle can be assessed in the standing position by having the patient attempt to heel-walk with the feet dorsiflexed and inverted. It can also be tested with the patient supine. Dorsiflex and invert the foot and have the patient resist efforts to pull the foot into plantar flexion. This is a powerful muscle and should be difficult or impossible to budge. Using the forearm against the dorsum of the foot is a good way to exact a significant testing force (Fig. 2–50).

L5 is represented by the extensor hallucis longus, the extensor muscles of the toes, and the gluteus medius. The extensor hallucis is the most easily recognized indicator of L5 radiculopathy. It is best tested with the patient supine. Place the great toe into extension and have the patient resist your efforts to flex it (Fig. 2–51). Be sure to contact the distal phalange only so as not to enlist the extensor hallucis brevis. The extensor muscles of the other toes can also be tested in this manner. These muscles should be very hard to beat. These tendons should stand out when the patient is attempting to heel-walk without inversion. The gluteus medius is tested by testing the strength of abduction (see Chapter 4 on Muscle Testing).

The peroneus longus and brevis, major evertors of the foot, are innervated principally by S1. The patient can be asked to walk on the medial border of the foot. They can be tested by placing the foot into eversion and attempting to invert against the patient's resistance (Fig. 2–52).

S1 and S2 innervate the gastrocnemius and soleus muscles, powerful plantar flexors, too strong to test manually. Have the patient toe-walk. Hoppenfeld[9] suggests having the patient jump up and down on the balls of the feet, one foot at a time. This puts enough force on the muscle to uncover weakness.

S2–3–4 innervate intrinsic muscles of the foot that are difficult to isolate. These nerve roots innervate the muscles of the

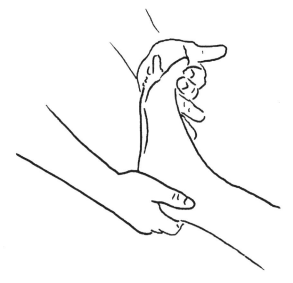

Fig. 2–51 Extensor hallucis longus—L5.

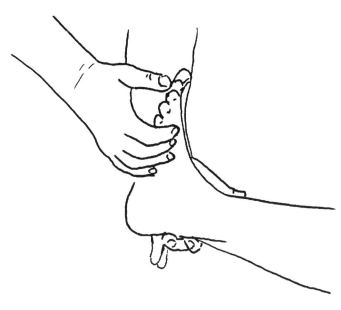

Fig. 2–52 Peroneus longus and brevis—S1.

bladder and any significant radiculopathy will show in bladder dysfunction.

Sensory Testing

Cutaneous innervation of the lower limb should be tested for altered sensation. Increased or decreased sensation should be noted. The most efficient way to assess the sensory system is to use double pinwheels and test bilaterally all the dermatomes. Figure 2–53 demonstrates the basic dermatome pattern. If any discrepancies are noted, a more detailed assess-

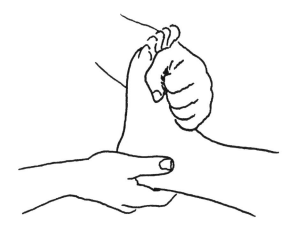

Fig. 2–50 Tibialis anterior test—L4.

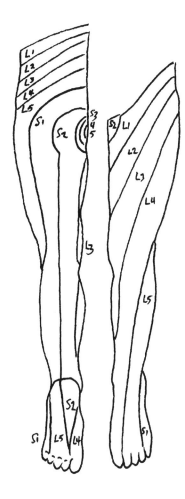

Fig. 2–53 Dermatome pattern.

ment can be done to differentiate sharp and light touch as well as vibratory sensation if necessary.

Visceral Examination

The chiropractor is the most likely physician to still have the palpatory skills to perform a thorough abdominal examination. The modern physician has come to rely on laboratory tests and high-tech diagnostic procedures, and at the most extreme, exploratory surgery to diagnose internal pathology. It seems likely that the "old school" doctors could, with a skilled physical exam, accurately diagnose and differentiate internal disorders, and would use lab and other procedures to back up their findings.

Modern physicians with the fear of malpractice on their minds have come to rely heavily on high-tech diagnostic procedures moving farther away from their trust in physical exams and the instincts that make physicians healers. Today, we tend to assume the worst probable diagnosis and work back to

the most likely. It has been said that today, 80% of medical costs are for diagnosis and only 20% go toward treatment.

The importance to the chiropractor of being able to differentiate between an organic pathology and a structural condition is clear. The detection and appropriate treatment of a patient's condition is the physician's responsibility. Understanding the interrelationship between visceral and structural pathology makes the chiropractor an important primary care physician and a qualified gatekeeper in the managed-care model. There are many patients who initially seek treatment from chiropractors.

Understanding visceral anatomy and function is important in the conservative management of internal disorders. There are many conditions that are treatable without medical intervention or, by patient choice, can be managed by means other than traditional intervention. Many common internal disorders are readily treatable by manipulation, nutritional therapy, and reflex techniques, which are within the scope of chiropractic. The important consideration is in being able to properly recognize the patient's condition and refer for appropriate treatment, if warranted. The early detection of serious pathology is often the chiropractor's responsibility.

Throughout his teaching, Dr. Logan stressed that every patient should have a thorough abdominal examination. The experience gained from the palpation of numerous abdomens, especially normal abdomens, prepares one for the easy recognition of abnormality. In his clinical experience, he detected several tumors in early stages, one that had been unnoticed in previous medical workups.

The abdomen is usually divided into four quadrants. It is generally considered that, in a normal abdomen, it is difficult to distinguish much of anything. The viscera that can sometimes be distinguished are the liver edge as it runs along the lower right rib cage, the large intestine, and the pulsating aortic and iliac arteries (Fig. 2–54).[10] The lower pole of the right kidney can be felt; however, the left is up under the ribs. In palpating, the examiner should be feeling for rigidity of the abdominal muscles, and any visceral structures that are discernible should be identified and considered for any abnormalities. If a significant gastrointestinal disorder is suspected, auscultation of the abdomen is important. The absence of sounds is a serious finding and may be a medical emergency.

Differential Diagnosis

Organic vs. Structural

There are numerous organic conditions that manifest back pain at some stage, usually early in the course of a disease. In considering a patient's complaints, it is essential to consider the age and sex of the patient and how these factors can relate to the more commonly found conditions. For instance, the role of osteoporosis in vertebral compression and femoral neck

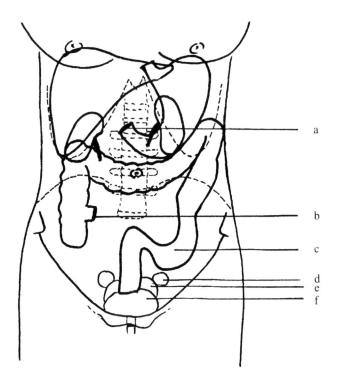

Fig. 2–54 Visceral palpation. a. pylorus, b. ileocacal valve, c. sigmoid colon, d. ovaries, e. uterus, f. bladder.

fractures in older postmenopausal women or prostate hypertrophy in older men. Any irregularities in organ function, such as digestion, bowel, or urinary habits and menstruation, should be noted.

Kidney infections cause low back pain of a dull nature in the earlier stages, becoming more pronounced with other unmistakable signs later. A patient unresponsive to initial treatment based on the working diagnosis should lead the clinician to further investigation. Cancer is a major concern, and the unresponsive patient who fits other criteria, considering their history, should be carefully evaluated. The classic sign of nocturnal back pain is found in cases of melanoma, or prostatic cancer, and the likely metastasis to the lower spine. The history of a gradual onset of pain with little evidence of likely structural problems or history of injury should cause concern and careful assessment.

Referred pain patterns can help in the diagnosis. The classic referred pain of renal colic or kidney inflammation to the lower back, usually over the Q-L muscle is well known, as is the referral of pain to the shoulder in liver, gall bladder, and pancreatic conditions—essentially an irritation to the diaphragm and the phrenic nerve. Rectal and uterine pain can be referred to the lumbosacral area.

Sir Zachary Cope[11] has emphasized the thorough understanding of the anatomy of the abdomen and pelvis. He believes that there are many anatomical relations between viscera and structure that can be used for diagnosis. For instance, there are often related irritations of adjacent muscles either by direct or reflex means. The psoas, Q-L, lateral abdominals, piriformis, obturator internus, and diaphragm can be affected by visceral disorders. They will often show signs of spasm, rigidity, or tenderness, with increased symptoms upon attempting to stretch them. This should be kept in mind when the patient's history is not clear as to a structural cause for symptoms.

Discopathy vs. Strain/Sprain

The signs and symptoms of strain/sprain and disk injuries can be difficult to differentiate. Damage to the connective tissue supporting the facetal joints has been shown to cause radiating pain into the buttock and posterior thigh that can resemble radiculopathy. It usually stays above the knee but a discogenic radiculopathy will more often travel into the calf or foot or both. Both types of injury can present with antalgia. Flexion and lateral lean are common. The classic antalgic lean away from the side of sciatica is indicative of a lateral disk protrusion and a lean into the side of sciatica is likely due to a central bulge. A strain/sprain injury will more often elicit palpatory pain to either side of the spinous, suggestive of facetal involvement.

A disk injury will more often be painful with direct anterior pressure over the spinous. This pressure seems to more directly influence the disk and the recurrent nerve that innervates the periosteum and inner disk structures. A vertebral fracture, especially a compression fracture, will elicit an exaggerated pain reaction when directly palpated. This type of response and a history of a prat fall or suspected osteoporosis should lead to a strong suspicion of vertebral fracture.

The correlation of these findings with the history, orthopaedic, and neurological findings should provide an accurate working diagnosis. A disk can be strained or sprained without protrusion or herniation, causing no discernible neurological symptoms. Conversely, the swelling of a facetal sprain can compress the structures in the intervertebral foramen and cause nerve root irritation. In determining the course of treatment in these situations, the initial therapy should be directed at reducing the inflammation and care should be exercised in the choice of manipulative techniques. A suspected disk injury should be handled carefully so as not to cause further damage.

Peripheral injuries in the hip can also cause radiating pain into the leg. The entrapment of the sciatic nerve in an injured piriformis can cause sciatic symptoms, the psoas can entrap lumbar nerve roots, and the lateral femoral cutaneous nerve can be trapped over the hip and anterior pelvic bones. Obviously, the clinical picture will show fewer signs of spinal involvement. The gluteus medius, when injured, can very closely resemble a sciatic radiculopathy, including neurological findings consistent with a discopathy. This muscle should be examined in all cases with sciatic symptoms.

In December 1994, the U.S. Department of Public Health and Human Services (DPHHS)[12] published the new guidelines for the assessment and treatment of acute low back problems. The Department defined acute as being episodes of lower back pain lasting less than four weeks. As ubiquitous as lower back pain is, there has been much scrutiny of the clinical approach. As with other recent studies (such as the Manga Report, a Canadian study demonstrating the effectiveness of chiropractic treatment in work-related low back injuries), there is a more general agreement that the conservative approach, including manipulation, in the assessment and treatment of lower back problems is best.

The DPHHS guidelines call for a more conservative diagnostic approach. If the clinical picture is that of "nonspecific back symptoms" and no potentially serious signs or symptoms exist, avoid aggressive diagnostic workups using imaging or lab testing. Treatment is conservative, with rest, manipulation, and simple pain relievers, such as aspirin. This seems to have the best results. Most cases will resolve within four weeks.

The guidelines point out several red flags in the initial assessment. The "potentially serious spinal condition" includes tumor, fracture, or a major neurologic compromise, such as cauda equina syndrome. Red flags for fracture are major trauma (or even minor in an older patient); for tumor or infection, age (over 50 or under 20), history of cancer, constitutional symptoms (fever, chills, unexplained weight loss), nocturnal pain, and recent history of systemic infection. Cauda equina symptoms would show saddle anesthesia, bladder dysfunction, or lower extremity neurological deficit. These signs and symptoms would warrant a more detailed assessment. Any clear sciatic symptoms that suggest nerve root compromise would also indicate a more serious situation and a more aggressive workup.

Assessment of the "Hot Low Back"

The patient who is carried into your office or presents with severe pain that makes a standard methodical history and exam difficult at best, is one that challenges all practitioners. These patients can barely move, cannot sit or stand, and find it agonizing to get on the exam table. Orthopaedic tests would all be positive for pain, and palpation is nearly impossible.

Initially, it is best to get the patient into the supine position, which best simulates the weight-bearing position. More information can be obtained by examining in this position first. A high–low chiropractic table can be helpful; however, great care should be exercised in lowering and raising the patient as sudden changes in weight-bearing especially raising the patient

can cause sudden excruciating pain. I have found it best to tell the patient what you want them to do and let them figure out how to do it. Stay close to assist them, but let them make the moves in their own way and in their own time. A pillow under the knees can often make the supine position more tolerable.

The history is important. How did this happen? Is it an exacerbation of a chronic condition, which would suggest inflammation. Did it happen while the patient was attempting to lift or set down a heavy object (recall that lifting may injure the psoas and lowering is likely to injure the gluteus maximus)? Is the pain a result of a slip/fall or prat fall? Is there any radiating pain? Most patients that present this way have had a sudden onset of severe pain. There are likely to be some similarities of signs and symptoms in all of these instances no matter what the underlying lesion or pathology. By addressing the acute factors, it is possible to reduce some of the pain and anxiety and gain the patient's confidence.

With the patient as comfortable as possible, assess the basic pelvic listings. Look for rotation. An AS ilium might suggest the iliacus or psoas is in spasm. Palpate the insertion on the medial thigh for pain. A PI ilium may involve the gluteus maximus. Compare the iliac findings with palpation findings in the lower extremities. Palpate the maximus origin and insertion for pain and spasm. Palpate the piriformis for abnormal pain, contraction, and any sciatic nerve entrapment. Palpate the Q-L and paravertebrals and determine their status.

Note the lumbar lordosis in the supine patient. Is it increased, suggesting hypertonic psoas, or is it flattened, suggesting gluteal and paravertebral hypertonicity? Palpate the hip joints for pain and edema. Palpate the sacroiliac joints and then support the ilia in varying directions as described earlier (see the section on Differentiating Joint and Muscle Dysfunction). Reduced sacroiliac pain with this test can provide indicators for ways to reduce severe symptoms.

Observe and palpate while the patient attempts to do an active SLR. Recall that the initial contraction of the contralateral Q-L and related muscles occurs first, followed by the abdominals in order to fix the pelvis. Actual lifting of the leg is accomplished by the psoas, iliacus, sartorius, rectus femoris, and TFL.

During the active SLR, note if the pelvis tilts anteriorly, indicating weak or nonfunctioning abdominals. Note if the lumbar spinouses rotate away from the active side indicating normal function of the contralateral support muscles. Note any deviation of the leg medially or laterally as it raises, which could indicate a problem with adductors or abductors.

By supporting the muscles that appear to be dysfunctioning and retesting, any reduced pain or increased ease of lifting the leg can indicate the muscles that need attention. By correcting these signs of dysfunction, the patient will likely experience a reduction in pain that is the first step in evaluating and treating the acute hot low back.

REFERENCES

1. Logan AL. *The Knee: Clinical Aspects.* Gaithersburg, Md: Aspen; 1994.

2. D'Ambrosia R. *Musculoskeletal Disorders: Regional Examination and Differential Diagnosis.* Philadelphia, Pa: Lippincott; 1986.

3. Manello D. Leg length inequality: A literature review. Presented at the Seventh Annual Conference of the Consortium for Chiropractic Research, California Chiropractic Association; Palm Springs, Calif: June 19–21, 1992.

4. Logan AL. *The Foot and Ankle: Clinical Aspects.* Gaithersburg, Md: Aspen; 1994.

5. Michele A. *Iliopsoas.* Springfield, Ill: Charles C Thomas; 1962.

6. Biron W., Welles B., Houser R. *Chiropractic Principles and Technique.* Chicago, Ill: National College of Chiropractic; 1939.

7. Friel, J. ed. *Dorland's Illustrated Medical Dictionary.* Philadelphia, Pa: Saunders; 1974.

8. Evans R. *Illustrated Essentials in Orthopedic Physical Assessment.* St. Louis, Mo: Mosby; 1992.

9. Hoppenfeld S. *Physical Examination of the Spine and Extremities.* New York, NY: Appleton-Century-Crofts; 1976.

10. Bates B. *A Guide to Physical Examination.* Philadelphia, Pa: Lippincott; 1974.

11. Cope Z. *The Early Diagnosis of the Acute Abdomen.* London: Oxford University Press; 1972.

12. U.S. Department of Health and Human Services. *Acute Low Back Problems in the Adult: Assessment and Treatment.* Rockville, Md; 1994.

Chapter 3

Imaging the Low Back

Joseph W. Howe, DC, DACBR, FICC

This chapter reviews diagnostic imaging of the most common abnormalities of the low back. Plain film radiography will be the major imaging method discussed, but appropriate use of advanced imaging will also be covered.

IMAGING METHODS

Plain Film Radiography

General Considerations

The minimum radiographic examination of the lumbosacral region should consist of coronal and lateral views,[1,2] the coronal view including the entire pelvis. By convention, the coronal view usually done for the low back is an anteroposterior (AP) view. However, Howe and others[3,4] advocate positioning the patient facing the film, a posteroanterior (PA) projection, which has geometric advantages and for female patients reduces the radiation to the ovaries. An angulated coronal spot film of the lumbosacral junction should nearly always be part of the routine lumbosacral series.[4,5] When including the entire

Special thanks to Terry R. Yochum, DC, DACBR for allowing the use of several illustrations from his book: *Essentials of Skeletal Radiology*, for sharing with me many films for my teaching file, some of which are used in this chapter, and for his continual efforts on behalf of the profession. Thanks also to Jeffrey Cooley, DC, DACBR for proofreading the manuscript and making suggestions that were helpful. My gratitude to my wife, Dee, for her patience while I neglected many projects she would have preferred I undertake. And particular thanks to Craig Sandberg, whose efforts contribute greatly to my practice and many other things in my life.

pelvis of a large patient, a 14 x 17 film will not allow the thoracolumbar junction to be visualized on the coronal view. An AP of the pelvis with the central ray at the top of the hip joints and a second coronal view (a PA using an 11 x 14 film is preferred) to see the lumbar spine to include the thoracolumbar junction is the optimal study. Oblique views are of value only under certain situations,[2] and a lateral spot film of the lumbosacral junction is only rarely indicated. It should be done only when the larger lateral view does not allow adequate visualization of the lumbosacral junction.[6]

Collimation limiting exposure to the area of interest and use of gonad shielding are important because low back radiography involves exposure of vital organs and gonads.

Upright vs. Recumbent Radiography

Most chiropractic radiographic facilities use an upright bucky or grid chamber and do not have the availability of a radiographic table to allow recumbent radiography. Because radiographs of a standing patient have specific value by depicting the upright posture (except for thin patients) diagnostic detail is not as good as is usually obtained when the patient is recumbent.[1] When a radiographic table is available, the optimum low back series takes advantage of both upright and recumbent radiographs. My personal preference is to do 14 x 17 coronal and sagittal views with the patient standing and the angulated coronal spot film (and obliques when done) on the table. With this procedure, the postural findings from the upright position and finer detail of bones and joints from the recumbent films are both obtained. Also, comparison of differences in spinal contours and alignment between upright and recumbent posture will be appreciated when present and may contribute postural information that may not be as well appreciated otherwise.

When only upright films are made, use of a compression band to both compress soft tissues and to help maintain stability so that no motion occurs during the exposure is helpful and is nearly mandatory in obese patients if adequate diagnostic detail is to be obtained. Use of the PA projection with the patient squeezing against the grid chamber is also helpful.

If postural information is to be of value from upright radiography, it is important that the floor or platform upon which the patient stands, the grid chamber, and the radiographic tube (therefore the tube column), be plumb, square, and level. It is equally important that the patient be carefully positioned to assure, as much as possible, that rotation of the pelvis and torso is not present to cause geometric distortion, which may be misconstrued as biomechanical abnormality.

The AP or PA View

For a standing coronal view, the patient should be placed with the feet directly under the hips. Having the feet more narrowly or broadly separated will cause a parallelogram effect that may produce pelvic unleveling (Fig. 3–1) that does not reflect the actual situation. The weight should be balanced between the legs, and the knees locked in extension. If the knees are bent unequally, a false unleveling of the pelvis will result with probable compensatory alteration of spinal alignment. As closely as possible (more easily accomplished with a PA than an AP projection), the S1 posterior tubercle should be at film midline with pelvic rotation eliminated to the extent possible. The central ray (CR) should be at the approximate level of L3,

perpendicular to film plane. When possible, the thoracolumbar junction and the bottom of the bony pelvis should be on the film. Use of a 60 in or 72 in Tube-Film-Distance (TFD) and a 14 x 17 film size will usually allow this, whereas with a 40 in (the usual standard) TFD in large patients it is often not possible to have both regions encompassed on a 14 x 17 film. Collimation laterally to the edges of the trochanters is optimal. Male gonad shielding should be employed.

If this radiograph is done with the patient recumbent, the prone position compresses the abdomen and gives better geometric visualization of the spine. If a supine position is used, the knees should be slightly bent with a roll placed under them, allowing some flattening of the lumbar curve.

The Angulated Coronal Spot View

This view is most easily accomplished with a PA projection because the CR can be located at the easily palpated L5 spinous process, whereas in an AP approach the positioning of the CR is less precise. A 25° to 30° angle of the CR is needed (more angulation is needed in a patient with an increased sacral base angle) with caudal tube tilt for the PA and cephalic tube tilt for the AP projection. An 8 x 10 film size is usually sufficient, but on large patients or the obese where palpatory landmarks are not as easily located, a 10 x 12 may be necessary. The object of this view is to see through the disk space at the lumbosacral junction. This view also allows optimal visualization of the sacroiliac joints. Optimally, the area seen includes L4 or even slightly higher. My preference is to do this radiograph with the patient prone on the radiographic table because that gives the best radiographic quality and also al-

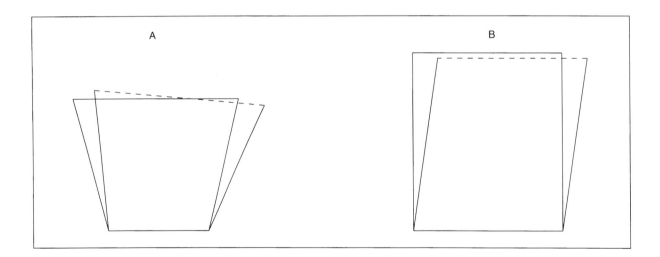

Fig. 3–1 (**A**) If in positioning a patient for an AP or PA view of the low back, care is not taken to be sure the hips are directly above the feet, lateral "sway" of the body will cause an apparent unleveling at hips and pelvis as this figure illustrates. (**B**) With the hips directly above the feet, a parallelogram is formed so that lateral sway does not cause geometric unleveling at the hips or pelvis. Therefore, with proper positioning, hips above feet and knees locked, any unleveling at hips and iliac crests seen on a coronal view of the low back should, in fact, indicate a short extremity on the low side.

lows any postural differences related to recumbency, as compared to that seen in the upright PA or AP view, to be noted. However, it can be easily accomplished with the patient standing (Fig. 3–2).

The Lateral View

A 14 x 17 film size, laterally collimated so that the field size is limited to the bony pelvis, is my preference because the radiograph should allow visualization of the sacrum and the thoracolumbar junction. Placing the patient to assure that there is as little rotation of the body as possible from a true lateral position is important because small amounts of rotation give false information regarding spinal relationships. The CR should be at the iliac crests. It is important to use a kilovoltage (kVp) high enough to penetrate the pelvis, allowing adequate visualization of the lumbosacral junction. A kVp approximating 90 will do this and will nearly always eliminate the need for a spot lateral view of the lumbosacral junction. The lateral spot view has continued to be routinely used in most medical radiology facilities and by a few chiropractors in spite of literature noting the futility of its use.[6] It was needed years ago when low powered equipment and lower kVp techniques would not allow adequate sagittal visualization of the lumbar spine and the lumbosacral junction on the same film. In my

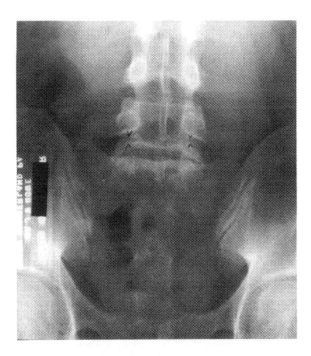

Fig. 3–2 Angulated coronal spot film. This film gives optimal visualization of the sacroiliac joints. Compare the appearance of the sacroiliac joints on this film to that on Figure 3–3, a standard AP view of the same patient. The L5/S1 disk space is also seen on this view and is only rarely seen on standard AP or PA lumbar films.

experience, there are very few occasions when the larger lateral view does not show the L–S junction adequately. By eliminating the lateral spot view, the radiation burden to the patient is greatly reduced.

Oblique Views

Oblique views allow optimal visualization of the facet joints, the partes interarticularis, and give another perspective on the vertebral bodies, disks, and paraspinal soft tissues.[1,2,3] These views are warranted when it is important to see those structures, especially when the coronal and lateral views suggest facet disease, or when pars defects are suspected. They are seldom of value in young patients unless needed to rule out fracture.[2,3] In older patients, especially those showing degenerative changes, they may demonstrate facet disease, facet imbrication, impingement of pars due to facet subluxation, or other findings not adequately appreciated from the coronal and lateral views. Rotation of the patient 45° with the CR at L3 is the appropriate positioning. Whether PA or AP obliques are used is up to the preference of the physician. I favor PA obliques because the positioning is easier and the geometry is theoretically better. Use of 10 x 12 films is usually adequate to capture the images of the lumbar vertebrae, but 11 x 14 films also allow the sacroiliac joints to be demonstrated and will include the thoracolumbar junction. In either case, lateral collimation is usually adequate at 10 in.

For more detailed information on specifics of these and other radiographic procedures please see other sources.[7–9]

Advanced Imaging

The use of advanced imaging procedures for evaluation of low back problems has great value in specific situations. However, their use should be limited to those circumstances where physical examination and plain film imaging does not give sufficient information to form an adequate diagnosis and treatment plan. The caveat that the justification for any imaging study—including plain film radiography—*must be* that the findings from the exam will influence the treatment of the patient. This should be the criterion for each and all decisions as to whether imaging should be done and what examination is best for the situation.

Computed Tomography

Computed tomography (CT) offers specific advantages in spine imaging.[10–15] The acquisition of axial images and the ability to see the structures in both bone and soft tissue windows allows evaluation of the spinal canal and intervertebral nerve root canals (intervertebral foramina), their bordering bony structures, the joints, and to some degree, the contents of the canals.[10–15] These findings cannot be gained from plain films. CT gives exquisite bone detail and demonstrates fractures and joint disease optimally. The ability to reformat the axial images to sagittal, coronal, and oblique planes is also of considerable value in most situations.[10–14]

In recent years, CT has largely been replaced by magnetic resonance imaging (MRI) for spine imaging, but CT still has definite value, especially in assessment of fractures and for evaluation of joint disease that may encroach upon neural structures.

Magnetic Resonance Imaging

Magnetic resonance imaging (MRI) has become the criterion imaging method for evaluation of disk disease, but because of its ability to allow visualization of soft tissues and to discriminate between various tissues, it has value in evaluation of nearly all spinal diseases.[10,14–17] MRI has the advantage of offering exquisite images in multiple planes and, with different pulse sequences, to differentiate various soft tissues—all without exposure to ionizing radiation. Unlike CT where axial images are acquired and other imaging planes must be obtained by reformatting the digital data, MRI can directly image any plane that is desired, resulting in greater clarity and lack of some distortion inherent in the reformatting process.[10,14–18]

MRIs allow visualization of the contents of the spinal canal and neural foramina, with the ability, using some pulse sequences, to discriminate the thecal sac from the epidural soft tissues, the nerve roots within the sac and as they exit from it, the conus medullaris, and the bony margins bordering the canal. Intra- and extradural masses, protrusions and extrusions of disk material, synovial cysts from facet joints, and other abnormalities that cannot otherwise be imaged can be demonstrated through MRI.[14,15,17,19] Bone and joint disease, abnormalities of paraspinal soft tissues, and evaluation of the postsurgical back by use of paramagnetic contrast media are other particularly significant advantages of MRI of the low back.[10,14,15,18]

Radionuclide Scanning

Radionuclide scanning (RN) has utility in imaging of the low back when infection is suspected,[10,14,19,20] when the age of a compression fracture is uncertain[10,14,19] (MRI is even more helpful in this instance,[10,14] but is considerably more expensive), in evaluation of disseminated bone or joint disease,[10,14,19] in certain tumors to determine activity, such as in the instance of an osteoid osteoma to verify an impression from plain films.[10,14,19]

RN scanning locates areas of increased or decreased bony metabolic activity and is very sensitive to early disease.[10,14,19] It is not at all specific, however, and can only be used to locate disease or to evaluate disease activity by sequential studies, not to form a diagnosis.[10,14,19] Technetium is the radionuclide usually used for spinal scanning, but when infection is suspected gallium may be used, usually as an additional procedure following a technetium scan.[10,14,19–21] Both contrast media are injected intravenously, and the areas of uptake are detected by a scintillation camera, which allows real time imaging. Single photon emission computed tomography (SPECT) is a more sophisticated method of RN scanning, allowing 3-D depiction of the skeletal structures, and giving much more sophisticated data that results in more discrete localization of subtle abnormalities.[14,19] Although RN scanning involves intravenous injection of radioactive material, the radiation burdens imposed are quite low. Short half lives of the radionuclides and low radioactivity result in equal or lower overall radiation to the patient than is incurred in most low back imaging procedures that use ionizing radiation.[10,14,19]

Myelography

CT and MRI have made lumbar myelography a nearly outmoded imaging procedure.[10] It is only infrequently used in recent years, more often than not at the request of a surgeon who has been comfortable with its use for many years and wants the reassurance of a familiar procedure. There are only a few situations where myelography will yield information that is not better seen by MRI, without the problems inherent in the invasive procedure of injecting an iodinated contrast medium into the subarachnoid space.

Discography

Discography, after many years of minimal use, has made a comeback in recent years.[22,23] It is a provocative procedure, and its advocates offer that it is the only imaging method that specifically isolates a symptom-producing disk. Injection of a contrast medium (occasionally it is done with saline rather than a contrast substance) into a disk, which causes replication of the pain, specifically locates the disk(s) that account for the patient's symptoms.[22–25] Radiography after the injection (when contrast medium is used) gives characteristic findings. A normal disk will show an H-shaped collection of the contrast medium in the nucleus of the disk, whereas radial annular tears and herniation of nuclear material will be depicted by extrusion of the contrast medium from the central portion of the disk.[14,22–25] MRI often shows several levels of disk degeneration or bulging or both or protrusion, and CT may show more than one level of disk protrusion. Discography allows the offending level to be specified in these instances.[14,22–25] A goodly number of people with no back or leg symptoms will show bulging disks on CT or MRI.[23,26] Discography, due to its provocative nature, is a discriminating procedure, although it is invasive and is painful.

SPINOGRAPHY

Historically, chiropractic physicians have used radiography to determine postural abnormalities, deviations of alignment, and specifically to locate or verify or both intervertebral subluxations. Although there are a number of spinographic systems advocated by adherents of certain chiropractic techniques and much anecdotal evidence of effectiveness of those techniques, there is little in the literature to verify the correlation of radiographically demonstrated subluxations and spinal distortions with symptoms. And there is even less peer reviewed published material to show that such findings can be improved by chiropractic adjustment or manipulation.

No attempt to be encyclopedic regarding spinographic analysis will be made in this chapter. The following are commonly accepted mensuration procedures that may have some significance in correlation with physical findings and palpation in the evaluation of low back disorders. The fact that a procedure is included should not be taken as a definitive statement that the procedure has proven clinical relevance. On the other hand, the omission of a spinographic procedure does not mean that it may not be relevant.

Sacral Base Angle (SBA; Ferguson's Angle)

This is a measurement of the angle of the sacral base to the horizontal.[27,28] It has a wide range of variation in asymptomatic individuals. There is no consensus regarding the significance of either an increased or a decreased SBA, but conventional wisdom suggests that a significant increase in the angle may be a mechanical factor in low back pain by increasing the stress on facet joints.

Lumbosacral Angle

The sacral base angle is often improperly referred to as the lumbosacral angle. Properly, the lumbosacral angle is the angle of the disk at the lumbosacral junction and is measured by the intersection of lines drawn along the margins of the vertebral end plates at the lumbosacral junction on the lateral view. Rowe,[29] properly, refers to this as the lumbosacral disk angle. Increase in this angle is evidence of hyperextension of the vertebral motion unit and has been linked to low back pain by imbrication of the facet joints. With decrease in the lumbar lordotic contour due to antalgia, this angle may diminish.[30]

Lumbar Lordosis

The angle between perpendiculars drawn from lines through the superior L1 end plate and the superior S1 end plate defines the angle of the lumbar lordosis. The range of this angle in asymptomatic individuals varies widely. Rowe[29] suggests an average for this angle to be from 50° to 60°. The significance of variation from the average value is controversial, opinions ranging from nil to considerable in relation to low back pain.[31]

Gravity Line (Ferguson's Line)

Ferguson noted that a vertical line from the center of L3 vertebral body should intersect the anterior one third of the sacral base.[27] Ferguson made his measurement from a lateral film done with the patient recumbent. One study,[30] however, suggests that it is irrelevant whether the patient is in an upright or a recumbent position. Significance is attributed when this line falls more than 10 mm anterior to the sacral promontory, due to increased shearing stress on the facet joints, or when it is shifted to the posterior, which suggests increased weight-bearing on the facets.[29]

Hadley's S Curve

Curvilinear lines drawn from the inferior of the transverse process along the margin of the inferior articular process to the apophyseal joint space and from there continuing along the outer margin of the superior articular process of the subjacent vertebra should result in a smooth S-shaped curve.[32,33] A discontinuous line at the joint space is evidence of facet subluxation. In 1970, I proposed that a more accurate determination could be made by a variation of this procedure using oblique views, again drawing a curvilinear line along the same path, discontinuity at the joint space being more readily visualized in this projection[34] (Fig. 3–3).

Lumbar Disk Angles

The angles made by intersection of lines drawn through the lumbar vertebral end plates can be measured and compared to standards noted in Yochum's authoritative text *Essentials of Skeletal Radiology*.[35] The angles vary at each level and are affected by alterations of posture, such as antalgia or muscular imbalance. The following are the mean values cited by Rowe[29]:

Disk level	Mean angle in degrees
L1/2:	08
L2/3:	10
L3/4:	12
L4/5:	14
L5/S1:	14

Intervertebral Disk Height

Normal disk height varies at different levels. In the lumbar spine, the L4/5 interspace usually exhibits the greatest height

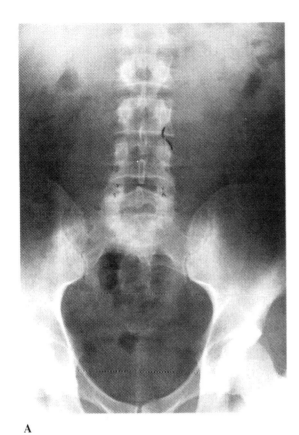

A

B

Fig. 3–3 Hadley's S curve. **(A)** This is an AP view of the same patient as Figure 3–2; the pars defects seen there are also seen here. *Comment:* Hadley's S curve is drawn in at the left L3/4 facet joint, demonstrating normal alignment. **(B)** This view of the same patient demonstrates the variation of Hadley's S curve as shown on an oblique.

and the interspace at L5/S1 the least height. Measurements are inexact at best so, in my opinion, visual evaluation is adequate. Particularly at L5/S1, where variation from normal anatomy is frequent, the presence of apparent decreased disk height is especially uncertain in significance unless accompanied by degenerative end plate changes.

Meyerding's Grading System for Spondylolisthesis

For this determination, the sacral base is divided into four quadrants and the degree of anterior translation of the last lumbar vertebra is judged by the quadrant in which a line down the posterior margin of that vertebral body falls.[36] In a grade one spondylolisthesis, the posterior margin of the vertebra is in the first quadrant; in a grade four it is in the fourth. When the vertebral body has slipped beyond the anterior sacral margin, it is called spondyloptosis (also noted as grade five).

Percentage of Slip in Spondylolisthesis

Because of limitations in Meyerding's grading, some prefer to grade spondylolisthesis by the percentage of slippage. The same quadrants used for Meyerding's system can be used, but a percentage assigned. This allows more accurate differentiation of the amount of slip because a 10% or a 24% slip would both be considered Meyerding Grade One, a 26% or a 49% slip considered Grade Two, etc.

Static Intervertebral Malposition

The Houston Conference in 1972 reached a consensus regarding the radiographic evidence of intervertebral subluxations following the inclusion of chiropractic care in Medicare coverage, which mandated that subluxations be demonstrated radiographically.[37] Although these classifications have never been universally accepted in chiropractic or by Medicare, they have some utility. There has never been peer reviewed published documentation that these malpositions are related to back pain or other disorders, nor that they can be corrected by chiropractic adjustment, but anecdotal evidence of their significance abounds. The following are those most demonstrable from routine radiography:

- Flexion Misalignment: On the lateral view, lines from the end plates diverge posteriorly, the spinous processes and facet joints diverge.
- Extension Misalignment: On the lateral view, lines from the end plates converge posteriorly, the facets imbricate and the spinous processes converge.
- Lateral Flexion Misalignment: On the AP (or PA) view, lines from the end plates converge on one side and diverge on the opposite.

- Rotational Misalignment: On the AP (or PA) view, the pedicles are asymmetrical, the pedicle on the anterior side being more lateral, the one on the posterior side being more central. The spinous process is deviated to the side of anteriority.

- Anterolisthesis (Spondylolisthesis): On the lateral view, there is anterior displacement of a vertebral body on the one below.

- Retrolisthesis: On the lateral view, there is posterior displacement of a vertebral body on the one below. In the lumbar spine this usually is due to considerable extension of the vertebral motion unit.

- Lateral Listhesis:On the AP (or PA) view, there is lateral displacement (overhang) of the vertebral body upon the one below. This accompanies marked vertebral rotation of the upper segment.

Cobb's Measurement of Scoliosis

On the AP (or PA) view, measure the angle formed by intersection of perpendiculars erected to lines across the superior end plate of the most superior vertebra in the scoliosis and the inferior end plate of the most inferior segment in the curvature.[38] It is important that the end vertebrae be noted so that for future comparison the same segments are chosen. This is the preferred method for scoliosis measurement when the end plates are easily visible (Fig. 3–4).

Risser-Ferguson Measurement of Scoliosis

On the AP (or PA) view, measure the angle formed by intersection of lines drawn from the centers of the superior and inferior end vertebrae to the center of the vertebra at the apex.[39] The end vertebrae must be noted for reference in future evaluations. This measurement gives values below those reached by the Cobb method, but is used when end plates are not easily seen to allow lines to be drawn across them.

Eisenstein's Method for Sagittal Spinal Canal Measurement

Except at L5, a reasonably close approximation of the sagittal diameter of the spinal canal can be made by measuring the distance from a line drawn connecting the superior and inferior tips of the articular processes of the same segment (representing the posterior of the spinal canal) and the midpoint of the posterior of the vertebral body.[40] At L5 the measurement is made from the spinolaminar junction to the posterior of the vertebral body. When this measurement is less than 14 mm, it suggests stenosis. Accurate determination of stenosis, however, requires axial imaging, either CT or MRI.

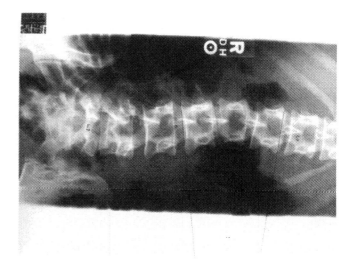

Fig. 3–4 Cobb's Measurements of Scoliosis. The lines needed to measure the Cobb angle of a scoliosis are demonstrated on this AP view of an anomalous spine (seven vertebrae with lumbar characteristics and congenital/developmental lateral wedging of L2). The end vertebrae should always be indicated when reporting a Cobb angle. The angle is measured by the intersection of lines drawn from the upper end plate of the selected superior vertebra and inferior end plate of the selected lower vertebra. The vertebrae selected should be those which will produce the largest angle. *Comment:* This film records a Cobb angle of 19° (L2–4). Also note that there is lateral flexion and rotational subluxation at L5/6 and L6/7.

Interpedicular Distance

On the AP or PA view, the coronal dimension of the spinal canal can be determined by measuring the distance between the innermost aspects of the pedicles. This measurement varies according to the patient's age among other significant factors.[41] In adults, Rowe[29] cites the average/minimum dimensions for this measurement to be 23/19 mm at T12, 25/21 mm at L1, 26/21 mm at L2 and L3, 27/21 mm at L4, and 30/23 mm at L5. Decrease of these measurements suggests possible stenosis, but it is best if this is considered in combination with a sagittal canal measurement. Significant increase in the coronal canal measurement may indicate a space occupying lesion in the canal (Exhibit 3–1).

Spinal Canal/Vertebral Body Ratio

The higher the ratio the smaller the spinal canal, possibly indicating spinal canal stenosis. This method has not been shown to be reliable.[40]

Intercrestal Line

A transverse line is drawn from the top of one ilium to the other. This is used to note the relationship of L4 and L5 to the

Exhibit 3–1 Spinal Canal/Vertebral Body Ratio

This ratio is derived by the formula $\dfrac{A \times B}{C \times D}$ *where:*

A = interpedicular dimension
B = sagittal canal dimension
C = transverse body dimension (width of the body from the AP view)
D = sagittal body dimension (AP dimension of the body at midpoint from the lateral view).

Normal ranges for this ratio are:

	minimum	maximum
L3:	1:3.0	1:6.0
L4:	1:3.0	1:6.0
L5:	1:3.2	1:6.5

top of the pelvis. Rowe[29] notes that the criteria for probable development of L4/5 degeneration are:

1. A high intercrestal line passing through the upper half of L4
2. Long L5 transverse processes
3. Rudimentary rib
4. Transitional vertebra

His criteria for probable L5/S1 degeneration are:

1. An intercrestal line passing through L5
2. Short L5 transverse processes
3. No rudimentary rib
4. No transitional vertebra

ANOMALIES AND NORMAL VARIANTS

The lumbosacral region is a frequent site of anomalies and variants from normal anatomy. Most of these do not significantly affect biomechanics of the low back, but some do have biomechanical significance. This is especially true where anatomical variations cause alterations of movement patterns producing asymmetrical stresses or transferring mobility to joints other than the usual locations. In such instances people with those anomalies may be predilected toward premature degeneration.[42,43] To chiropractic physicians, spinal anomalies and variants have particular significance in that they may confuse palpatory discrimination if their presence is not known. And, with asymmetrical anomalies or alterations of segmentation, associated altered movement patterns may necessitate a different approach to spinal adjusting than is routinely applied.

The scope of this chapter is not such that an encyclopedic review of lumbosacral variants is feasible, so only the most common, or those that may be diagnostically confusing, or those with potential biomechanical/clinical significance will be covered.

Block Vertebrae

Nonsegmentation of lumbar vertebrae is not uncommon. The lack of segmentation may be at the vertebral bodies, facet joints, posterior arch structures, or all of these. Asymmetry of block vertebrae is not unusual. The nonsegmentation may be complete on one side and incomplete on the other. Regardless, the segments in a block vertebra cannot move on one another, necessitating transfer of the motion that would ordinarily take place at that vertebral motion unit to those above or below or both. Such alteration of motion patterns frequently causes asymmetrical or unusual stresses to articulations above or below the anomaly or both, which often results in premature degeneration.[33] Chiropractors adjusting a spine in which there are block vertebrae must change their usual approach to accommodate for the differences in mobility resulting from the nonsegmentation (Fig. 3–5).

Butterfly Vertebrae

These most commonly occur in the thoracic region, but occasionally will be found in the lumbar spine. A butterfly vertebra results from nonunion or incomplete development of the primordia for the vertebral body resulting in two half vertebral bodies with a cleft or partial cleft at the center.[44,45] The appearance resembles the wings of a butterfly. Although the appearance is striking, when this is an isolated anomaly, the significance of a butterfly vertebra is negligible. With spinal dysraphism there may be multiple butterfly vertebrae, the

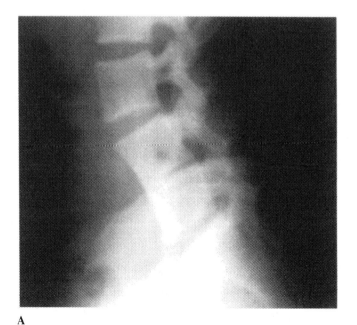

A

Fig. 3–5 Block Vertebrae. (**A**) This block vertebra representing L4–5 has anterior nonsegmentation, constricting the anterior of the vertebral bodies producing a relatively typical "wasp-waist" appearance.

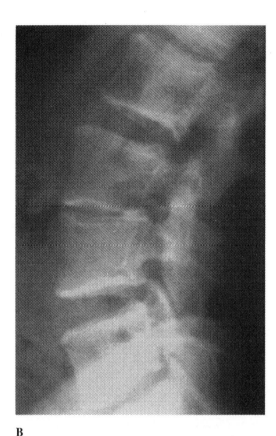

B

Fig. 3–5 (B) Block vertebra, posterior non-segmentation. This unusual block vertebra has posterior nonsegmentation. *Comment:* The lack of separation of the apophyseal joint structures has also resulted in a hypoplastic disk.

dysraphic problem being of great clinical significance[46] (Fig. 3–6).

Hemivertebrae

Absence or nondevelopment of part of a vertebral body, usually one side, but rarely the anterior or even more rarely the posterior portion of the body, results in a significant anomaly that causes a structural spinal curvature.[44,45,47] Lateral hemivertebrae cause structural scolioses. Occasionally a shift in segmentation will result in lateral hemivertebrae on opposite sides of the spine at different levels that can offset the asymmetry so that the resulting scoliosis is minimal. Posterior hemivertebrae cause a localized kyphos and can be mistaken for pathological vertebral collapse. The extremely rare ventral hemivertebra causes less spinal deformity than other forms of hemivertebrae,[46] and is very easily misdiagnosed as pathology. Hemivertebrae are known to coexist with block vertebrae and are also found in those with diastematomyelia, meningocele, and spondylothoracic dysplasia.[45] Dorsal hemivertebrae are found in achondroplasia and other severe forms of dwarfism[48] (Figs. 3–7 and 3–8).

Transitional Vertebrae

Vertebrae at the transition from one spinal region to another may take on characteristics of the adjacent region. Thoracolumbar and lumbosacral transitional segments are relatively common anomalies.[33,44–46] There may be increase or decrease in the number of vertebrae with usual lumbar characteristics when a transitional segment is present at either end of the lumbar spine.

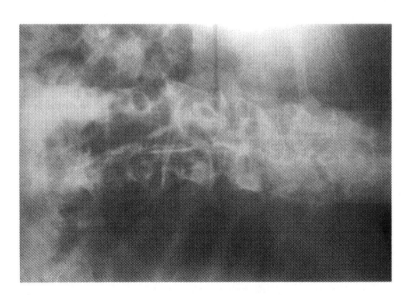

Fig. 3–6 Butterfly vertebrae. T12 is a butterfly vertebra and corresponding anomalies at T11 and L1 are present. L3 is a partial butterfly, the central cleft which produces the butterfly appearance is incomplete. Note also that there are only four lumbar vertebrae.

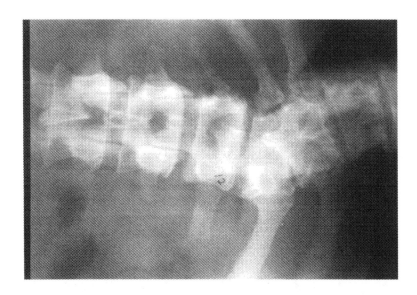

Fig. 3–7 Lateral hemivertebra. A lateral hemivertebra is present at T11 which is unusual in that it has ribs present bilaterally. Note the asymmetry of the T12 ribs. *Comment:* The T11 hemivertebra and congenitally wedged vertebrae at other levels produce a structural scoliosis.

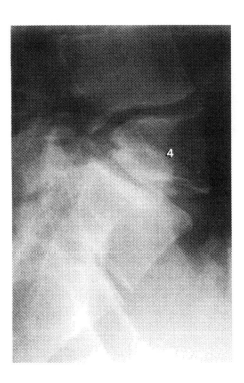

Fig. 3–8 Ventral hemivertebra. L5 is a transitional segment with a developmentally narrow disk at L5/S1. L4 is a ventral hemivertebra, the posterior arch structures not having developed. *Source:* Reprinted with permission from T.R. Yochum, *Essentials of Skeletal Radiology,* © 1987, Williams & Wilkins.

At the thoracolumbar junction, L1 may have small rib processes, unilaterally or bilaterally, rather than typical lumbar transverse processes, and contrariwise T12 may have lumbar type transverse processes rather than small ribs. Transitional segments at the T–L junction are biomechanically and clinically insignificant.

Lumbosacral transitional vertebrae are common and may be either symmetrical or asymmetrical. When L5 assumes some sacral characteristics (sacralization), the effective lumbosacral junction is shifted cephalically and the "sling" mechanism at the lumbosacral junction that is afforded by the ilio-lumbar ligaments allowing a "universal joint" mechanism at the junction is not present. When S1 takes on lumbar characteristics, often called lumbarization, it also alters biomechanics at the lumbosacral junction. (See "Intercrestal Line" in the spinography section of this chapter.) Asymmetrical transitional segments have greater potential for altering biomechanics than do symmetrical ones.[33,49] It is quite common for degenerative changes to be found in those with transitional lumbosacral segments (especially those that are asymmetrical) where accessory articulations are present between the spatulated transverse processes of the most caudal lumbar vertebra and the subjacent sacral ala[33,43,49] (Fig. 3–9).

Agenesis or Hypogenesis of a Pedicle

The absence of a pedicle is a potentially significant finding. Pedicular agenesis or hypogenesis must be differentiated from pathological destruction of the pedicle. Pedicular destruction

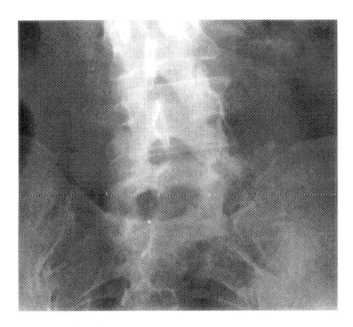

Fig. 3–9 Asymmetrical transitional lumbosacral vertebrae. The large spatulated left transverse process forms an accessory articulation with the subjacent sacral ala. *Comment:* Currently, the author and others consider it to be more reasonable when encountering such transitional vertebrae to simply designate the anomaly as a transitional segment and note its main functional characteristics, rather than to try to determine whether it is a sacralized lumbar segment or a lumbarized sacral vertebra.

---

is not infrequent in carcinoma metastatic to bone and has grave significance, whereas congenital pedicular absence is usually of little clinical significance.[33,50] When a pedicle fails to develop or is rudimentary, there is usually hypertrophy of its contralateral counterpart that is frequently sclerotic due to increased biomechanical stress placed upon it. The congenital absence of a pedicle is also manifest by a large intervertebral foramen[33,50] (Fig. 3–10).

Facet Tropism

Many years ago, Ferguson[27,28] postulated that the lumbar facets should be sagittally faced except at L5/S1 where they should be coronal. Although this may be the ideal, it is rarely realized. Asymmetry of facet facings, which has been called tropism, is very common, and in fact truly sagittal or coronal facet facings are extremely uncommon because the facet joints are not planar but are curvilinear. The clinical significance of tropism is uncertain and remains controversial.[50]

Facet-Lamina Joints

Occasionally large inferior articular processes form accessory joints with the subjacent lamina.[51] Such anomalies limit

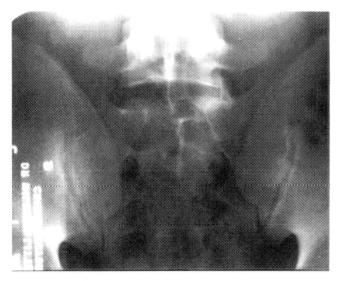

A

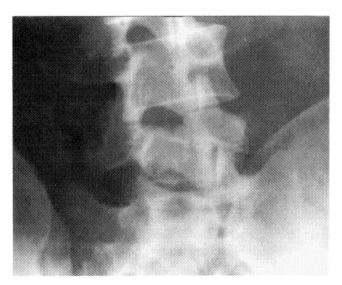

B

Fig. 3–10 Agenesis of a pedicle. **(A)** AP view. **(B)** Oblique view. The right L5 pedicle and inferior articular process are agenetic. Note the hyperplasia of the contralateral structures. Courtesy of Dr. William E. Litterer, Elizabeth, New Jersey.

---

extension of the vertebral motion unit and may interfere with other intervertebral motions. Facet-lamina joints frequently show degenerative changes, sclerosis and irregularity of the articulating margins, and when such changes are present, there are usually associated symptoms (Fig. 3–11).

Intraarticular Ossicles

Failure of union of accessory ossification centers at the superior, or more commonly the inferior, aspects of inferior articular processes.[33] These have been called Oppenheimer os-

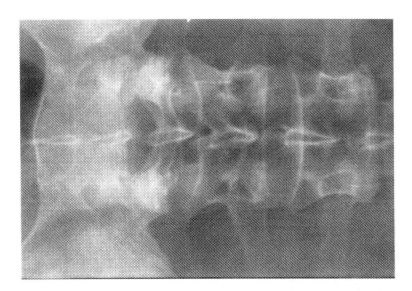

Fig. 3–11 Facet-lamina joint. A large facet-lamina joint is present at L4/5 on the right. Such anomalous joints often become degenerative, as is true with this one, and limit ability of the vertebral motion unit to extend and/or rotate. *Comment:* This film also demonstrates tropism at L3/4 and L4/5. The right L3 facet is coronally faced, the left sagittally faced. The opposite orientation is seen at L4/5.

sicles and can be mistaken for fractures of the articular processes, especially in the posttraumatic back. In the lumbar spine, they may be unilateral or bilateral (Fig. 3–12).

Spina Bifida Occulta and Vera

Occult spina bifida (SBO) is so common at S1 as to often be overlooked from radiographs. At other levels, spina bifida occulta is more notable, but regardless of location, it is nearly always clinically insignificant.[52,53] Absence of spinous pro-

cesses occasionally accompanies SBO at the thoracolumbar junction, and although not a clinically significant finding, to palpation the absence of one or more spinouses may be of concern until radiography identifies the abnormality. Spina bifida vera (SBV) is rarely found in the low back except in children with severe spinal dysraphism. Unlike SBO, which is a small defect in the posterior arch due to congenital lack of closure, SBV takes place when failure of closure of the posterior arch extends over more than one segment, essentially unroofing the spinal canal. To be labeled SBV, there must be protrusion of

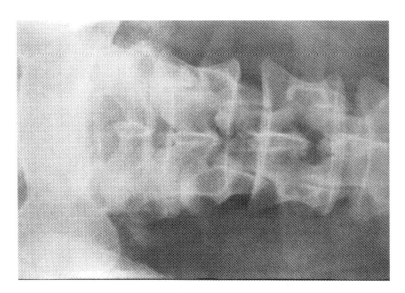

Fig. 3–12 Oppenheimer ossicle. An ununited accessory ossicle is present at the inferior of the right inferior articular process of L3. *Comment:* These ossicles are normal variants which may be mistaken for fractures.

the contents of the canal through the defect[50] (Fig. 3–13).

Knife-Clasp Deformity

This relatively common anomaly found at the lumbosacral junction has been so named for its resemblance to a folded jackknife.[28,51] An enlarged L5 spinous process is received into a multilevel SBO defect in the posterior arch of S1 and S2, occasionally even S3. The knife blade, the enlarged spinous process, is probably due to coalescence of the L5 spinous with the posterior tubercle(s) of the upper sacrum leaving a gap in the sacral posterior arch where the tubercles should have been. When a knife-clasp deformity is accompanied by pain on extension due to the protrusion of the "knife blade" into the sacral spinal canal, it is called a "knife-clasp syndrome"[50] (Fig. 3–14).

Bone Islands (Enostomas)

Bone islands are clinically insignificant collections of dense bone found within medullary (cancellous) bone and are asymptomatic. They may be small or large and can be found in any bone, but are frequent in the upper femurs, pelvic bones, and not uncommon in vertebrae.[54,55] Bone islands can be confused with osteoblastic lesions. Characteristically, bone islands are homogenous and have a serrated or "brush" border.[54,55] A few may increase in size, and those that do may be "hot" on bone scans, making differentiation from an osteoblastic lesion difficult[56,57] (Fig. 3–15).

FRACTURES AND DISLOCATIONS

Traumatically induced fractures or dislocations in the lumbar spine and pelvis are not commonly encountered in the acute stage in chiropractic practice because most will present to the emergency room or to orthopaedic surgeons. A few, however, particularly fractures of lumbar transverse processes that have not been previously diagnosed in a recently trauma-

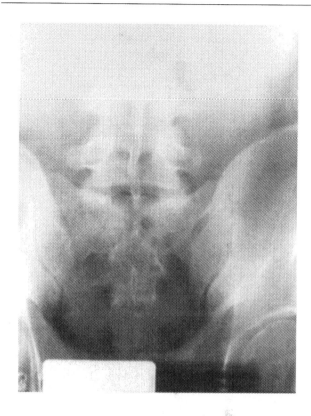

Fig. 3–14 Knife-clasp deformity. A classical knife-clasp deformity is present at the lumbosacral junction. The elongated L5 spinous process (actually that process fused with the tubercle of S1) extends caudally into the open posterior arch at S1 and S2.

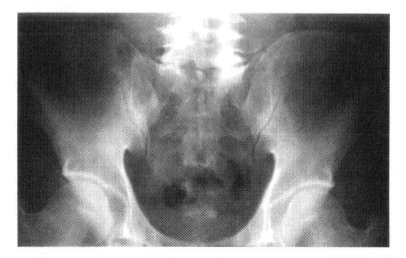

Fig. 3–13 Partially unossified posterior arch simulating occult spina bifida. Somewhat unusual appearances simulating occult spina bifidas are present at S1 and S2. The posterior tubercles are ossified, but there is radiolucency on both sides of those tubercles indicating that the posterior arches are cartilage which has not ossified.

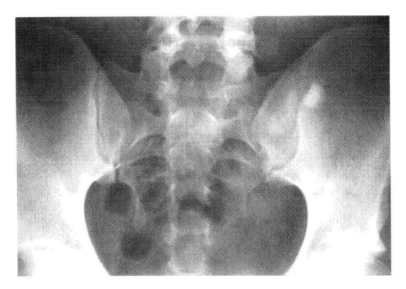

Fig. 3–15 Iliac bone island. A homogenous radiopacity in the ilium with a "brush border" represents a benign bone island. *Comment:* It should not be mistaken for an osteoblastic lesion.

tized patient may be encountered by chiropractic physicians.

Spinal and pelvic fractures, on the other hand, are something that every primary care physician needs to be alert to find in older patients, especially postmenopausal women, those who are immunocompromised, and those who are long-term users of catabolic steroids, such as those with disseminated joint disease, chronic respiratory disorders, etc.

This chapter will cover only those fractures and dislocations in the lumbosacral spine and pelvis that are most likely to be encountered in chiropractic practice. Pars interarticularis fractures and spondylolisthesis will be dealt with separately from other spinal fractures.

Fractures of Transverse Processes

Transverse process (TP) fractures are the second most common fractures in the lumbar spine, only compression fractures being more frequent. Due to overlying intestinal gas subsequent to trauma, TP fractures can be easily missed. The L2 and L3 TPs are the most frequently fractured, multiple fractures being common.[58,59] Fractures of the L5 TPs often accompany pelvic fractures or disruptions of the sacroiliac joint. When horizontal TP fractures are found, close inspection for a Chance fracture is important.[58] Hemorrhage accompanying TP fractures may obscure the psoas shadow. Renal or ureteral damage or both may also accompany these fractures. Examination of the urine for occult or manifest blood is mandatory in patients with TP fractures[58] (Fig. 3–16).

Chance (Lap Seat Belt) Fractures

In 1948, Dr. Chance documented a horizontal fracture completely through the vertebral body and neural arch, resulting in

splitting the vertebra horizontally.[60] Surprisingly, only about 15% of those who have suffered this type of fracture develop neurological deficit.[58] The most common site for this fracture is from L1–3. Because Chance fractures most frequently occur from automobile trauma in which the injured person was wearing a lap seat belt, there are usually bruises or abrasions or both on the upper abdomen in the area where the seatbelt was positioned[58] (Fig. 3–17).

Lumbar Fracture Dislocations

Most lumbar fracture dislocations are serious and accompanied by neurological abnormalities[58] that make them unlikely to be encountered in chiropractic practice except in a late stage situation. Fracture dislocation in the low back is usually in the thoracolumbar area following violent trauma. The only type of low back fracture dislocation likely to present to a chiropractor in an acute situation is a fracture of an articular process with associated facet dislocation, and even that is unlikely.

Compression Fractures

Compression fractures are not as common in the lumbar spine as in the thoracic spine, but do occur from flexion and axial compression forces.[59,61,62] They are more commonly found in the geriatric population, especially in those with osteoporosis, such as postmenopausal women, but with sufficient forces, can be found even in young active individuals. The most common sites for low back compression fractures are T12, L1, and L2.[58] Radiographic signs of compression fractures are: (1) anterior wedge deformity that may be subtle and may take several days following the traumatic incident to become apparent, (2) an anterior "step defect" where there is

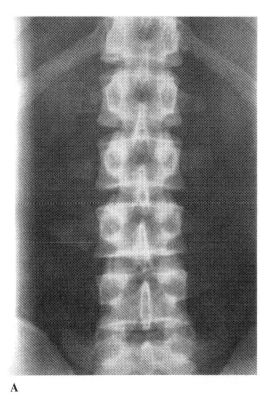
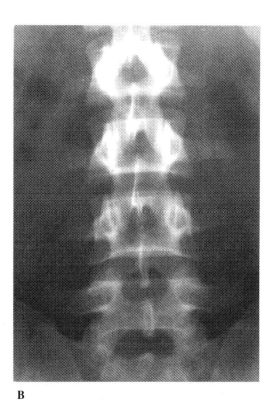

A   **B**

Fig. 3–16 Transverse process fractures. **(A)** There are displaced fractures of the L1, L2, and L3 transverse processes on the reading left. **(B)** A subtle fracture of the L3 transverse process on the reading right is shown to be a radiolucent line traversing the process from top to bottom. There is no displacement of the fracture. Courtesy of Dr. John A.M. Taylor, Gresham, Oregon.

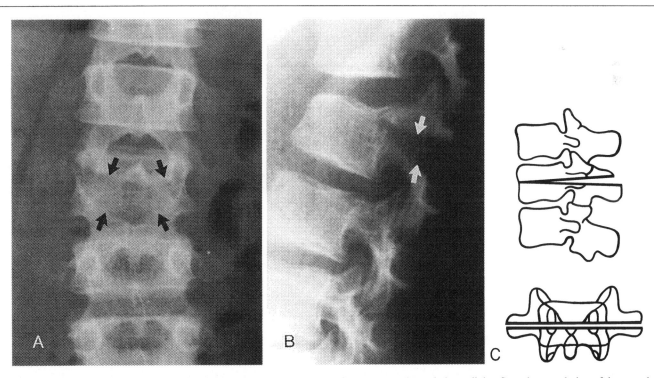

Fig. 3–17 Chance fracture. The AP and lateral radiographs show splitting of the vertebra through the pedicles. Superior angulation of the superior portion of the fractured vertebra is best seen by the separation of the upper and lower portions of the posterior arch structures on the lateral view. The schematic depicts a horizontal splitting fracture, a variant of a Chance fracture. *Comment:* These fractures result from a lap seat belt acting as a fulcrum where the force from a severe auto accident splits the vertebra immobilized by the seat belt. *Source:* Reprinted with permission from T.R. Yochum, *Essentials of Skeletal Radiology,* © 1987, Williams & Wilkins.

violation of the anterior cortical line of the vertebral body, usually associated with depression of the end plate, (3) a linear zone (white band) of condensation adjacent to the end plate, (4) invagination of the end plate, and (5) paraspinal edema.[58] It is far more common for the compression to affect the superior of the vertebral body/end plate, but there are rare occasions when the compression deformities are found at the anteroinferior aspect of the vertebra. Abdominal ileus is usually evident at and for some time following the trauma, associated with the pain.[58]

The radiographic manifestations of compression fractures are often very subtle early on, and may not be radiographically evident for a few days following the traumatic incident. In a spine that is severely osteoporotic or otherwise weakened by some pathological process, compression fractures may occur with minimal trauma or even with no apparent trauma.[58,59] It is sometimes difficult to determine whether compression deformity of a vertebra represents old or recent collapse. The linear radiopaque line under the damaged end plate is not a constant finding, but when present, identifies an area of impaction of the damaged trabeculae. This becomes more evident as callus formation occurs, and disappears with healing. The "step defect" is also an early finding that is no longer evident after healing takes place. Both these signs are evidence of a fracture that is less than two months old.[58,63] When there is a question as to the age of a compression deformity, a radionuclide bone scan may be helpful. The uptake at the fracture site will be increased, the scan showing a "hot" focus, during active bony repair, but the scan may remain positive (hot or warm) for as long as 18 months to 2 years.[63] In a patient who has been previously injured, a bone scan may be confusing rather than helpful (Figs. 3–18 and 3–19).

Burst Fractures

Violent axial compression trauma may create a burst fracture. The vertebral body literally "explodes" with severe compression and often a vertical fracture line is seen on the coronal view.[64] Comminution of the vertebral body with marked invagination of superior and inferior end plates is best appreci-

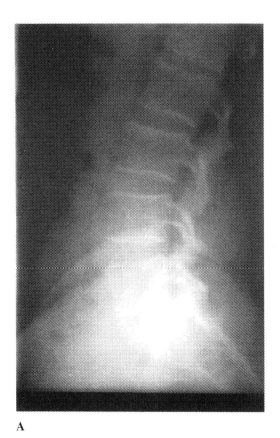

A

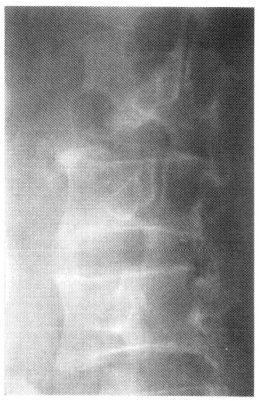

B

Fig. 3–18 Early L3 compression fracture. A slight anterior "beak," seen better on the oblique view than on the lateral, and associated sclerosis with slightly thickening of the superior end plate are evidence of a new compression fracture, subsequently proven when greater deformity was documented a month later. *Comment:* These films, of only fair quality, confirm the need for excellent radiographic quality. The finding was not detected from these films but when further films (not available to present) were done a month later the fracture was evident.

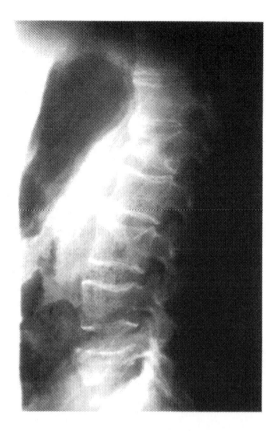

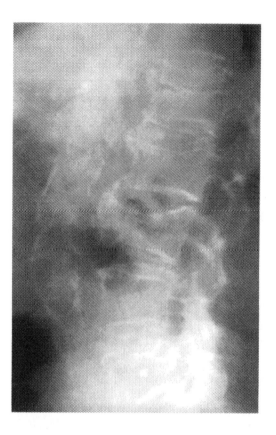

Fig. 3–19 There is compression deformity of the L1 vertebral body with decreased anterior but not posterior height. The superior end plate is mildly invaginated and there is "dome like" invagination of the inferior end plate. Although the anterior vertebral body margin is altered in contour, the bone is now normal in composition. This is an old healed compression fracture that is now stable. L3 also shows marked invagination of its superior end plate representing collapse of trabeculae in the spongiosa. *Comment:* The patient is a 61-year-old male, recovered alcoholic, and exhibits relatively advanced osteopenia. Extensive atherosclerotic aortic and common iliac calcification is obvious, demonstrating aortic tortuosity. Note the relationship of the aorta to the spine. Such advanced aortic changes are due to deposition of calcium in necrotic tissues of the vessel. While the appearance suggests vascular rigidity, in fact the vessel is "rotten" due to the necrosis and can be damaged by excessive force.

Fig. 3–20 Burst fracture, L3. This 79-year-old male fell onto his buttocks. In addition to compression, there has been fracture completely through the body from top to bottom displacing the anterior fragment. Note also that there are compression deformities of the vertebral bodies above, indicating partial collapse of these segments. *Comment:* The fracture at L3 probably represents re-fracture of a vertebra that had previously been fractured or had partially collapsed from osteoporosis.

ated on the lateral view. Posterior displacement of a fragment may damage the conus or cauda equina (Fig. 3–20).

Horizontal Sacral Fractures

Transverse fractures of the distal sacrum are fairly common following direct trauma to the sacrum. They are often very difficult to visualize on coronal views due to overlying gas and fecal material and the diagnosis is usually made from lateral views. A cleansing enema is usually necessary if the fracture is to be adequately appreciated from a coronal perspective. Upper sacral transverse fractures are less common and usually result from severe trauma[58] (Fig. 3–21).

Vertical Sacral Fractures

These are rarely isolated injuries, and trauma sufficient to cause them is usually indirect and so severe that the patient is not ambulatory. They are usually detected by noting disruption of the sacral struts, the transverse sacral foraminal lines. A coronal tilt view may demonstrate the fracture, but tomography or CT may be necessary.[58,65]

Coccygeal Fractures and Coccygeal Dislocation

Fractures of the coccyx, like those of the lower sacrum, are usually obliquely transverse. The lateral view makes the diagnosis. They are rarely appreciated from the coronal view. Coccygeal dislocation/subluxation is usually to the anterior, but posterior dislocation can occur. Variations in sacro-coccygeal morphology can be confusing and may result in misdiagnosis by an inexperienced observer.

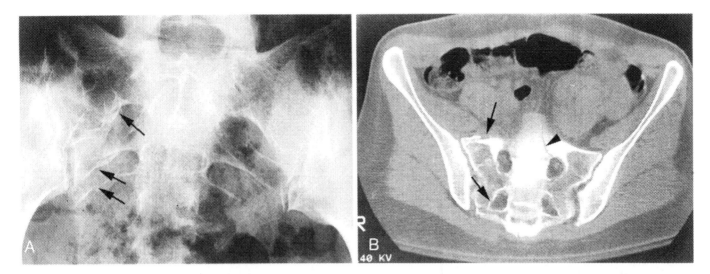

Fig. 3–21 Sacral fracture, disruption of foraminal lines. On the frontal view no definite fracture line is evident, but the foraminal (arcuate) lines are disrupted (arrows). The CT scan shows the fracture lines at the foramina and also demonstrates a contralateral vertical fracture line. *Comment:* Disruption of foraminal lines may be the only radiographic sign of sacral fracture. Courtesy of John C. Slizeski, Arvada, Colorado.

Iliac Wing Fractures

These result from direct trauma and are stable.[58] The fracture line is usually best appreciated from an oblique view and displacement is minimal due to the attachments of large muscles.

Avulsion Fracture of the Anterior Inferior Iliac Spine (AIIS), of the Anterior Superior Iliac Spine (ASIS), and of the Ischial Tuberosity

Avulsion of the origin of the rectus femoris causes a fracture at the AIIS, but avulsion of the sartorius origin fractures the ASIS. Hamstring avulsion causes fractures of the ischial tuberosity. These are injuries suffered through various strenuous athletic activities and their diagnoses are straightforward (Fig. 3–22).

Acetabular Fractures

Most acetabular fractures result from automobile accidents or pedestrian vs. auto trauma. The mechanism of injury is usually from indirect trauma, the femoral head jammed into the acetabulum, the position of the femur at the time of injury dictating the type of fracture.[66] Fractures of the posterior acetabular rim often accompany posterior hip dislocation. Anterior column fractures disrupt the ischiopubic line and medially displace Kohler's teardrop. Central fractures are the most common acetabular fractures and the most severe, the femoral head punching through the acetabulum, effectively splitting the innominate bone into upper and lower portions. Although on occasion a patient with an undiagnosed anterior or posterior column fracture may consult a chiropractor, the severity

of a central acetabular fracture makes it highly unlikely that a chiropractor will see one as the initial doctor.

SPONDYLOLYSIS AND SPONDYLOLISTHESIS

Spondylolysis and spondylolisthesis are such common entities that they are considered separately in this chapter.

There remain those who question whether some pars defects (spondylolyses) are congenital or whether all are, in fact, pars fractures.[67,68] Let the question be laid to rest because no instance of pars defects have been documented in the newborn. Wiltse,[69] who is recognized as the preeminent authority on spondylolisthesis has shown that the theory that the pars defect is due to nonunion of two separate ossification centers or due to a defect in cartilagenous development is fallacious because no evidence has been produced to verify those theories.

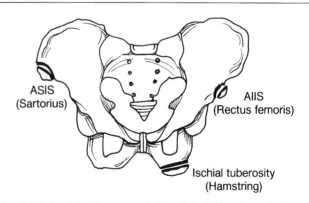

Fig. 3–22 Avulsion fractures of the pelvis. This schematic demonstrates the three most common sites of avulsion fractures of the pelvis. *Source:* Reprinted with permission from T.R. Yochum, *Essentials of Skeletal Radiology,* © 1987, Williams & Wilkins.

The most common proposed etiology regarding pars defects is that they are due to stress fractures. Wiltse[69] has postulated that these occur as a result of recurrent mechanical stress and this is supported by an in vitro study done in 1978 by Cyron and Hutton.[70] On rare occasions an acute pars fracture may occur from trauma. This is more likely if the bone is brittle from a dysplasia, such as osteopetrosis, or in advanced osteoporosis.

Spondylolisthesis is uncommon in the case of unilateral spondylolysis, and there are occasions when there may be bilateral pars defects with no anterolisthesis.

Oblique views are frequently needed to adequately visualize pars defects, but it is not uncommon that the defects can be seen without the additional exposure from obliques. The determination as to whether obliques should be done when there is an obvious anterolisthesis and the lateral or the coronal views or both show evidence that pars defects are present, or probable, should (as should be true in any decision regarding whether radiographs should be done) be based on whether or not the additional views will influence treatment (Figs. 3–23, 3–24, and 3–25).

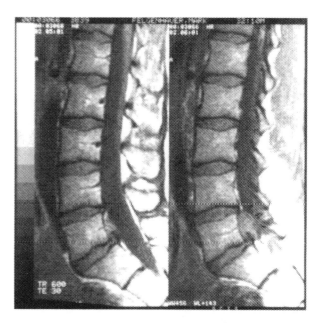

Fig. 3–24 Spondylolisthesis, MRI scan, disk extrusion. T1 weighted Mid- and parasagittal images of different patients with an L5 spondylolisthesis demonstrate associated disk extrusion. The mid-sagittal image shows disc material extending above the inferior L5 end plate, but the parasagittal image shows huge extruding disk material extending cephically to the upper L5 end plate. The interrupted posterior common ligament is seen as a linear dark structure extending upward from the posterior of the S1 body. *Comment:* Posterior disk protrusion is a frequent finding with symptomatic spondylolisthesis. This case is an extreme example, but MRI should be considered when radicular symptoms accompany spondylolisthesis. Courtesy of Dr. Stephen L.G. Rothman, Torrance, California.

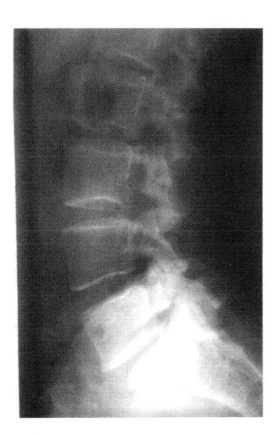

Fig. 3–23 Pars defects, multiple levels. In this lateral view, pars defects are present at L2, L3, and L5. There is a slight spondylolisthesis of L5 on S1.

The most commonly used classification of spondylolisthesis lists five types:[69]

1. Dysplastic: These are due to a congenital abnormality in the upper sacrum or the L5 neural arch that allows the displacem]ent to occur.
2. Isthmic: There are three subcategories under this classification:
   (a) Lytic—pars defects due to stress or fatigue fracture. This is the most common type of spondylolisthesis.
   (b) Elongation of intact partes interarticularis.
   (c) Displacement due to acute pars fractures.
3. Degenerative: These are found mainly in women in the sixth decade or later and are due to chronic disk and facet degeneration. The pars are intact. The majority of degenerative spondylolistheses are found at L4. Many of these are not particularly symptomatic, but displacement beyond the usual (10% to 15%) can result in spinal canal stenosis with the attendant symptoms.
4. Traumatic: This classification is reserved for those anterolistheses where a neural arch fracture other than

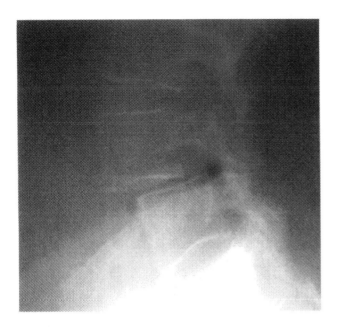

Fig. 3–25 Degenerative spondylolisthesis. A 25% degenerative spondylolisthesis of L4 on L5 is shown. There appears to be slight elongation of the isthmus on this radiograph, but oblique films did not demonstrate pars defects. *Comment:* The symptoms of degenerative spondylolisthesis may be negligible as in this patient, but entrapment of nerves may lead to radicular or cauda equina symptoms.

at the pars interarticularis allows the displacement. These are very rare in the low back.

5. Pathological: These occur with bone disease, either localized or generalized, which allows the displacement to occur. The most common pathologies to result in such subluxations are metastatic carcinoma, Paget's disease, and osteopetrosis. Yochum notes that a sixth type called postsurgical or iatrogenic spondylolisthesis is also feasible.[71] This could result from either a stress fracture of the pars above or below an area of spinal fusion, or from surgery where too much bone is removed during laminectomy or facetectomy causing instability.

DEGENERATIVE SPINAL DISEASE

Spinal degeneration is an inevitable consequence of aging, but it is accelerated by trauma, repetitive stress, systemic disease, inactivity with resultant wasting of supportive tissues and bone, and probably other factors. It is so frequently seen in nonsymptomatic individuals that there is question in the literature as to its relationship to those who do have back symptoms.[72–76] The debate as to whether degenerative spinal changes have relevance to back pain exhibits lack of understanding of several important aspects related to the genesis of the several types of spinal degeneration and the cause/effect

role that degenerative changes play in spinal biomechanics. From the viewpoint of the chiropractor, the altered spinal function that attends spinal degeneration transcends the simplistic question of the relationship of back pain to spinal degeneration. The concept that dysfunction in any portion of the musculoskeletal system has effects on all other body systems through alteration of neural integration is basic to chiropractic thinking and to that of others who espouse a wholistic approach to many aspects of health and disease.

It is not within the scope of this chapter to go into great detail regarding the pathogenesis of spinal degenerative changes, but some consideration of that subject cannot be avoided if one attempts to relate imaging findings to clinical circumstances. In this discussion of spinal degeneration, a functional approach to the consequences thereof will be taken because this explains, or at least postulates, the relevance of many things we can see through imaging. This is also in keeping with the concepts and teachings of Roy Logan that this book attempts to portray.

Although all spinal degenerative changes are integrated with one another, there are differences in origin and mechanical consequences of those changes that make discussion of different degenerative aspects of the degenerative process worthwhile.

Degenerative Disk Disease

As the disk loses water, fissuring of internal annuli occurs with protrusion of nuclear material into those fissures.[33,43–45] MRI has enabled noninvasive in vivo demonstration of disk degeneration, the decreased hydration within the disk being shown as decreased signal intensity of T2 weighted images[23,77] (Figure 3–26). As the hydrostatic function of the disk is altered, subtle alterations of intervertebral movements occur. These changes in biomechanics result from degeneration, but also cause further degeneration to occur at the primary site and also at those other articulations that are affected by the altered mobility. Unfortunately, although degenerative changes can be demonstrated by imaging, the sometimes subtle biomechanical alterations that attend such changes are usually not well understood from the images. In 1972, after chiropractic had been included in Medicare with the unfortunate mandate that for reimbursement of chiropractic services spinal subluxations had to be demonstrated by radiography, I testified to HCFA that only about 10% to 15% of subluxations that could be found clinically could be shown radiographically. My opinion in that regard has not changed.

Resnick[78] has called degeneration beginning in the nucleus (intervertebral chondrosis), which causes loss of resiliency in the nuclear material resulting in changes in the adjacent bone, intervertebral osteochondrosis, and he calls degeneration of the outer annulus, which is manifested by marginal osteophytic changes, spondylosis deformans (more commonly simply called spondylosis).

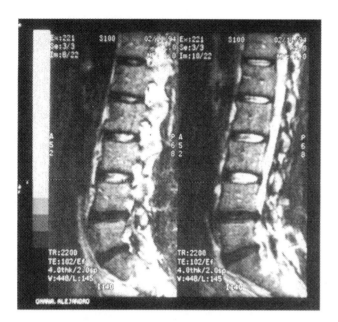

Fig. 3–26 Disk degeneration, MRI scan. T2 weighted images through levels of the neural foramina and parasagittal regions show severely decreased disk signal intensity at L4/5 and L5/S1, whereas the other visualized disk interspaces show bright signal intensity. *Comment:* The decreased signal intensity is evidence of decreased water content within the disk associated with proteoglycan degeneration. These images show the protruding disk material occluding the inferior portion of the L4/5 neural foramen and extending into the lateral recess.

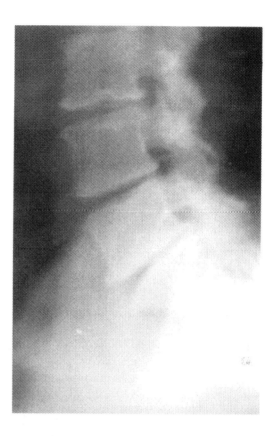

Fig. 3–27 Intervertebral osteochondrosis, L4/5 and L5/S1. The narrow disk interspaces, the intradiscal gas (vacuum phenomenon) at L5/S1, and the sub-chondral sclerosis abutting the end plates are the stigmata of this type of disk degeneration. *Comment:* A Schmorl's node is seen in the inferior L3 end plate with a very shallow Schmorl's node opposite it indenting the superior L4 end plate.

Intervertebral Osteochondrosis (IVOC)

As nuclear degeneration progresses, fissuring of the inner annulus and migration of nuclear material into the fissures, as well as its conversion to less elastic tissue, results in progressive narrowing of the interspace. Gas frequently accumulates within the fissures and is demonstrated radiographically as radiolucency within the interspace.[78–80] The gas collections are known as vacuum phenomena. These are usually central within the disk, but may extend to the outer annulus. Concomitantly with loss of disk height, the annulus bulges and traction on the attachment of the annulus to the vertebral margin causes small osteophytic lipping (Fig. 3–27).

Spondylosis Deformans

Anterior and anterolateral osteophytes (spondylophytes) at vertebral body margins are the most common radiographic manifestation of disk degeneration.[78–80] These occur from disruption of the attachments of the outer annulus to the vertebral margins decreasing anchorage of the disk to the vertebral body, allowing displacement of the disk which excites bone formation at the discovertebral margins. Spondylotic hypertrophy is mainly seen where the anterior longitudinal ligament attaches to the discovertebral junction, thus the anterolateral location. Spondylophytes are oriented roughly parallel to the vertebral end plate at their origins, but as they enlarge may curve upward from the more inferior vertebral body margin or downward from the margin of the more superior vertebra. Their horizontal origin differentiates spondylophytes from the syndesmophytes and parasyndesmophytes of inflammatory spinal diseases (to be discussed later), which are more vertically oriented, paralleling the outer aspect of the disk annulus[80–81] (Figs. 3–28 and 3–29).

The marginal osteophytes of spondylosis deformans are greater in size than the small osteophytes that accompany the later stages of IVOC. However, the degenerative process is a continuum, and these processes are not entirely separate.[78,80]

Intervertebral Disk Displacement

Displacement of disk material has been called herniation, but that term is so nebulous as to be confusing rather than helpful. For purposes of this discussion, herniation will be

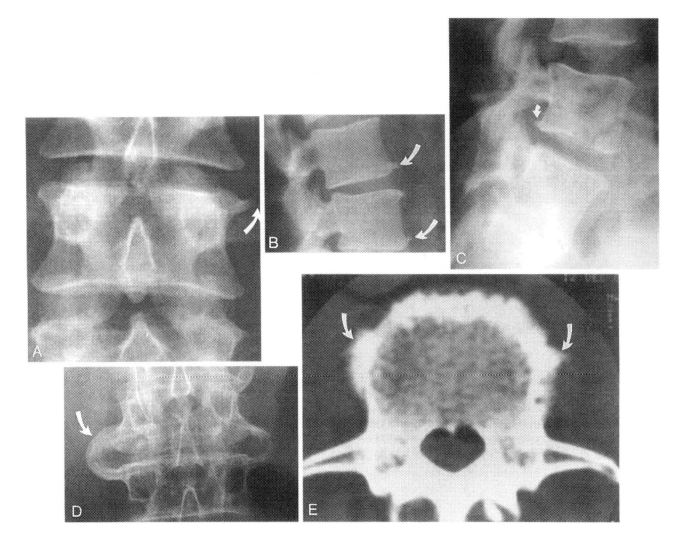

Fig. 3–28 Spondylophytes. (**A**), (**B**), and (**C**) These are non-marginal spondylophytes that are essentially horizontal in orientation called traction osteophytes. (**D**) These "claw" osteophytes, which nearly bridge the disk interspace, are also usually non-marginal, but are large, curve vertically, and, as in this case, may approximate one another and even fuse to immobilize the vertebral motion unit. This is an axial CT image of claw osteophytosis. *Comment:* Spondylotic changes, as this image demonstrates, are found in the area where the anterior longitudinal ligament attaches to the vertebral body. They are rarely found posterolaterally. *Source:* Reprinted with permission from T.R. Yochum, *Essentials of Skeletal Radiology*, © 1987, Williams & Wilkins.

used in a generic sense and more specific terminology will be used in alluding to the several types and sites of disk displacement.

With the exception of Schmorl's nodes in some instances, for displacement of disk material to occur some degenerative disease must be present. In light of the above discussions of IVOC and spondylosis, anterior and anterolateral disk protrusion from those disease processes will not be repeated. I will attempt, while being simplistic in describing the various other types of disk displacement, to use terminology that is widely accepted avoiding as much as possible the generic term herniation.

Schmorl's Nodes

Superior or inferior displacements of disk material or both that herniates through the cartilagenous vertebral end plate into the spongiosa of a vertebral body are designated as Schmorl's nodes.[44,80] Schmorl's nodes may be idiopathic, usually occurring in childhood; may accompany Scheuermann's disease, infection, metabolic or endocrine disease, neoplasm; or may result from trauma.[78,80] They are recognized as radiolucent lesions within the vertebral body, usually communicate with the disk interspace, and have sclerotic borders that may be thick or thin (Fig. 3–30).

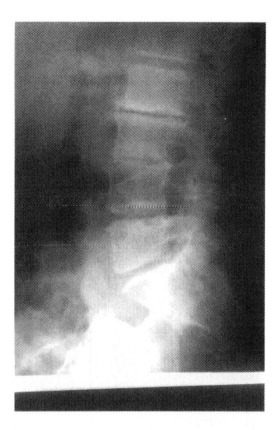

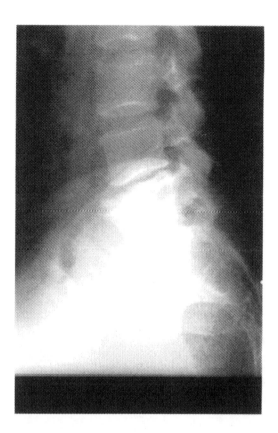

Fig. 3–29 Intervertebral osteochondrosis and spondylosis deformans. At L2/3 the narrow disk interspace, end plate sclerosis, and vacuum phenomena are indicative of IVOC, but at L2/3 and L4/5 the spondylophytes are more typical of spondylosis deformans. At L3/4 the indistinctness and irregularity of end plates is suspicious of infectious discitis, but more probably is simply advanced degeneration. *Comment:* This case is presented to make the point that spondylosis deformans and IVOC are frequently found together, and in fact are simply different manifestation of the process of disk degeneration.

Fig. 3– 30 Schmorl's node. A "giant" Schmorl's node is present at the anterosuperior corner of L5. *Comment:* Schmorl's nodes are infrequently found at the margins of vertebral end plates, but when they do occur in those location, as in this case, a portion of the end plate margin may be displaced. This occurs prior to skeletal maturity and the avulsed fragment of the limbic apophysis becomes a limbus bone (also known as limbus vertebra).

Limbus Bones

Protrusion of disk material in childhood, interrupting a portion of the limbic apophysis and displacing a fragment of bone from that apophysis, results in a characteristic appearance that has been called a limbus vertebra,[33,44] but more properly should be termed a limbus bone. This is most common at the anterior superior corner of a vertebra, but may occur anteroinferiorly and on a few instances posteriorly. Limbus bones are usually incidental findings in adults and, in adults, even posterior limbus bones usually have little clinical significance except in individuals with congenitally small spinal canals[78,82] (Fig. 3–31).

Posterior and Posterolateral Disk Displacement

That which is usually referred to as disk herniation is posterior or posterolateral displacement of disk material or both. Any and all of the following have been called disk herniation

in the literature.[15–17] More specific terminology is needed if the severity and significance of the displacement is to be understood. The following descriptive nomenclature is preferred by some,[15–17] although there is no present standard terminology.

- Annular Disk Bulge: Bulging of the annulus may be diffuse and circumferential, or localized. In a bulging disk, the annular fibers remain intact[15–17,43] although both nuclear and annular degeneration are probably necessary for bulging to occur. However, magnetic resonance images may show disk bulging with minimal decrease in disk signal intensity.[15–17,43] Annular bulges may protrude into the spinal canal, lateral recesses, and intervertebral nerve root canals (neural foramina) and efface and occasionally impinge upon neural structures.

- Disk Protrusion (Prolapse): When nuclear material extends through at least some of the annulus, but the outer annulus is not violated, it is best referred to as diskj protrusion.[15–17] Such protrusions may be central, and, de-

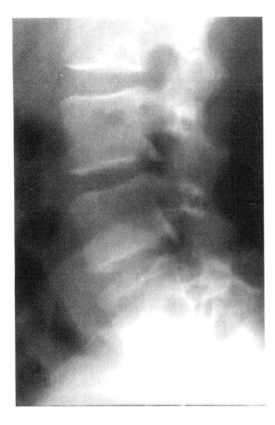

Fig. 3–31 Posterior limbus bones. Posterior limbus bones are demonstrated at the inferior end plates of L3 and L4. *Comment:* These are quite uncommon. Such findings have potential to cause neurological symptoms, but such symptoms occur in a surprisingly few instances.

pending on the size of the protrusion, may efface or compress the thecal sac. Paramedian protrusions may also displace the exiting nerve root. Posterolateral protrusions, again dependent on size, may fill the lateral recess and extend into the entrance of the nerve root canal. Far lateral protrusions into the nerve root canal that may compress the nerve root or ganglion or both have been demonstrated by CT and MRI and explain why prior to the time when axial imaging was available myelography would not show such abnormalities[15-17] (Fig. 3–32).

- Disk Extrusion: These are protrusions of nuclear material that have completely penetrated the annulus but are still contained by the posterior longitudinal ligament (PLL).[15-17] Because the PLL is a central structure, this classification refers only to central and paramedian protrusions. Extruded disks are usually of such size that the thecal sac is compressed and one or both exiting nerve roots may be displaced. The protruding material may extend above or below the vertebral end plates or both at the affected interspace.[15-17]

- Disk Sequestration (Free Fragment): When the protruding nuclear material detaches from the parent disk and either penetrates through the PLL into the epidural space or moves up or down for some distance under the PLL, it is termed a sequestered or free disk fragment.[15-17,43] Sequestered disk fragments, even though large at times, have been shown to regress or even disappear given time,[15,43,83] although some of the apparent regression may be due to resorption of hemorrhage.

Facet Joint Degeneration (Facet Arthrosis; DJD)

Facet joints are arthrodial (synovial) articulations and degenerative disease affecting them does not differ in its pathological progress from that of degenerative joint disease in peripheral joints. The hallmarks of sclerosis of articular surfaces, marginal osteophytes, and eventual bony hypertrophic changes that result from the breakdown of articular cartilage and its effects on the contiguous bone are demonstrable radiographically. In the lumbar spine, these are often better appreciated on oblique radiographs than on coronal and lateral views. Axial

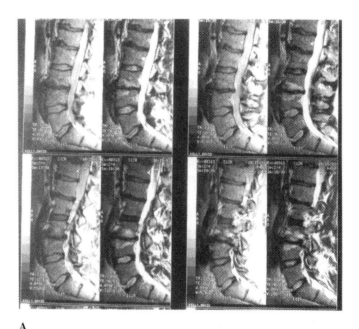

A

Fig. 3–32 Disk protrusion and reactive marrow degeneration, MR scans. (**A**) Side by side first and second echo (proton density and T2 weighted) mid-sagittal and just parasagittal images show severely decreased disk height and signal intensity at L3/4 with posterior protrusion and with reactive marrow changes on both sides of the interspace. Disc narrowing with Schmorls nodes and decreased signal intensity is also seen at L1/2 and L2/3. Remarkably normal disk heights and signal intensity at L4/5 and L5/S1 is most unusual with the extensive degeneration above. Courtesy of Dr. Stephen L.G. Rothman, Torrance, California.

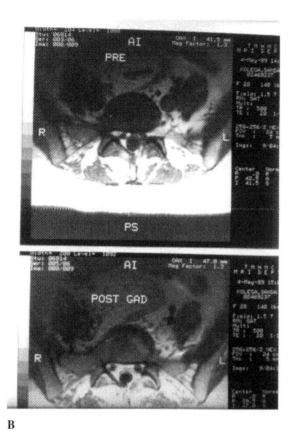

B

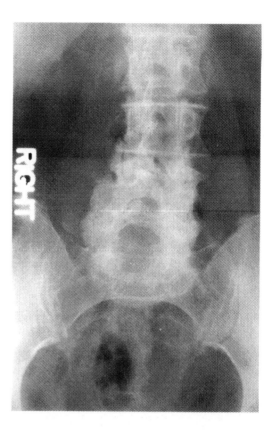

Fig. 3–32 (B) T1 weighted pre- and post-gadolinium axial images at the lumbosacral junction demonstrate the efficacy of obtaining paramagnetic contrast images in symptomatic post-surgical patients where there is question whether recurrent disk protrusion or post-surgical scar causes the pain. *Comment:* The pre-image shows a large mass of material encompassing the left nerve root. The post-gadolinium image shows enhancement of that area, indicating that the material is vascularized and therefore represents scar tissue rather than disk which would not enhance. Courtesy of Dr. Stephen L.G. Rothman, Torrance, California.

Fig. 3–33 Hypertrophic degenerative facet joint disease. There is severe hypertrophic degenerative facet joint disease at L3/4, L4/5 and L5/S, more severe on the right. Facet-lamina joints are evident at L3/4 and particularly at L4/5, on the right at both levels. *Comment:* The bony bridging at the lateral aspects of the T12/L1 disk interspace and on the right at L1/2 suggest ankylosis, which is confirmed on the lateral view.

imaging is superior to plain film radiography in demonstrating facet disease and additionally allows visualization of the ligamenta flava, which form part of the joint capsules, and when hypertrophic or buckled may protrude into the spinal canal or lateral recess sufficiently to produce stenosis. Synovial cysts accompanying facet degeneration may also protrude into the spinal canal or lateral recess causing stenosis.[10,17,18]

Degenerative facet disease is usually associated with disk degeneration, but is occasionally found without obvious accompanying disk disease. Isolated or unilateral facet disease bespeaks previous specific trauma.[15,33,44,80] More commonly, facet arthrosis results from prolonged stresses, such as those from chronic postural faults, scoliosis, or repetitive tasks that impact the low back (Fig. 3–33).

Diffuse Idiopathic Skeletal Hyperostosis (DISH; Forrestier's Disease)

DISH is a degenerative spinal disease, which in some aspects resembles inflammatory disease. Its cause is uncertain,[78,80,81] but it is a bone forming pathology, an enthesopathy, and is characterized by hyperostotic bony proliferation at tendinous or ligamentous attachments (entheses). In the low back, it is most commonly found in the upper lumbar region, but may affect the entire lumbar spine.[78,80,81] The bony proliferation may be quite large. Resnick's criteria for the diagnosis of DISH requires that four contiguous segments be involved.[78] However, for practical purposes, a smaller area of spinal involvement may still represent DISH. Frequently, ankylosis occurs at the superior portions of the sacroiliac joints,[78,80,81] as opposed to ankylosis of the lower or synovial portions, which is seen in inflammatory spinal disease (Fig. 3-34).

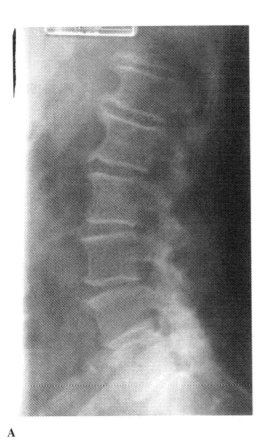

A

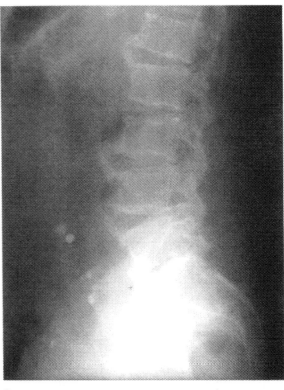

B

Fig. 3–34 Diffuse idiopathic skeletal hyperostosis (DISH). (**A**) Hyperostotic bony changes at the anterior of the T11/12, T12/L1, L1/2 and L3/4 with lesser similar changes at L2/3 are evidence of DISH. *Comment:* Resnick's criterion for DISH is involvement at 4 contiguous levels, but for practical purposes, the diagnosis is valid when fewer contiguous segments are found but the hyperostosis is relatively typical. (**B**) Extensive anterior hyperostosis at L1/2, L3/4, L4/5 and lesser changes at L5/S1 are compatible with DISH although the contiguous nature of the abnormal findings is interrupted. *Comment:* Scattered radiopacities in the soft tissues anterior to the spine are due to barium retained in colonic diverticulae, residual from a previous gastrointestinal study.

Neurotrophic Spondylopathy

Neurologic deficits that cause loss or impairment of pain sensation or proprioception or both may cause destructive arthropathy, which may affect the spine. The major diseases causing neurotrophic spinal arthropathy are tabes dorsalis and diabetes mellitus.[80,81,84] In the spine, the hypertrophic pattern of destruction is found, rather than the atrophic form, which may occur in peripheral joints.[80,81,84] The lumbar spine is the most common site for spinal neuroarthropathy, and the end-stage destruction may be spectacular with deformity, severe subluxations, dislocations, and even fractures occurring, marked sclerosis being a hallmark. The early signs are those of degeneration with disk narrowing, vacuum signs, sclerosis, and osteophytes that may become exuberant. This progresses rapidly to the severe destructive stage. In contrast to peripheral neuroarthropathy, spinal disease may be accompanied by significant pain[80,81,85] (Fig. 3–35).

INFLAMMATORY SPINAL DISEASE

Inflammatory diseases of the spine have very serious clinical implications. These diseases will be presented in the order of the severity of the problems they cause.

Infectious Spinal Disease

Spinal infection, other than iatrogenic, is not common. Infection other than that which results from direct inoculation (iatrogenic or otherwise) occurs from blood borne pathogens or by direct extension from adjacent septic tissues. The vascular route is more frequent.[84,86] The pathogens lodge in small vessels in vertebral bodies, usually close to vertebral end plates, or occasionally subjacent to the sacroiliac joint surfaces. Because the enzymes that occur with infection are more strongly chondrolytic than osteolytic, the disease moves rapidly to the disk or joint surface and results in erosions and ir-

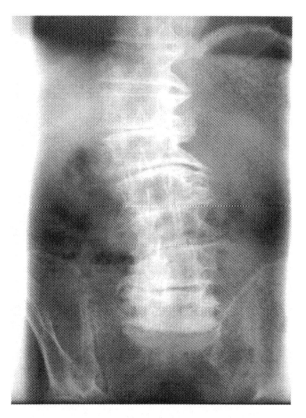

Fig. 3–35 Neurotrophic arthropathy (tabes dorsalis). Extensive hypertrophic spondylophytes, disk narrowing at many levels, multiple subluxations, and a short double scoliosis are present in this patient with tabes dorsalis. *Comment:* Neurotrophic arthropathy in the spine, as elsewhere, is characterized by extensive joint destruction and instability.

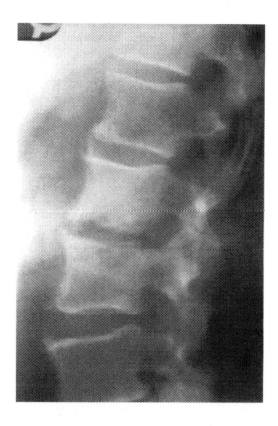

Fig. 3–36 Infectious discitis. This 62-year-old man had been diagnosed as having degenerative spinal disease. The erosion of the vertebral end plates at L2/3 was seen and a diagnosis of infectious discitis made.

regularities of end plate or articular margins that are ragged and often mildly sclerotic from the debris.[84,86] Spreading across the joint to involve the other joint surface/end plate and the adjacent bone is common but not invariable.[84,86] Soft tissue involvement frequently occurs, and may produce paraspinal abscesses that may spread the infection to adjacent tissues.[84,86] Prompt diagnosis so that treatment can begin early is extremely important because suppurative infections move rapidly with destruction proceeding over a few days to a few months,[84,86] depending on the virulence of the pathogen, the resistance of the patient, and the effectiveness of treatment. Staphylococcus aureus accounts for 90% of suppurative infections, but in immunocompromised individuals other, more exotic, bacteria may be found. More indolent infections, such as tuberculosis, although slower in their action may still cause radiographically visible changes within a few weeks.[84,86] Tuberculous spondylitis most commonly involves the lower thoracic or upper lumbar vertebrae or both and frequently causes a paraspinal abscess.[84,86] A psoas abscess may allow gravitation of caseous material caudally into the inguinal area or even into the upper leg (Figs. 3–36 and 3–37).

The end result of suppurative spondylitis is ankylosis.[84,86] Tuberculous spondylitis, however, most frequently causes vertebral body collapse that may result in gibbus formation.[84,86]

Rheumatoid Arthritis and Rheumatoid Variants Affecting the Spine

Rheumatoid arthritis (RA) involvement of the lumbar spine is almost unknown. Rheumatoid arthritis affects synovial joints, so that if it is found in the lumbar spine, the facet joints would be the site of involvement. Very rarely, RA may affect a sacroiliac joint, in which case the involvement is unilateral, whereas in other areas of the body RA is bilateral and usually symmetrical.[80,87]

Low back involvement with the rheumatoid variants: systemic lupus erythematosus (SLE), progressive systemic sclerosis (scleroderma), and dermatomyositis is so infrequent that they will not be discussed in this chapter.

The Sero-Negative Spondylopathies

The following inflammatory spinal diseases are characterized by a lack of the rheumatoid factor in the serum, but have

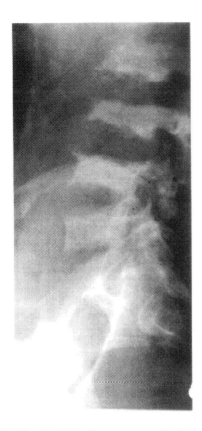

Fig. 3–37 Multilevel discitis. Extreme case of infectious discitis affecting all lumbar disks. *Comment:* The disk heights appear to be maintained due to the severe erosion of the affected vertebral bodies. (Courtesy: Dr. Stephen L.G. Rothman, Los Angeles). Courtesy of Dr. Stephen L.G. Rothman, Torrance, California.

increased probability of having a positive HLA-B-27 (90% in ankylosing spondylitis, 75% in psoriatic arthropathy and Reiter's syndrome).[80,88–92]

Ankylosing Spondylitis (AS)

Ankylosing spondylitis is not infrequently found in patients who seek chiropractic care. Its usual onset is in young adults, and it is predominantly a male disorder.[33,44,80,89,90] The usual stigmata are bilateral and relatively symmetrical sacroiliitis, squaring of vertebral bodies anteriorly, and syndesmophytes that are thin and usually symmetrical, involving both sides of the spine. The sacroiliac inflammation affects the synovial portions (lower two thirds) of the joints and may begin unilaterally or bilaterally, but not symmetrically. However, early on, the inflammation will become bilateral and symmetrical and at advanced stages may ankylose the fibrous portions of the joints as well as the synovial sections.[33,44,80,90] Pseudowidening of the joint spaces due to erosions of articular surfaces and obliteration of the "white line" that should be found on the iliac side of the joint are early signs. The progression through irregularity and sclerosis of joint margins to eventual ankylosis may take years. The earliest spinal involvement is usually

thoracolumbar or sometimes lumbosacral and the changes may progress caudally or cephically, or in both directions.[80,90] Erosions at the discovertebral junctions at the corners of the vertebral bodies, the Romanus lesion, cause the appearance of "squaring" of bodies.[80,88,90] As the erosions heal, sclerosis at vertebral body corners known as the "shiny corner sign" becomes evident.[46,80] Progression to ossification of the outer annulus causes bony bridging of the interspace, these shell-like ossifications being called syndesmophytes, contrasted to spondylophytes that are due to degenerative changes at end plate margins. Syndesmophytes are parallel to the disk borders, whereas spondylophytes are relatively parallel to the end plates. Eventually, the ligamentous structures at facet joints, termed the "trolley track sign,"[80] and even the inter- and supraspinous ligaments may ossify. This distinctive appearance has been called the "dagger sign."[80]

The disease may advance to involve much of the spinal column, but it may stop spontaneously at any point in time.[33,44,80,90] Ankylosis, of course, is accompanied by hypomobility, and osteoporosis from lack of movement is often prominent and may occur early. Biconcavity of vertebral bodies in ankylosed areas is not infrequent. Due to the fragility of ankylosed portions of the spine, fractures may occur that are characteristically transverse and have been called "carrot stick fractures."[80] These are less common in the low back than in the cervical or thoracic regions and in the lumbar spine may not be accompanied by severe symptoms.[80,90] Failure to reankylose after such fractures occurs and results in a pseudoarthrosis that may require surgical stabilization.[80,90]

Approximately 50% of AS patients will also develop arthritic changes in peripheral joints, most commonly in hips, shoulders, and the calcaneus.[80,88,90] These are erosive and enthesopathic lesions and may be quite destructive. (Figs. 3–38, 3–39, and 3–40).

Enteropathic Spondylopathy

When disease of the gastrointestinal tract is accompanied by spinal changes identical to those of AS, it is called enteropathic spondylopathy. The findings in the spine cannot be distinguished from those of AS.[80,93]

Psoriatic Arthropathy

Psoriatic arthritis resembles rheumatoid arthritis in some respects in the peripheral skeleton and has some resemblance to AS in the spinal column. Sacroiliitis, which is usually bilateral but asymmetrical, is found in 30% to 50% of people with psoriatic arthritis.[80,91] Occasionally, unilateral involvement is found. Spinal involvement is more common; up to 60% of those with skin lesions exhibit some spinal disease.[80,91] Asymmetrical nonmarginal syndesmophytic changes are the most common manifestation and occur most frequently in the upper lumbar and thoracolumbar region.[80,91] These parasyndesmophytes begin off from the vertebral end plate and initially appear as fluffy or thin curvilinear paravertebral calcifications

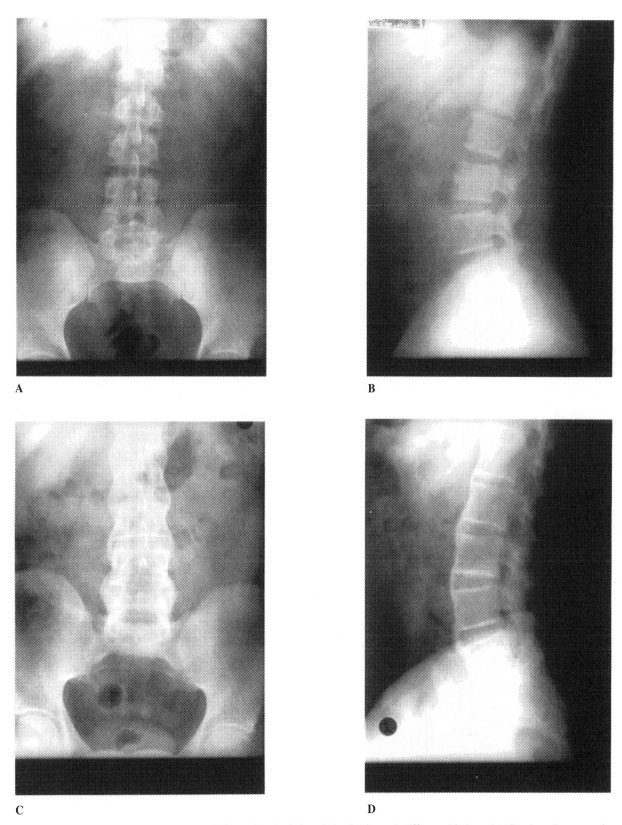

A

B

C

D

Fig. 3–38 Ankylosing spondylitis. **(A)** Although the patient had chronic backache and stiffness, this lateral (AP) view shows no signs of the disease except for early "squaring of vertebral bodies. **(B)** No sacroiliac disease or syndesmophytes are apparent at this time. **(C)** and **(D)** are the same patient ten years later. **(C)** In this lateral View, The typical stigmata of Ankylosing spondylitis are seen with syndesmophytic changes bridging the disk interspaces throughout the lumbar region. **(D)** The AP now is also typical of the disease, complete ankylosis of the sacroiliac joints having occurred and the typical "bamboo spine" appearance seen.

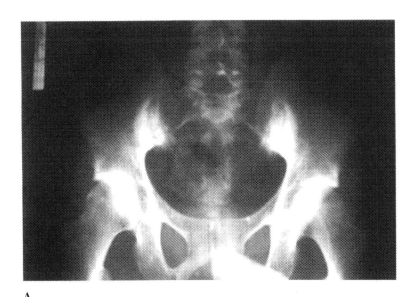

A

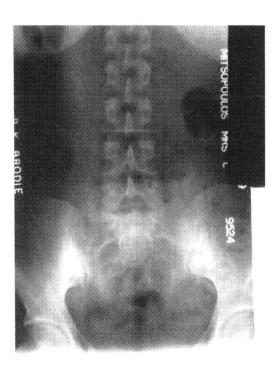

B

Fig. 3–39 Sacroilitis vs. osteitis condensans ilii. It is sometimes difficult to differentiate between bilateral symmetrical sacroilitis and osteitis condensans ilii. This depicts extensive bilateral symmetrical sacroilitis. Both sides of the joints are affected, the joint margins are irregular with erosions, and sclerosis affects the sacrum as well as the ilii. Osteitis condensans ilii may simulate sacroilitis, but only the iliac sides of the joints are affected. *Comment:* The sclerosis may be florid, or mild, but is confined to the ilii, is usually symmetrical and typically has a triangular configuration. The joint margins are not eroded. OCI is usually found in multiparous women and in most instances regresses after years, especially after menopause.

that eventually become relatively thick bony excresences arising from the vertebral body near the end plates. They may or may not bridge the disk interspace. A parasyndesmophyte that bridges the interspace but shows cleavage between itself and the vertebral bodies is called a "Bywater's–Dixon " or floating syndesmophyte.[80] Quite infrequently psoriatic syndesmophytes may simulate those of AS, but the corner changes that are found in AS are not seen with psoriatic spondylopathy (Fig. 3–41).

Reiter's Syndrome

A triad of conjunctivitis, urethritis, and polyarthritis is the criterion for Reiter's syndrome. The several entities that comprise the syndrome may not all be present simultaneously.[80,92] The skeletal manifestations of Reiter's are found in the thoracolumbar and lumbar spinal regions, in the sacroiliac joints, and in the lower extremities. Sacroiliac involvement may be present in as many as 50% of those with the disease.[80,92] Rowe and Yochum report that radioisotope studies have indicated

that up to 70% of those with the disease have sacroiliac involvement that may resolve without visible plain film findings.[80] Sacroiliac disease in Reiter's usually is predominantly iliac and is seen as erosions, variable sclerosis, and alteration of the joint space. Involvement may be unilateral or bilateral, with bilateral involvement tending to be asymmetrical. Ankylosis is not as frequent as with AS. Spinal changes tend to be parasyndesmophytic, indistinguishable from those seen in psoriatic spondylopathy. Spinal involvement is not as frequent as is sacroiliac disease[80,92] (Figs. 3–42 and 3–43).

DEPOSITION DISEASES INVOLVING THE SPINAL COLUMN

Gout

Gouty arthritis infrequently affects the spine or sacroiliac joints,[80,94] but when it does, the manifestations are similar to those it produces in other articulations. Joint spaces are usu-

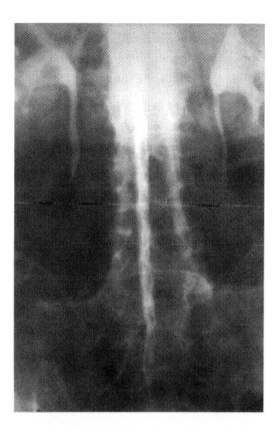

Fig. 3–40 Late ankylosing spondylitis. In late stage AS there may be ankylosis of facet joints and spinous processes as is shown in this film. *Comment:* The spinous ankylosis has been called the "dagger sign" and when it is accompanied by facet ankylosis, the term "trolley track sign" has been used.

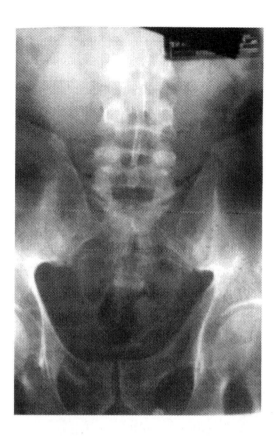

Fig. 3–41 Asymmetrical sacroilitis (psoriatic arthropathy). Ankylosing spondylitis is manifest by bilateral symmetrical sacroilitis, although in the early stage the finding may be asymmetrical. This radiograph of a person with psoriatic arthropathy illustrates moderately advanced asymmetrical sacroilitis. This radiograph of a person with psoriatic arthropathy illustrates moderately advanced asymmetrical sacroilitis.Asymmetrical sacroilitis beyond an early stage, however, should suggest one of the other seronegative spondyloarthropathies. Psoriatic arthritis and Reiters disease both frequently manifest with asymmetrical sacroiliac disease.

ally preserved. Erosions adjacent to joints that eventually may destroy the joint, soft tissue, or even interosseous tophi, chondrocalcinosis, and sclerosis associated with avascular necrosis, are radiographic signs accompanying the disease.

Hydroxyapatite Deposition Disease (HADD)

Hydroxyapatite deposition in degenerated or inflamed tissues or both is common in peripheral joints accompanying bursitis, tendinitis, and necrosis. In the spine, it may occur in the nucleus pulposus or annulus fibrosus.[80,95] It is also encountered in tendons and ligaments attaching to the pelvis and the femoral trochanters.

Deposition in the nucleus in children is usually accompanied by acute symptoms of fever, pain, and restricted motion. Increase in the disk space is usual and symptoms usually resolve in about two months.[80,95]

Nuclear calcification in adults is usually asymptomatic and mostly is secondary to degeneration, sequestered disk fragments, block vertebrae, or metabolic disease.[80,95]

Annular calcification is usually degenerative and is more common than is nuclear calcification.[80,95]

Calcium Pyrophosphate Dihydrate Deposition Disease (CPPD)

Spinal involvement with CPPD is infrequent. The most common findings are disk space narrowing, vacuum phenomena, marked vertebral body sclerosis, and osteophytes. Annular calcification may resemble syndesmophytes, being thin calcifications along the margins of the disk. Nuclear calcification is uncommon.[80,96] Calcification of the ligamenta flava occurs and may be visible radiographically, but is better seen on CT images.[80,96]

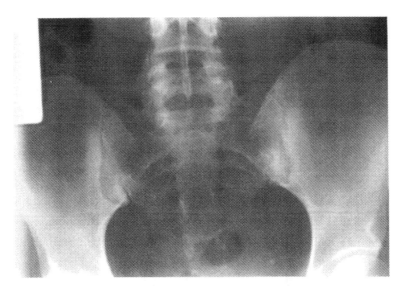

Fig. 3–42 Asymmetrical sacroilitis (Reiter's disease). There are no radiographically differentiating features to distinguish sacroilitis from Reiter's disease from that of psoriatic joint disease. Clinical findings are the differentiating factors.

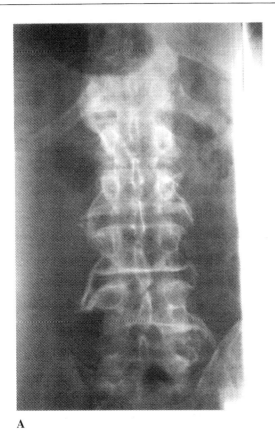

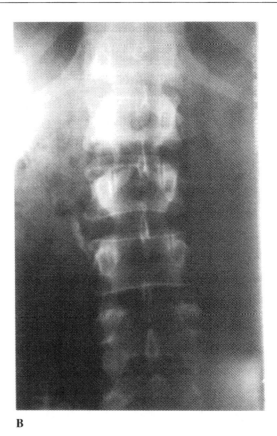

A   B

Fig. 3–43 Parasyndesmophytes. (**A**) Thick osteophytic changes arising from above and below the vertebral end plates and parallel to the disk margins occur in psoriatic arthropathy and Reiter's disease. *Comment:* These may cause ankylosis or may not completely bridge the interspace. They differ from the spondylophytic changes of disk degeneration which are parallel to the end plates, and differ from the thinner syndesmophytes of ankylosing spondylitis which arise from end plate margins and conform to the margins of the disks. The florid parasyndesmophytes seen here were found in a patient with Reiters disease although spinal manifestations are more commonly found in psoriatic disease than with Reiters. (**B**) Occasionally a parasyndesmophyte, such as is seen here, develops which is not attached to one or both vertebral bodies. These may occur in either psoriatic arthropathy or Reiter's disease, but are more common with psoriatic disease. *Comment:* Interestingly, the patient depicted here had Reiter's.

Ochronosis

This is a rare hereditary disease in which absence of homogentisic acid oxidase results in deposition of homogentisic acid in tissues causing joint disease. The spinal manifestations are characteristic.[80,97] Heavy plate-like calcifications within interspaces parallel to the end plates accompany vacuum phenomena, narrowing of disc spaces, with minimal marginal osteophytic changes. Multiple levels are involved and eventually ankylosis may occur, which may somewhat resemble AS, [80,97] although disk narrowing and lack of syndesmophytes are distinguishing factors. The sacroiliac joints are unaffected. Facet joint and interspinous calcification are eventual findings. Excretion of homogentisic acid in urine that turns black with standing is an identifying feature of the disease[80,90] (Fig. 3–44).

DISEASES CAUSING OSTEOPENIA IN THE LOWER SPINAL COLUMN

Osteoporosis

In the spine, osteoporosis is characterized by decreased bone density. Radiolucency, per se, does not connote os-

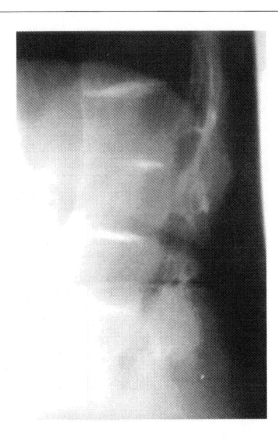

Fig. 3–44 Ochronosis. This is a rare disease in which ankylosis occurs due to calcification of disks. Its radiographic manifestations are occasionally similar to those of ankylosis spondylitis, but in most instances should not be confused.

teoporosis because osteomalacia, hyperparathyroidism, and other diseases which diminish bone mass are also causes of radiolucency. The descriptive term osteopenia is appropriate as a general designation of radiolucency with osteoporosis reserved as a specific diagnostic term.

Because of the extensive discussions needed to elaborate on the several causes of osteoporosis, the imaging manifestations will be discussed in a general manner, not specifically noting the several causes, except in passing.

Decrease in bone substance occurs with age and with disuse and disease. In osteoporosis, bone quantity diminishes, but the quality of the remaining bone remains normal. This is in contrast to osteomalacia where the quantity of bone remains, but quality is reduced. Generalized osteoporosis is most commonly a result of aging, especially in postmenopausal females. Generalized osteoporosis may also be found in malignancy, especially multiple myeloma, in which it may be the only radiographic manifestation until late in the disease, in prolonged use of catabolic steroids, in Cushing's disease, in those on long\-term heparin therapy, in acromegaly, and in anemias.[98-101] Regional osteoporosis occurs with disuse, such as in immobilization, and in migratory and transient osteoporosis as well as in reflex sympathetic dystrophy (RSD) also known as Sudek's atrophy.[15,98,99] Focal osteoporosis is seen adjacent to severe diseases, such as infection, inflammatory arthritides, and neoplasms.[98,99]

In osteoporosis, the cortical margins, while thinned, remain relatively radiopaque as compared to the decreased cancellous trabecular bone in vertebral bodies. As bone loss occurs, trabecular loss takes place first in the trabeculae that are not under (postural) stress. The decrease in these trabeculae makes those remaining more visible. The appearance of osteoporotic vertebral bodies is often somewhat "pale" or "washed out" with vertical striations in the spongiosa and thin cortices that appear to be sclerotic in contrast to the decreased opacity in the bodies. Biconcavity of vertebral bodies due to invagination of end plates is common. Compression deformities with wedging of vertebral bodies and even collapse to a "vertebra plana" configuration can occur as osteoporosis progresses.[98,99] Isolated depressions of vertebral end plates are also found due to localized fractures with invagination of disk material at the fracture sites. Spinal contours may also be altered, especially with thoracic vertebral collapse, which increases the thoracic kyphosis and causes compensatory alteration of the lumbar configuration. Osteoporosis is manifested in the pelvis by essentially the same appearances due to trabecular loss and relatively greater cortical opacity (Fig. 3-45).

It is important to remember that in cancellous bone it takes at least 30% and sometimes more that 50% loss of bone substance before it is visible radiographically.[1,3,98,99] For this reason, it is risky to diagnose osteoporosis from radiographs unless it is blatant, remembering that if the disease has progressed to the point where it is obvious, it is quite ad-

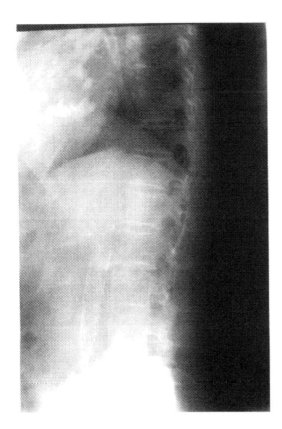

Fig. 3–45 Advanced osteoporosis. Decreased bone density which is not much greater than the opacity of the soft tissues and thin cortices are the specific stigmata of advanced osteoporosis. *Comment:* It is important to realize that at least 30%, and often greater than 50%, loss of bone density is necessary before it is evident from radiographs. Therefore the diagnosis of osteoporosis from radiographs cannot be made until it is fairly far advanced. Note the extensive atherosclerotic calcification in the aorta. It should be remembered that when there is atherosclerotic calcification in a peripheral vessel, the likelihood that there is also such disease in coronary and/or cerebral arteries is quite high.

vanced. Quantification of bone mass by means of single or dual photon radionuclide or radiographic absorptometry or by quantitative CT allows not only comparison to the present status of bone quantity but also by serial examinations can trace the progress or lack thereof with passage of time.[15,98,99] Particularly in older women where there is clinical suspicion of osteoporosis, periodic bone mass evaluation is a worthwhile procedure.

Cushing's Disease and Steroid Osteopenia

Cushing's disease and bone disease from prolonged steroid use both have all the usual manifestations of osteoporosis. In Cushing's disease, osteonecrosis is not common, but it is in prolonged therapeutic steroid use.[98,102] Both entities commonly cause biconcave vertebral bodies, and compression

fractures are frequent. Hazy interbody sclerosis accompanying compression fracture due to hypertrophic callus formation is more common in these diseases than in vertebral body collapse from other causes of osteoporosis.[98,102] A finding in compression fractures due to steroid use that is not found in other situations is an intervertebral vacuum cleft sign where gas is found within the collapsed vertebral body.[98,102]

Hemolytic Anemias

The hemolytic anemias, sickle cell anemia, thalassemia, and hereditary spherocytosis, due to marrow proliferation or secondary effects of the diseases or both, may cause visible osteopenic spinal changes. The changes in thalassemia are the most severe of those attributed to these diseases. Generalized osteoporosis with coarsened trabeculae and enlarged vascular channels, widening of the cancellous portions of the vertebral bodies with thinning of cortices may progress to a "honeycomb" appearance affecting multiple segments. The honeycomb pattern may also be seen in the pelvic bones.[100,101] Particularly in sickle cell disease, unique end plate deformities with central depressions produce the H-shaped or "fish vertebra" appearances of vertebral bodies that are nearly pathognomonic of these diseases.[100,101] Infarcts in bone are common in the hemolytic anemias, and in the spine massive infarction may cause vertebral body collapse that, fortunately, may be restored to normal height with only mild residual sclerosis remaining.[100,101] For unknown reasons, those afflicted with hemolytic anemias have a predilection for salmonella osteomyelitis, and spinal involvement may occur. *E. coli* and *H. influenzae* bone infection has also been documented (Fig. 3–46).

Osteomalacia

In contrast to osteoporosis, osteomalacia is characterized by decreased bone quality, but preservation of bone quantity until very late in the disease. Osteomalacia is due to insufficient deposition of calcium in osteoid tissue and literally means "soft bone." Osteomalacia in children is rickets. In adults there are many causes. Radiographically, bone is radiolucent, and trabecular patterns are coarse. There is loss of cortical definition, and pseudofractures are not uncommon.[98,103] Spinal manifestations are consistent with bone softening, radiolucency with invaginated end plates, vertebral body collapse, alterations in spinal contours due to vertebral body deformities. The diagnosis of osteomalacia from spinal films is hazardous.

Hyperparathyroidism (HPT)/Renal Osteodystrophy

Hyperparathyroidism is actually a form of osteomalacia. Primary and secondary (renal osteodystrophy) hyperparathyroidism produce osteopenia, which results from increased osteoclastic activity, especially in subperiosteal locations. Wid-

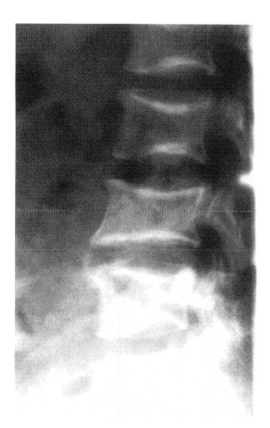

Fig. 3–46 Sickle cell anemia. The proliferation of hematopoetic marrow causes osteopenia, and the resorption of vertical (weight-bearing) trabeculae allows invagination and compaction of the end plates. The trabeculae are coarse in appearance. The configuration of the vertebral bodies may be altered, as is illustrated here, with loss of height and mild increase in horizontal dimensions.

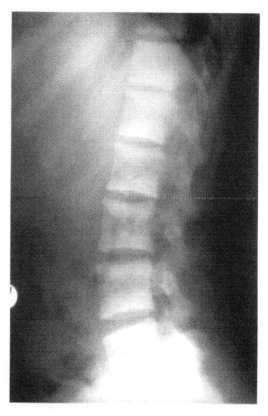

Fig. 3–47 Hyperparathyroidism (HPT), rugger jersey spine. In hyperparathyroidism resorption of calcium in the vertebral spongiosa and retention and even reinforcement adjacent to the end plates may result in the "striped" appearance of vertebral bodies that has been called the rugger jersey spine.

ening of sacroiliac joint spaces and irregular joint margins are relatively common findings in HPT, and similar changes may be found at the symphysis pubis.[98,104] Loss of cortical definition and accentuation of trabeculae are common and invagination of vertebral end plates occurs in many instances. Soft tissue calcification may be present and may be extreme [98,104] (Figs. 3–47 and 3–48).

TUMORS AND TUMOR-LIKE CONDITIONS OF BONE

Fortunately, spinal tumors are not frequently encountered in chiropractic practice. However, some patients with such pathology will invariably seek chiropractic care, and there will be few practices that do not find at least one over the years. With an aging population, the frequency of such incidents is nearly certain to increase. In this presentation, there will be no attempt to discuss all known tumors or tumor–like processes that can be found in the low back. Only those that are more

common will be covered. It is also worth stating that the job of the chiropractor as a primary health provider is to find, not necessarily to make a definitive diagnosis of, such abnormalities as tumors and those entities resembling them.

Malignant Bone Tumors

Metastatic Bone Tumors

Approximately 70% of all malignant bone tumors are metastatic[105,106] usually from carcinoma. In the spine, the percentage of metastasis is probably even higher because the spine is a major target region for most visceral malignancies. The most common primary malignancies that metastasize to the spine are: breast, prostate, lung, kidney, thyroid, and bowel.[105,106] Sarcomas, such as Ewing's and osteosarcoma, on occasion, may also metastasize to the spine or pelvis.[105,107,108,109] The discovery of metastasis to the spine is grave, signifying that the disease is well advanced. Not infrequently, the first real pain associated with a visceral carcinoma occurs with metastasis to bone. Bone pain is severe, although the tumor in a viscus may

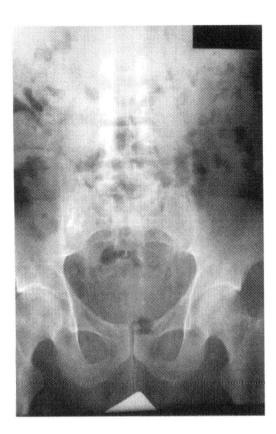

Fig. 3–48 Hyperparathyroidism, pseudowidening of the sacroiliac joints. In HPT, periosteal resorption of calcium may result in pseudowidening of the sacroiliac joints as is illustrated here. Another frequent finding with HPT is extensive vascular calcification, seen her in pelvic soft tissues.

cause few symptoms until far advanced. In females, breast carcinoma accounts for up to 70% of bony metastasis, with the spine the most frequent site.[105,106] Thyroid, kidney, and uterine malignancies account for most of the rest,[105,106] but as lung cancer increases in women, metastasis from that source will also increase. About 60% of bone metastasis in males is from prostate cancer, the lung accounting for about 25% more.[105,106] The spine and pelvis are by far the most commonly affected areas. The most frequent route is through the blood stream, the metastatic emboli depositing in vascular/marrow-rich areas, such as a vertebral body or the pelvic bones. Other pathways for metastatic spread are by direct extension or through lymphatic channels. Metastatic lesions tend to be multiple and not necessarily in contiguous areas of the skeleton, but most are axial.[105,106]

Metastasis to the spine, with the exception of that from the prostate is nearly always osteolytic.[105,106] In females, osteoblastic metastasis is usually from the breast.[105,106] It must be remembered that with routine radiography at least 30% and often more than 50% of destruction of cancellous bone must have taken place before it is visible. Cortical changes are visible with much less destruction, but cortical involvement in

metastasis does not usually occur until medullary disease is well along. Metastasis to the cortex directly is rare, and the usual primary tumor metastasizing to cortical bone is bronchogenic carcinoma.[105,106,110,111] Whereas radiography is not sensitive for visualizing early bone destruction, radionuclide (RN) imaging will detect such changes at an early stage. Routine Technetium 99m bone scans have been cited as being able to detect 3% to 5% of alterations in bone metabolism.[105,106,112,113] SPECT scans are even more sensitive and more succinctly define the lesion(s).[105] Because bone scans allow whole body imaging, when metastasis is suspected, and particularly when it is known to exist, RN scans should be used to document the areas of involvement. CT is useful in evaluation of metastatic lesions, being considerably more sensitive than radiography in depicting lesions and more specific in defining the involvement. MRI is even more sensitive than RN, and has the advantage that soft tissue involvement is very well demonstrated.[15,105] However, whole body MRI is not presently an option so that RN imaging is more applicable to find and locate involvement, with MRI used to evaluate specific lesions.

Lytic bone destruction takes place from pressure of tumor material destroying the surrounding trabeculae, with osteoclastic activity not particularly involved.[105,107] On radiographs, this results in patterns of destruction that have been termed "motheaten" or "permeative." A motheaten pattern is characterized by ragged areas of destruction that resemble a wool cloth that has been riddled by moths.[105,114,115] This pattern of destruction can also be found in osteomyelitis. The appearance described as permeative is more subtle and more lethal. Permeative means that the lesion has "gone clear through" the affected bone. It has been likened to the appearance of many tiny drill holes through the affected area. This may result in simply a hazy indistinct look to the bone. In both motheaten and permeative destruction, the margins of the lesions are usually poorly defined, even indistinct (called a long zone of transition) because the tumor material is invading the adjacent bone (Fig. 3-49).

An unusual manifestation of metastasis to bone occurs occasionally with lung, thyroid, or kidney carcinoma when a large expansile "bubbly" bony lesion is found rather than multiple poorly defined lesions that are more common. These are called "blow-out" lesions.[105] Similar appearing lesions may occur with giant cell tumor or with a solitary plasmocytoma.

Osteoblastic metastasis is much less common than is osteolytic disease. The increased bone density seen with osteoblastic metastatic disease is not a manifestation of the tumor material itself, but is reactive sclerosis in the affected osteoid[105,106] (Fig. 3–50). Because of this, mixed osteoblastic and osteolytic lesions are often seen. Increasing radiopacity in a lesion or spread of osteoblastic activity is a sign of great concern, indicating that in spite of the body's attempt to repair the diseased bone, the cancer is progressing.[105,106]

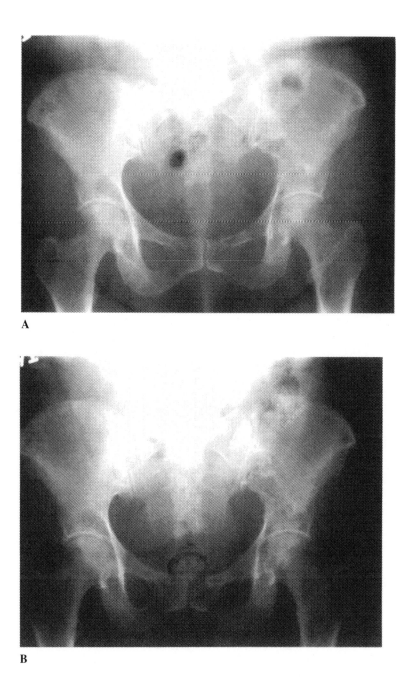

Fig. 3–49 Osteolytic metastatic carcinoma. (**A**) Osteolytic lesions are present in the lateral aspect of the right iliac crest, and have destroyed the margin of the left pelvic brim. There is also osteolytic destruction in the left pubic body and superior ramus. (**B**) In two months the osteolytic destruction has progressed significantly and left supra-acetabular destruction is now visible which was questionable on the earlier radiograph.

Because of the mechanism of involvement in metastasis to the spine, there are specific areas of predilection for the lesions. The most common site is the vertebral body because that is where the greatest accumulation of marrow is found and the vascularity is greatest. Metastasis to the vertebral body may be osteoblastic or osteolytic; osteolysis is definitely seen more frequently. A severely osteoblastic vertebral body has been termed an "ivory vertebra"[105,106] (Fig. 3–51). In addition to metastatic carcinoma, ivory vertebrae may be due to Paget's disease, lymphoma (Hodgkin's disease), myelosclerosis, or mastocytosis.[105,116,117] Another frequent site for metastasis is a pedicle. An affected pedicle may be osteoblastic or, more commonly, osteolytic[105,106] (Fig. 3-52). The absence of a pedicle is not a certain sign of a metastatic focus because

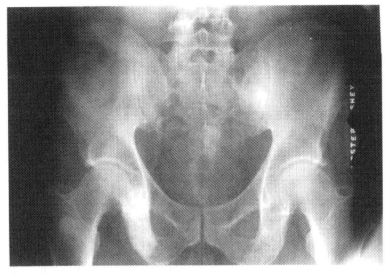

A

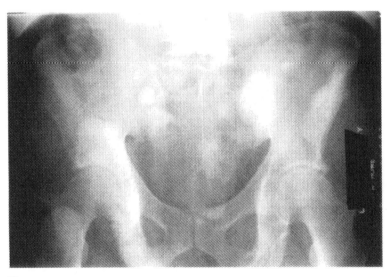

B

Fig. 3–50 Osteoblastic metastasis. **(A)** This patient with prostate carcinoma shows osteoblastic foci in the right ischium, the intertrochanteric portion of the right femur, and a questionable focus in the left ilium at the sacroiliac joint. **(B)** six months later, the lesions seen previously have advanced grossly and new lesions have appeared in numerous locations.

agenesis of pedicles occurs, but with pedicular agenesis or hypogenesis there is usually reactive enlargement and increased radiopacity of the opposite pedicle[105] (Fig. 3-53). Where a missing pedicle is found and reactive changes are not seen on the opposite side, metastasis must be considered until disproven. In patients under 30 years of age, pedicular destruction may be due to aneurysmal bone cyst (ABC) or osteoblastoma rather than to metastasis.[105,107] A neural tumor extending through a neural foramen is another possible cause for a missing or eroded pedicle.[105,118]

Primary Malignant Bone Tumors

Multiple Myeloma

Multiple myeloma (MM) is the most common primary bone tumor.[105,119,120] It is rarely found before age 40, and its incidence increases markedly with age. Multiple myeloma occurs more frequently in males with an approximate 2:1 ratio.[105,119–121] The "classical" radiographic appearance of MM has been described as multiple small punched out lesions, but in the spine punched out lesions are extremely uncommon. In many,

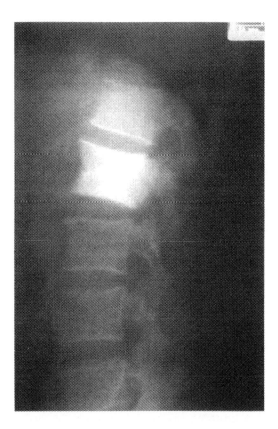

Fig. 3–51 Ivory vertebra. Dense sclerosis of a vertebra may occur with Paget's disease, osteoblastic metastasis, lymphoma of bone, or idiopathically. With Paget's there is usually expansion of the vertebra and the margins are usually more sclerotic than the center of the vertebral body. With lymphoma frequently there is scalloping of the anterior of the vertebral body due to pressure from enlarged lymph nodes. Osteoblastic metastatic and idiopathic ivory vertebrae have no distinguishing characteristics. The ivory vertebra found in this patient was idiopathic. No primary neoplasm was found, there were no other sites to suggest Paget's, and the patient did not have lymphoma. Biopsy was done and only sclerotic bone was found.

if not most, cases the only radiographic findings may be osteoporosis, which at first may be fairly minimal but as the disease progresses can be severe enough that bone density in vertebral bodies is not much greater than that of the disks[105,119,120] (Fig. 3–54). Vertebral collapse is inevitable and may occur at one or many levels. The pedicles are less likely to be involved than the vertebral bodies because they contain little marrow, and when there is vertebral body collapse without pedicle involvement, it is known as the "pedicle sign of multiple myeloma"[46,105] (Fig. 3–55). This is not an invariable situation, many cases of pedicle involvement having been reported.[105] In the pelvis, sharply defined, purely osteolytic, lesions of varying size, but usually small and multiple, occur with MM. Femurs are favored sites for MM lesions, and in lumbosacral ra-

diographs that include the femoral heads and necks, lesions may be visible. Rarely (less than 3% of those with MM), sclerotic lesions may occur.[105,119–121] These may be single or multiple, and the spine has been known to be involved. A single ivory vertebra has been seen with MM, and the differential diagnosis from other causes of ivory vertebra may be nearly impossible without biopsy.[105,119] Radionuclide scans are not sensitive to lesions of MM because the bone changes are osteolytic. Except in the rare instance of osteoblastic MM, the only positive RN findings would be at fracture sites.[105,119,122] CT depicts lesions that are not visible on plain film radiographs as well as those that are.[15,105,119] MRI, due to its ability to image marrow, is very sensitive in detection of MM lesions, revealing low signal intensity in marrow fat on T1 weighted images and increased signal intensity with T2 weighting.[15,105,119]

Solitary plasmacytoma is a localized form of plasma cell proliferation that is much less common than MM and that fre-

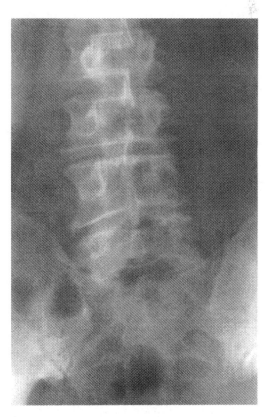

A

Fig. 3–52 Missing pedicle. (A) The left pedicle of L4 is missing, having been destroyed by osteolytic metastasis. This has been described as the "one eyed pedicle" sign. *Comment:* The pedicle is a common site for osteolytic metastasis. The constriction of blood vessels in a pedicle allows cancer cells in the blood stream to lodge and cause destruction as they proliferate.

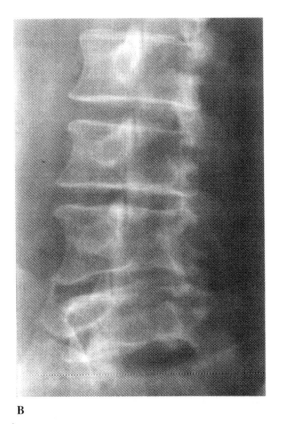

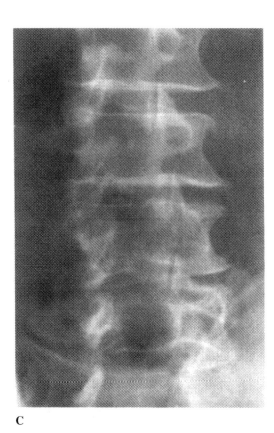

B

C

Fig. 3–52 (**B**) and (**C**) The oblique views show the intact pedicles on the patients' right side and the missing pedicle on the left.

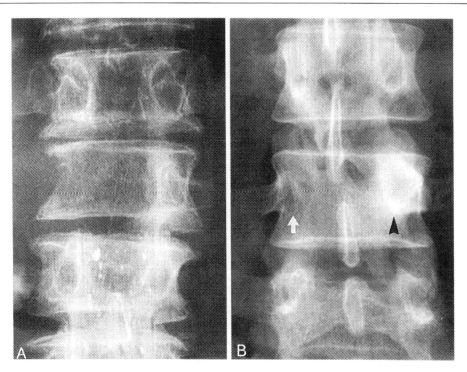

Fig. 3–53 Missing pedicles, congenital vs. neoplasm. (**A**) Obliteration of the right pedicle of L1 resulting from osteolytic metastasis. The lamina and spinous process have also been destroyed. Note that the opposite pedicle shows no evidence of reactive sclerosis or hypertrophy. (**B**) The left pedicle is missing, but the opposite pedicle is sclerotic and has hypertrophied. This is a reactive change due to the altered biomechanical stresses from the long-standing alteration of anatomy. *Source:* Reprinted with permission from T.R. Yochum, *Essentials of Skeletal Radiology,* © 1987, Williams & Wilkins.

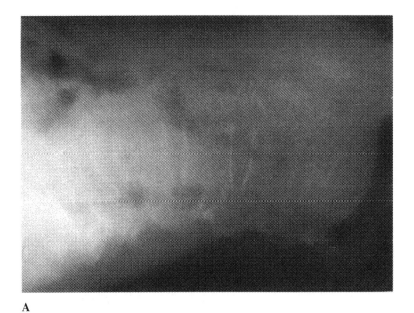

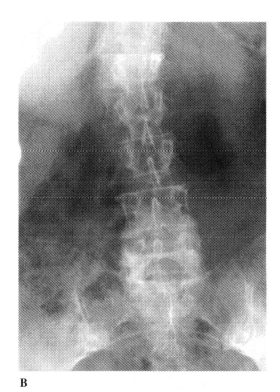

Fig. 3–54 Multiple myeloma (MM). (**A**) Generalized osteopenia and compression deformities at L1 and L5 are non-specific findings, in this patient who has multiple myeloma. *Comment:* MM, especially in the spinal column, often has no radiographic manifestation except for osteopenia. The presence of multiple compression fractures, particularly if noncontiguous, in an older osteopenic patient should raise the possibility of MM. (**B**) AP view of same patient.

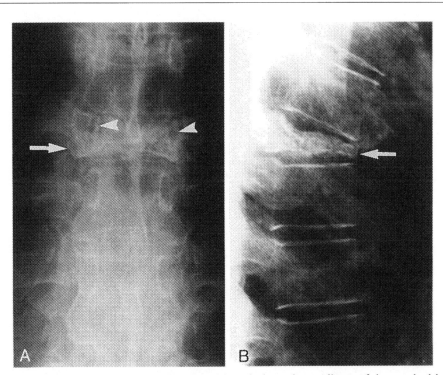

Fig. 3–55 Multiple myeloma, the pedicle sign. (**A**) and (**B**) AP and lateral views show collapse of the vertebral body but the pedicles are preserved. Note that even the posterior of the vertebral body has been destroyed while the pedicles have been spared. *Comment:* In MM marrow proliferation may, as in this case, leads to bony collapse. The pedicles, having minimal marrow, remain viable. *Source:* Reprinted with permission from T.R. Yochum, *Essentials of Skeletal Radiology,* © 1987, Williams & Wilkins.

quently occurs at an earlier age[105,119–121] (Fig. 3–56). A patient with plasmacytoma is expected to have the disease progress to full blown MM over time with lethal consequences, although with radiation treatment or surgery or both a small percentage of patients survive. The lesion of plasmacytoma is a solitary geographic, usually expansile, osteolytic lesion with "soap bubble" characteristics, often appearing to be benign. The differential diagnosis includes aneurysmal bone cyst, the pseudotumor of hemophilia, fibrous dysplasia, brown tumor of hyperparathyroidism, and giant cell tumor. The spine is infrequently the site of these lesions, the pelvis more commonly affected.

Osteosarcoma

Osteosarcoma is a primary malignant bone tumor with five distinct clinical types (central, multicentric, parosteal, secondary, and extraosseous).[105,107,109,121] Of these, the central and secondary varieties are the only ones found in the spinal column with any frequency. Central osteosarcoma is the second most common primary malignant tumor of bone.[105,107,109,121] It occurs mainly by or before age 25, but a few cases of primary osteosarcoma have been documented in older patients. Osteosarcoma in older patients is usually secondary, representing malignant degeneration in a lesion of Paget's disease, fibrous dysplasia, in an osteochondroma, or in an area of bone irradiated for another malignant tumor.[105,107,109,116,118,121] Central osteosarcoma only very rarely affects the spine itself, but has been found in the sacrum and other pelvic bones. Because osteosarcoma is derived from undifferentiated connective tissue, the radiographic appearance varies according to the predominant tissue being proliferated. If the histologically predominant tissue is collagenoblastic or chondrogenoblastic, the lesion will be mainly osteolytic, but, if osteoblastic, the lesion will be densely sclerotic. Mixed osteolytic and osteoblastic lesions are common. Expansion of the lesion is rapid, and metastasis to the lungs ("cannonball metastasis") is early and lethal.[105,107,109,121]

Multicentric osteosarcoma is a rare manifestation of this tumor variety. It is not entirely certain whether the lesions in this form of the disease are distinct simultaneous foci or multiple metastatic lesions, although there has been inability to identify a primary lesion from which the others are derived[105,107,121] (Fig. 3–57). Only a few cases of this entity have been reported, but some have involved the spine.

Chondrosarcoma

Chondrosarcoma may arise in any bone, but is distinctly uncommon in the spine.[105,107,121,123] Chondrosarcomas may be primary or secondary and either central (arising in the medullary portion of bone) or peripheral (arising from the cortex). Rarely, a chondrosarcoma may arise in extraosseous soft tissues. Most chondrosarcomas occur after age 40, and there is a 2:1 predominance in males.[105,107,121,123] The most common sites of involvement for chondrosarcoma are the pelvis and proximal femur,[105,107,123] both of which are usually shown on lumbosacral radiographs. Secondary chondrosarcomas occur in preexisting cartilaginous tumors, such as enchondroma, rarely osteochondroma, and also from lesions of Paget's disease or fibrous dysplasia. There is a much higher rate of malignant degeneration to chondrosarcoma in benign cartilaginous tu-

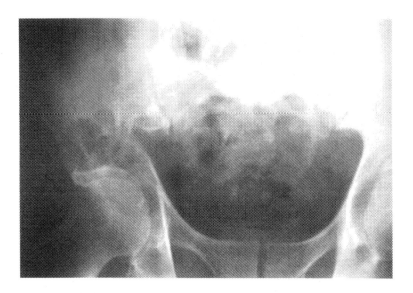

Fig. 3–56 Plasmacytoma. A large septated radiolucent lesion above and medial to the acetabulum is a solitary plasmacytoma, a precursor to multiple myeloma. Large lytic lesions such as this in older patients, even though the margins appear to be discrete, should be considered to have grave potential.

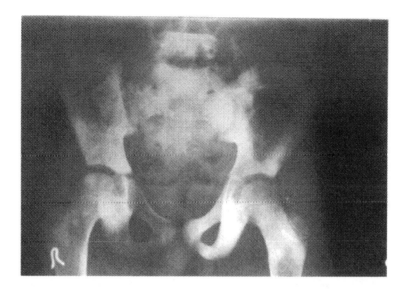

Fig. 3–57 Osteosarcoma. This is a rare case of multicentric osteosarcoma. *Comment:* Osteosarcomas are the most poorly differentiated skeletal sarcomas and proliferate bone, cartilage, and fibrous materials, accounting for the varying radiographic characteristics. Courtesy of Dr. William E. Litterer, Elizabeth, New Jersey.

mors that are in or near the axial skeleton than those that are more peripheral.[105,107,121,123] Chondrosarcomas are destructive proliferative lesions and calcification occurs in the tumor matrix in two thirds of these tumors [105,107,121,123] (Fig. 3–58). The appearance of "rings and arcs" in the matrix is an indication of a cartilage tumor and all cartilage tumors, especially in the axial skeleton, should be considered potentially malignant.[105,107,121] Chondrosarcoma, especially in comparison to osteosarcoma and Ewing's sarcoma, is fairly slow growing, but metastasis to the lungs is not uncommon.

Ewing's Sarcoma

Ewing's is a highly malignant connective tissue tumor that is usually found in males (2:1 male:female ratio) between the ages of 10 and 25. It is rare before 5 years of age or after 30, but a few cases have been reported in the elderly.[105,107,108,121] It is classified as a "round cell tumor" along with MM and non–Hodgkins's lymphoma. Lesions in the axial skeleton are more likely in those over 20.[105,107,108] There is a predilection for flat bones, the innominate bones a target site, with the sacrum less commonly involved.[105,107,108] Vertebral lesions are rare. The usual radiographic presentation is mixed lytic and blastic and a permeative pattern is frequent (Fig. 3–59). Especially clinically, differentiation from infection or lymphoma may be a problem. The "onion skin" appearance of periosteal proliferation, which is frequently seen in long bones, may be present in the pelvis. Ewing's is the most common bone tumor to metastasize to bone with metastasis to the spine common.[105,107,108,121] Cannonball metastasis to the lungs may occur.

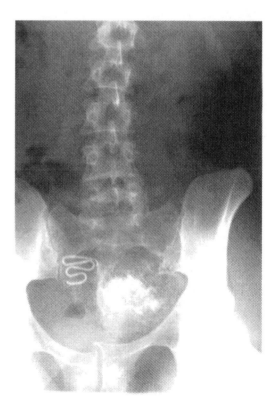

Fig. 3–58 Chondrosarcoma. In chondrosarcoma the neoplastic activity proliferates fibrous as well as cartilaginous material. Irregular calcification within the neoplastic cartilage is frequent and may be quite dense. The radiographic appearance of "arcs and rings" in the lesion is characteristic of a cartilage based tumor.

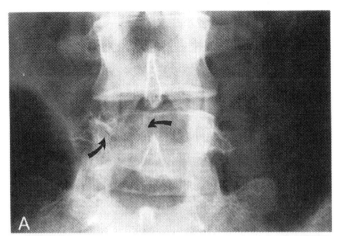

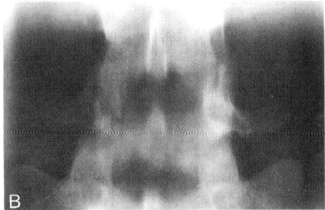

Fig. 3–59 Ewing's sarcoma. (**A**) and (**B**) A plain film and a tomogram illustrate osteolytic destruction of the L5 pedicle and a portion of the vertebral body; *Comment:* Ewing's is uncommon in the spine, when present, usually affecting the sacrum or lumbar spine. *Source:* Reprinted with permission from T.R. Yochum, *Essentials of Skeletal Radiology,* © 1987, Williams & Wilkins.

Fibrosarcoma and Malignant Fibrous Histiocytoma

Fibrosarcoma is a malignant tumor that is osteolytic because it proliferates collagen. It is usually found in adults and, although usually a primary tumor, may complicate a preexisting benign lesion.[105,107,121,124] It is uncommon in the spine, occasionally found in the pelvis. Radiographically, it presents as a permeative area of destruction, usually with a soft tissue component that may be large (Fig. 3–60). Secondary fibrosarcoma may be found in malignant degeneration in Paget's disease, fibrous dysplasia, and chronic infection.[105,107,116,118,121,124] Malignant fibrous histiocytoma is a radiographically indistinguishable "first cousin" of fibrosarcoma, which is known to occur in bone infarcts.[105,107,121] Fibrosarcomas are usually relatively slow in their progress and metastasize late although there are a few very aggressive tumors that metastasize early. Metastasis to lung and liver is common. Selective lymphatic metastasis also occurs.[105,107,121,124]

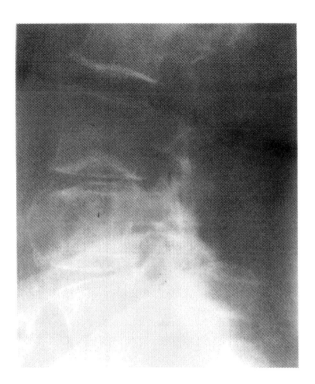

Fig. 3–60 Fibrosarcoma. This expansile radiolucent lesion in the L4 vertebral body is a fibrosarcoma. *Comment:* Fibrosarcoma is the most differentiated of the skeletal sarcomas, producing malignant fibrous material but not cartilage or bone, so that its radiographic appearance is purely lytic. Its occurrence in the spine is rare. *Source:* Reprinted with permission from T.R. Yochum, *Essentials of Skeletal Radiology,* © 1987, Williams & Wilkins.

Chordoma

Chordoma is a rare primary malignant bone tumor arising from notochordal remnants. It is a slow-growing, locally aggressive, expansile tumor that usually has a large associated soft tissue component. Metastasis is uncommon. Because its origin is notochordal, it occurs in the axial skeleton, predominantly in the sacrococcygeal and cervicocranial regions[105,107,121,125] (Fig. 3–61). It is reported to make up at least 40% of sacral tumors.[105,107,121] Most chordomas are found in persons between ages 40 and 70, but can occur at any age. There is a 2:1 male predilection.[105,107] Clinically, the tumor may reach large size before being discovered. The symptoms are usually due to the effects of the slowly enlarging tumor on the adjacent tissues. Sacral tumors may be eccentric, but classically should be midline. The radiographic appearance of a sacrococcygeal chordoma is an expansile tumor containing calcification and incomplete septa with areas of lytic destruction and a considerable soft tissue component that may contain calcification. Due to rectal gas and feces, adequate visualization of the sacrum/coccyx is often difficult, especially in a coronal projection. Cleansing of the lower intestine prior to

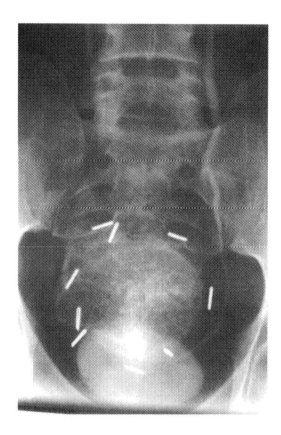

Fig. 3–61 Chordoma. This expansile tumor; seen above the opacified bladder in this film from an excretory urogram has mixed radiopacity due to amorphous calcification within the matrix. *Comment:* Chordomas are usually osteolytic but frequently contain amorphous calcification. The sacrococcygeal area is a predilected site for these rare tumors which arise from notochordal remnants.

radiography, or use of conventional or computed tomography may be necessary to adequately evaluate the tumor. Very rarely, a vertebra may be the site of a chordoma and an ivory vertebra related to chordoma has been reported.[105,107] Vertebral chordomas may be either lytic or blastic and have no radiologic characteristics to distinguish them from myeloma or metastasis. Chordoma is one of a very few tumors that may involve contiguous segments, destroying the intervening disk.[105,107]

Non–Hodgkin's Lymphoma of Bone (Reticulum Cell Sarcoma) and Hodgkin's Lymphoma of Bone

Like myeloma and Ewing's sarcoma, Hodgkin's and non–Hodgkins lymphomas are round cell tumors. The majority of lymphomas found in bone are secondary to malignant lymphomas in other locations, but a small percentage arise primarily in bone.[105,107,121,126] In non–Hodgkin's lymphoma of bone, the majority of cases have been found in persons before age 40, particularly between ages 20 and 40, but a goodly number

have been reported in those above 50 years of age. There is a 2:1 male preponderance.[105,107,121,126] Pelvic bones and vertebrae are sometimes involved, but the majority of bone lymphomas are found in extra-axial locations. Lymphomatous lesions in bone are usually lytic with a permeative pattern of destruction, but may be blastic. Vertebral or sacral collapse may occur, the features indistinguishable from involvement with metastasis or plasmacytoma. Up to 20% of patients with Hodgkin's lymphoma develop lymphomatous bone disease, primarily in the lower thoracic and upper lumbar vertebrae.[105,107,126] Most such lesions are osteolytic but may be blastic with an ivory vertebra appearance. Scalloping of the anterior or lateral aspects of the involved vertebral body is a characteristic but unusual feature.[105,107,126] The pelvic bones are occasionally involved.

Giant Cell Tumor (GCT), the Quasi-Malignant Tumor of Bone

Giant cell tumor is a relatively common bone tumor that may affect the spine, the sacrum being the most common site. GCT is the most common benign tumor of the sacrum.[105,107,121,127] The bones of the pelvis are occasionally affected, and rarely a vertebra may be involved. Approximately 20% of GCTs have malignant characteristics and, therefore, all should be considered malignant until proven otherwise, especially because some very benign appearing lesions have metastasized with fatal results.[105,107,121,127] Biopsy is necessary to determine malignancy or benignancy. There is a 3:2 female predominance with benign GCTs, but a 3:1 predilection for males in the malignant variety.[105,107,127] The usual age range is 20 to 40, with few occurring before 20 or after 40.[105,107,121,127] Giant cell tumors are expansile radiolucent lesions with thin cortices and wide zones of transition from abnormal to normal bone, suggesting malignancy. A "soap bubble" appearance is common. As in the extremities, iliac GCTs tend to be subarticular, occurring near the sacroiliac joints or acetabuli[105,107,121,127] (Fig. 3-62). The more aggressive lesions tend to be purely lytic, and a soft tissue mass may be present. Vertebral GCTs resemble osteoblastoma or aneurysmal bone cysts and radiographically cannot be differentiated from these.[105,107,127]

Benign Bone Tumors

Only those benign tumors that are commonly found in the spine and pelvis will be discussed.

Hemangioma

Hemangioma is the most common benign spinal bone tumor.[105,107,128,129] Many small hemangiomas cannot be detected by plain film radiography, but CT, and especially MRI, are sensitive in their detection.[105,107,129] Nearly all are asymptomatic, but with the rare expansile lesions, fracture, or hemor-

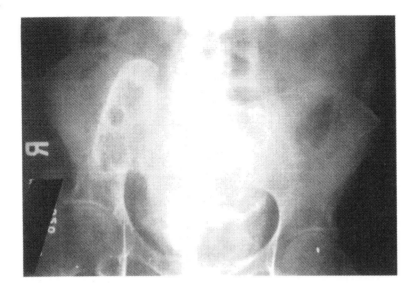

Fig. 3–62 Malignant giant cell tumor of the sacrum. This grossly expansile sepated tumor was found to be a malignant giant cell tumor. *Comment:* GCTs rarely reach this size although most are expansile. GCT is the most common benign tumor of the sacrum, but GCTs are quasi-malignant tumors and the possibility of a malignant nature must always be considered. The sacrum is the most common site for spinal GCT. Courtesy of Dr. William E. Litterer, Elizabeth, New Jersey.

rhage, symptoms may occur.[105,107,129] Most spinal lesions are solitary, but multiple lesions have been reported. The radiographic appearance is characteristically a striated or "corduroy cloth" mildly radiolucent vertebral body or portion thereof, but occasionally the neural arch structures are affected (Figs. 3–63 and 3–64). Other disease processes that result in a striated appearance of bone similar to that seen in hemangioma are Paget's disease and moderately advanced osteoporosis.[99,105,116] Distinguishing features are that the cortical thickening and bony expansion that typify Paget's are not found in hemangioma, and osteoporosis is a more generalized finding. Hemangiomas can be found anywhere in the spine and occasionally in the pelvis.

Osteochondroma and Hereditary Multiple Extostosis (HME)

Osteochondromas are exostoses arising from the surface of bone. They are composed of bone with a cartilage cap and represent displaced growth cartilage that proliferates to form a benign tumor mass. Osteochondromas are the most common benign bone tumors, but are not common in the spine. They are, however, not infrequent in pelvic bones[105,107,129] (Fig. 3–65). Although osteochondromas arise in childhood, most are not detected until adulthood. Except in the spine, unless large enough to cause an obvious deformity or lump, or located where they interfere with joint function, they are usually found serendipitously. Spinal osteochondromas usually occur near secondary ossification centers and may be radiographically spectacular, but unless they alter function or cause neurological abnormality due to compression, are usually nonsympto-

matic. However, if large, they may cause serious vascular or neurological damage or both.[129] Malignant degeneration of solitary osteochondromas is rare[105,107,129] (Fig. 3-66).

Multiple hereditary exostosis, also called osteochondomatosis or diaphyseal aclasis, is a hereditary disorder where osteochondromas of varying sizes occur in many locations. There is no male or female preponderance, but males seem to be more severely affected.[105,107,129] It is usually discovered in childhood, nearly always before age 10, and may be the cause of obvious deformities or abnormal joint function or both. Pelvic lesions may be particularly large and deforming. Spinal lesions may cause spinal cord compression.[105,107,129] Malignant degeneration may occur in up to 25% of those affected[105,107,121,129] (Fig. 3–67).

Osteoid Osteoma

Osteoid osteomas (OO) are benign, but frequently very painful, bone tumors that usually occur in persons between the ages of 10 and 25, but have been known to be present in those beyond 30. Males are affected about twice as often as females.[105,107,130] OO in the spine are often difficult to be demonstrated, many times requiring multiple imaging exams. Pain from OO may precede any radiologic manifestation. The pain related to OO may be attributed to mechanical problems, spinal strain/sprain, or disk disease, thus delaying diagnosis, especially when the lesion is not easily appreciated from radiographs.[105,107,130] Spinal OO is usually found in a neural arch, the pedicle a preferred area, and the lumbar spine is the most common location with the sacrum the next most common axial site.[105,107,130] Plain films are frequently inadequate to demon-

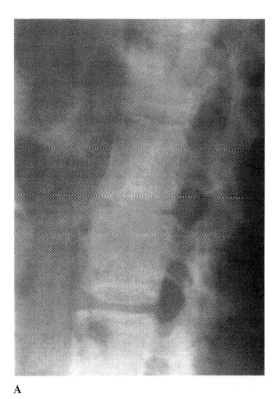
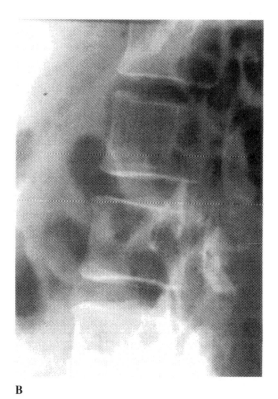

A   B

Fig. 3–63 Small hemangioma. The lesion in the L2 vertebral body is characteristic of a hemangioma, displaying vertical striations within a radiolucent lesion (the "corduroy cloth" appearance). *Comment:* Hemangiomas, when small, may not be visible on plain film radiography, and are frequently seen on CT and MRI exams when not detectable on radiographs of the same patient. Hemangiomas are the most common benign tumors of the spine, probably more common than is realized since many are undetected radiographically.

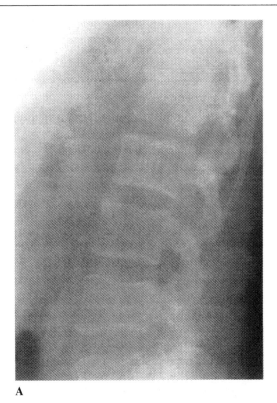
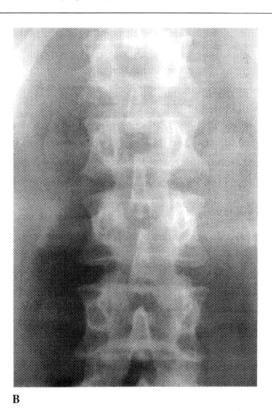

A   B

Fig. 3–64 Hemangioma. Another hemangioma, also found in L2. This occupies a grater portion of the vertebral body and is therefore more easily seen.

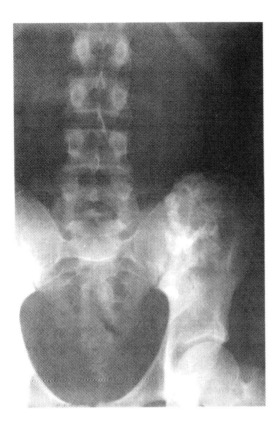

Fig. 3–65 Osteochondroma, ilium. The characteristics of this large cauliflower-like tumor are typical of cartilage based lesions with arcs and rings of calcified material mixed with radiolucency. *Comment:* The size and irregular nature of this lesion make further investigation of possible malignancy necessary since all cartilaginous lesions except for enchondromas in hands or feet, have malignant potential.

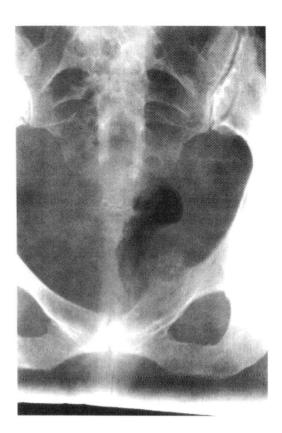

Fig. 3–66 Malignant degeneration of an osteochondroma. A sessile osteochondroma arising from the left superior pubic ramus has an indistinct border superiorly, and the appearance at the top of the lesion suggests an aggressive nature. *Comment:* This was proven to be degeneration of an osteochondroma to a chondrosarcoma.

strate a subtle spinal lesion[15,105,107] (Fig. 3-68). CT is particularly helpful in locating the radiolucent nidus, which may not be demonstrable with plain films. The sclerosis surrounding the nidus is reactive rather than due to tumor bone and may be mild or severe.

Bone Island (Enosteoma)

Bone islands are not truly tumors, but their radiographic appearance resembles tumor activity, especially osteoblastic metastasis or osteoid osteoma. Bone islands are discrete areas of compact lamellar bone in a location where there should be cancellous bone. Because they are actually normal bone in an abnormal location, no symptoms are associated. Their appearance is that of a homogenous sclerotic focus. Sizes vary from a few millimeters to possibly several centimeters, especially in the pelvic bones, with variable shapes (Figs. 3–69 and 3–70). The "brush border," a serrated or slightly spiculated appearance of the margins of the lesion, is characteristic. They are found in all bones, the vertebral body in the lumbar region

being the most common spinal location. Neural arch, and particularly pedicle locations, may simulate OO, but the lack of symptoms makes differentiation fairly obvious.

Osteoblastoma

These are rare true bone-forming tumors and are most commonly found in the spine.[105,107,131] Histologically, but not radiographically, they resemble OO, and for many years were considered to be giant osteoid osteomas. These are painful lesions, usually found in the neural arch. Although the age range has been noted as 3 to 78, most occur between 10 and 20. There is a 2:1 male preponderance.[105,107,131] These are expansile lesions with a thin cortical margin. Most are purely radiolucent, but a mottled blastic and lytic appearance may be found. The usual size is 4 to 6 cm, but some are larger and have a soap bubble appearance, making the differentiation from aneurysmal bone cyst difficult.[105,107,131] Osteoblastomas that are mainly sclerotic do occur, making the diagnosis less troublesome.

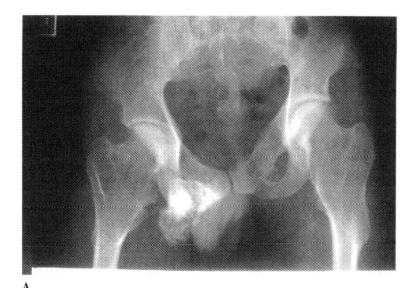

A

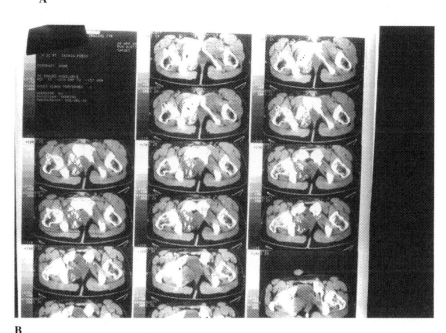

B

Fig. 3–67 Malignant degeneration of an ischial osteochondroma in a patient with hereditary multiple exostosis (HME). (**A**) The deformities of the femurs make identification of HME an easy diagnosis. The aggressive appearance of the right ischial lesion and irregular calcification at the cartilaginous margin of the lesion inferiorly are manifestations of a highly malignant transformation of this lesion. *Comment:* The percentage of malignant degeneration in HME has been reported to be as high as 25%. (**B**) In this CT scan of the same patient, the images define the lesion and depict its margins and characteristics better than does plain film radiography. Note the extent of the non-calcified cartilage within the lesion and the random distribution of the calcified areas within. Courtesy of Dr. Steven Foreman, Woodland Hills, California.

Enchondroma and Enchondromatosis (Ollier's Disease)

Enchondromas are cartilage-based tumors that develop from growth cartilage that is displaced. They are, therefore, found near physes and occur during growth, but most solitary lesions are found in the third decade. There is no male or fe-

male preponderance.[105,107,132] Enchondromas are not found in the spine, but do occur in the pelvic bones.[105,107,132] The appearance is that of a geographic expansile radiolucent lesion with well-defined margins and an intact, but possibly thin cortex. Fifty percent show calcification that is stippled or punctate. Pelvic lesions without internal calcification must be differentiated from fibrous dysplasia, osteoblastoma, and giant cell tu-

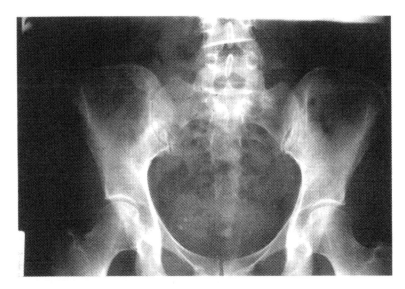

Fig. 3–68 Sacral osteoid osteoma. This patient had pin point pain in the right upper sacral area. The lesion is subtle and is indicated by pencil marks. The radiolucent area around the small radiopaque nidus blends with the adjacent foramen. *Comment:* The usual characteristics of osteoid osteomas in tubular bones are an area of reactive sclerosis with a nidus which may be difficult to visualize. In flat bones or in the cancellous portion of tubular bones there may be little to no sclerosis, making the lesions difficult to identify. Courtesy of Dr. J.F. Winterstein, Lumbard, Illinois.

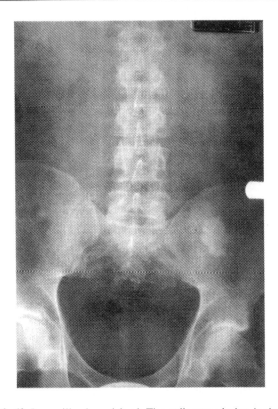

Fig. 3–69 Large iliac bone island. The radiopaque lesion in the left ilium has distinct but serrated margins, typical of a bone island. *Comment:* The differentiation of a lesion of this sort from an osteoblastic focus may be difficult. The homogenous matrix and the serrated margins are helpful in making the right diagnosis, but when there is uncertainty, a bone scan may help. It must be remembered, however, that in a small percentage of bone islands will show increased activity on radionuclide examination.

mor.[105,107,132] Ollier's disease or enchondromatosis are terms used when there are enchondromas in multiple sites. Malignant degeneration in enchondromatosis has been stated to be as high as 50%.[105,107,121,132] Cartilaginous tumors near the axial skeleton have a greater predilection for malignant degeneration than those that are more peripheral.[105,107,121,132]

Aneurysmal Bone Cyst (ABC)

Aneurysmal bone cysts are not true tumors but consist of a cystic cavity filled with blood. They are expansile soap bubble lesions and were named for their radiographic appearance rather than their histology.[105,107] Most occur secondarily in preexisting or coexisting lesions.[105,107,121] The radiographic appearance is that of an eccentric, rapidly expanding radiolucent lesion with a thin "blown out" outer margin. The cortex is intact. Vertebral lesions are predominantly in the neural arch, but vertebral body lesions do occur, usually associated with a neural arch lesion (Fig. 3–71). The radiologic appearance may make differential diagnosis from osteoblastoma difficult.[106,107,133] Pelvic ABCs are typically "blow out" lesions and may be very large (Fig. 3–72).

Tumor-Like Conditions of Bone

Paget's Disease

Paget's disease is a common disease of bone that varies in incidence according to geography and may have a familial predisposition. Differing hypotheses for its prevalence in some geographic regions and populations and paucity of cases in others have been advanced without conclusive answers.

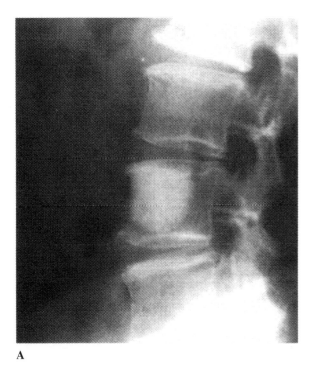

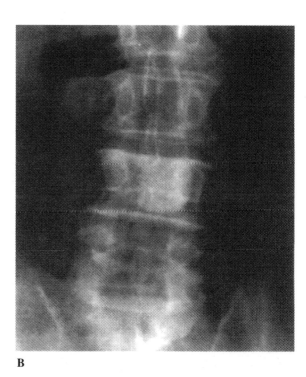

A   B

Fig. 3–70 L4 vertebral body bone island. To determine whether a lesion of this sort is a bone island or an osteoblastic focus may be difficult. The serrated margins of the lesion suggest bone island, but further imaging and possibly a biopsy may be necessary to make a definite diagnosis. *Comment:* The history and symptomatology are vital to making the decision whether to proceed with extensive and expensive further investigation. Comparison with previous films, if available, is very important. Depending on the clinical picture, a period of watchful waiting may be the wisest approach.

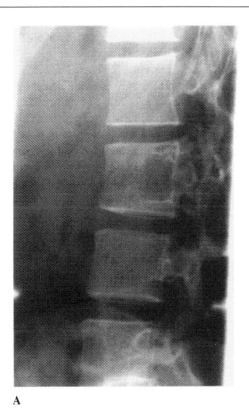

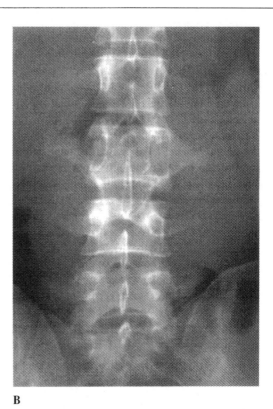

A   B

Fig. 3–71 L3 aneurysmal bone cyst (ABC). An expansile lucent lesion in the posterior arch, transverse processes, and posterior of the vertebral body was proven to be an ABC. Courtesy of Dr. William E. Litterer, Elizabeth, New Jersey.

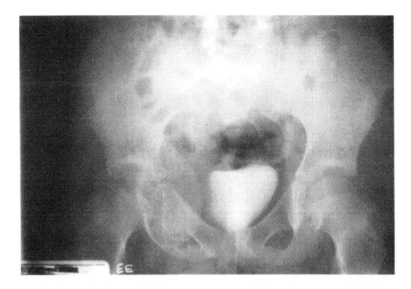

Fig. 3–72 Ischial aneurysmal bone cyst. A large radiolucent "blow out" lesion of the right ischium compresses the lateral aspect of the opacified bladder. *Comment:* The continuous border with a grossly expansile radiolucent lesion is characteristic of an ABC. Courtesy of Dr. Larry Cooperstein, Pittsburgh, Pennsylvania.

Older patients are affected. Paget's is rare in those under 40 years of age, and the incidence rises with age. There is a 2:1 male preponderance.[105,116,134] Most patients with Paget's disease do not have associated symptoms. In those who do, the origin of pain is mechanical, associated with the bony deformities and softening of bone. Any bone may be affected and involvement of multiple bones is usual although monostotic Paget's does occur. The spine and pelvis are common sites of involvement, and the radiographic manifestations are similar to those in other bones, with a few findings that are typical of vertebrae and pelvis[105,116,134] (Fig. 3–73). The third and fourth lumbar vertebrae seem to be predilected sites for involvement as are the pelvic bones.[105] Pelvic involvement may be of a single innominate bone or the entire pelvis including the sacrum. Sacral Paget's without innominate involvement is relatively common[105,116,134] (Figs. 3–74 and 3–75). In the lumbar spine, a "picture frame vertebra" is a distinct presentation where the thickened cortex with relatively radiolucent spongiosa results in the unusual appearance[105,116] (Fig. 3–76). Bony expansion is common with squaring of the vertebral body, especially seen on the lateral view. Accentuation of vertical trabeculae may simulate the appearance of hemangioma.[105,116] Dense vertebral sclerosis, especially in monostotic spinal Paget's, may present as an ivory vertebra. In the few instances where the Pagetic bone has not expanded, the differentiation of a Pagetic ivory vertebra from one due to osteoblastic metastasis or Hodgkin's lymphoma (when scalloping of the vertebral margin is not present) may be difficult.[105,116] Due to the expansile nature of Pagetic bone, spinal stenosis may eventuate with resultant neuropathy.[105,116] In the pelvis, the "brim sign," where trabecular thickening and sclerosis occur along the margin of the pelvic rim obliterating Kohler's teardrop, is a well-known manifestation, but is not pathognomonic for Paget's because osteoblastic metastasis may also obliterate the teardrop. Trabecular thickening and irregularity with bony expansion are the hallmarks of Paget's disease.[105,116,134] Paget's disease and fibrous dysplasia are known as the "great imitators of bone disease," and Paget's must be considered in nearly any presentation of sclerotic bone.[105,116] Paget's disease degenerates malignantly in a small percentage of those afflicted. The malignant transformation may be to osteosarcoma, chondrosarcoma, or fibrosarcoma, and the prognosis is poor.[105,107,121] Malignant degeneration is indicated by visible change in a Pagetic lesion. The alteration is usually lytic, but may be sclerotic or mixed, and is accompanied by localized pain.

Fibrous Dysplasia

Fibrous dysplasia is a bone abnormality of unknown origin, which may be monostotic or polyostotic. It is a relatively common affliction of bone, but rarely affects the spine.[105,118,135] The pelvis, however, is occasionally involved (Fig. 3–77). This may be a monostotic focus, but pelvic lesions are more frequently found in polyostotic disease. The rare instances of vertebral fibrous dysplasia are associated with the polyostotic form, and the vertebral body is affected rather than the neural arch.[105,118,135] Monostotic fibrous dysplasia is usually manifest at about age 14; polyostotic disease without associated endocrine disorders at about 11, and polyostotic disease with endocrine disorders at about age 8. Polyostotic disease with associated endocrine disorders is predominantly a female affliction,

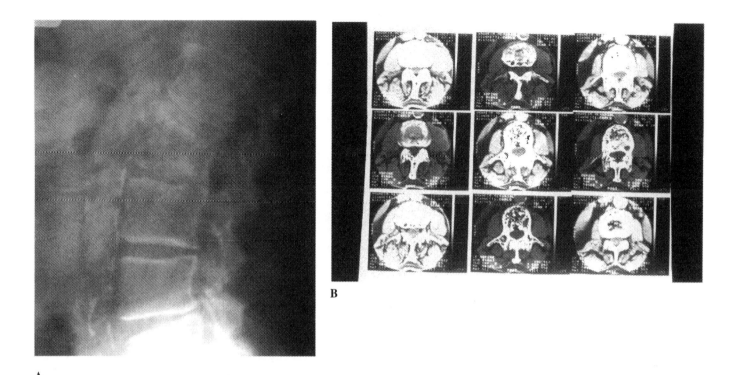

Fig. 3–73 Paget's disease. (**A**). There is expansion of the L2 vertebral body with grossly irregular trabeculae and a striated appearance which extends into the posterior arch as well as the vertebral body. Much less evident striation within the L3 and L4 vertebral bodies is also present. *Comment:* These findings are consistent with Paget's disease, but the vertical striations are reminiscent of hemangioma as well. Note the extensive atherosclerotic calcification in the aorta and the degenerative disk narrowing and facet arthrosis at L4/5. (**B**) This CT scan of another patient with Paget's disease in the lumbar spine is presented to show the abnormal trabeculation within the affected vertebral body.

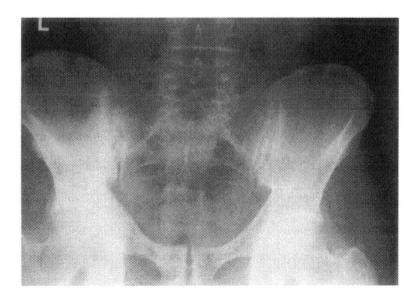

Fig. 3–74 Paget's disease, innominate bone. Increased radiopacity and coarse trabeculation in the ischium and pube of the right innominate are findings typical of Paget's.

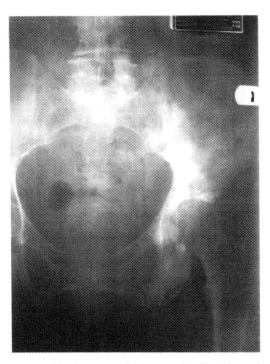

Fig. 3–75 Paget's disease, innominate bone vs. osteoblastic metastasis. Increased radiopacity and coarse trabeculation in the ilium and ischium of the right innominate with obliteration of Kohler's teardrop as show in this patient could represent either Paget's or osteoblastic metastasis. *Comment:* The lack of bony expansion suggests metastasis, but the distribution is more typical of Paget's. Determining whether there are other areas of involvement, and if so their characteristics, is important and may determine the diagnosis without further tests. The final diagnosis in this case was Paget's disease.

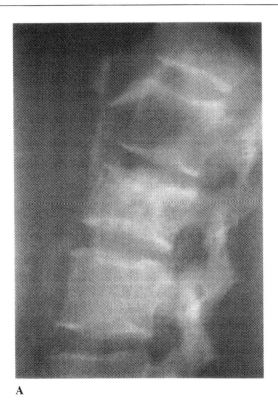

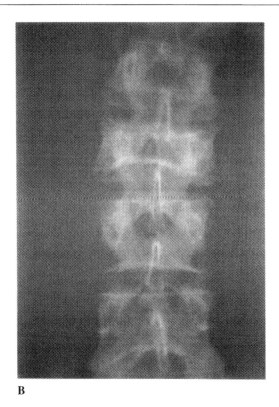

A   B

Fig. 3–76 Paget's disease, picture frame vertebra. L2 has thickened sclerotic trabeculae at the margins of the vertebral body, particularly adjacent to the end plates, causing a "picture frame" or nearly "bone within a bone" appearance. *Comment:* In an older patient, such as is shown here, these findings are indicative of Pagets disease.

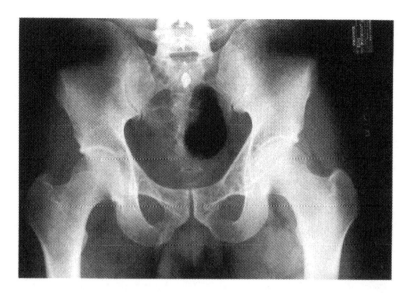

Fig. 3–77 Fibrous dysplasia, left innominate bone. A septated radiolucent, "smoky" or "ground glass" appearance in the tri-radiate area and superior public ramus of the left innominate bone represents a lesion of fibrous dysplasia. *Comment:* Note the residual contrast medium (pantopaque) in the sacral spinal canal from a previous myelogram. Pantopaque is no longer in use as a myelographic medium due to its slow absorption and the potential to cause arachnoiditis. The non-ionic contrast media used today are absorbed and excreted in a short time, but side effects are still encountered occasionally. With the sophistication of MRI, myelography is now a procedure that is only infrequently used.

but the other forms of the disease have no male or female preponderance.[105,118,135] Café-au-lait skin manifestations with irregular borders (coast of Maine appearance) are frequent in fibrous dysplasia. These differ from the café-au-lait spots of neurofibromatosis, which have more smooth, regular margins (coast of California appearance).[105,118] The radiologic hallmark of fibrous dysplasia, as with all fibrous lesions of bone, is a radiolucent "smoky" or "ground glass" appearance within the lesion. Fibrous lesions characteristically have a sclerotic margin called a "rind of sclerosis."[105,118] Areas of sclerosis and areas of greater lucency within lesions of fibrous dysplasia may simulate the appearance of a mixed metastatic focus. Septations within fibrous lesions produce a soap bubble appearance. Bony expansion is not uncommon, and can be differentiated from Pagetic expansion by lack of coarse trabecular accentuation and cortical thickening. Because fibrous tissue is replacing bone in this disease, bony deformity is common.[105,118,135] As with Paget's disease, fibrous dysplasia must be considered with nearly any sclerotic bony abnormality and with many radiolucent lesions. Symptoms in patients with only bony manifestations of fibrous dysplasia are those associated with mechanical difficulties due to the bone softening and deformity. The lesions themselves do not produce symptoms unless fractures occur.

Neurofibromatosis

Neurofibromatosis is an inherited disorder that frequently affects the spine. Café-au-lait spots, multiple soft tissue cutaneous tumors, and bone changes characterize the disease with 50% of those afflicted having skeletal abnormalities. Although the abnormalities are present at birth, they are usually not discovered until early childhood. Neurofibromatosis affects males and females equally.[105,118,136] Spinal manifestations are kyphoscoliosis, usually in the lower thoracic spine, posterior scalloping of vertebral bodies, and enlargement of neural foramina. Posterocentral vertebral scalloping may extend over several segments due to dural ectasia. Eccentric unilateral scalloping occurs from neural tumors (dumbbell tumors) that arise within the spinal canal from nerve roots and extend through and enlarge neural foramina[105,118,136] (Fig. 3–78). There are many extraspinal manifestations of the disease, which will not be discussed here. Spinal findings other than in the low back are more common than those in the lumbopelvic region. There is about a 5% incidence of malignant degeneration in neurofibromatosis.[105,118,136]

SIGNIFICANT INCIDENTAL FINDINGS

It must always be remembered that problems which affect the low back may be related to visceral or vascular disease although the symptoms may seem to be of a musculoskeletal nature. Such entities as aneurysms of the aorta or other vessels, cholecystitis or gallstones or both, urinary stones or urinary tract disease or tumors, liver disease, gastrointestinal disease or tumors, must be considered in evaluation of low back pain. Some of these may have radiographic manifestations that can be seen on radiographs or other imaging studies of the lumbosacral region (Figs. 3–79 and 3–80). Proper evaluation

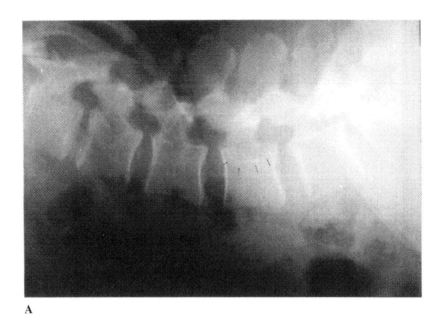

A

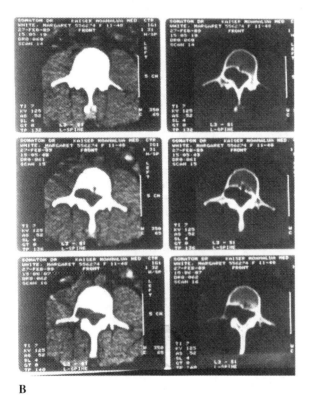

B

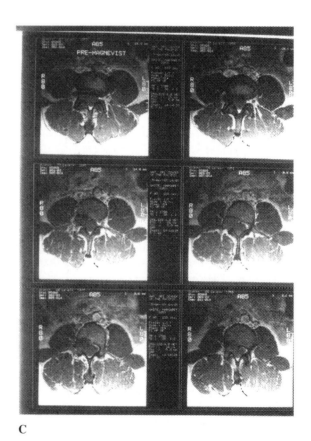

C

Fig. 3–78 (**A**) Neurfibroma. (**B**) and (**C**) Scalloping at the posterior of the L4 vertebral body led to the CT and MRI scans which revealed a large neural tumor ("dumbbell tumor") that had eroded the vertebral body and enlarged the neural foramen as it protruded through.

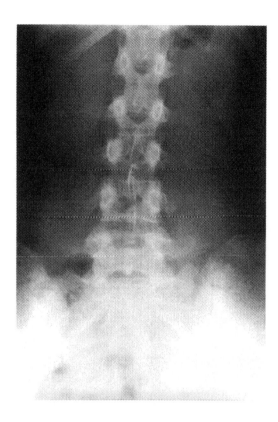

Fig. 3–79 Abdominal cyst. Faint cyst-wall calcification in the left upper abdomen was found in this patient whose radiographs were taken as part of his workup for back pain. *Comment:* The cyst was an incidental finding, unrelated to the presenting symptoms, but demanded further evaluation. It was determined to be a pancreatic cyst.

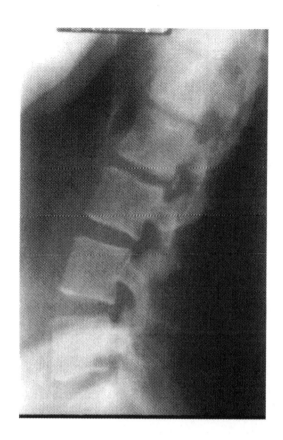

Fig. 3–80 A radiopacity seen in the L2/3 neural foramen adjacent to the posterior of the vertebral body was found lateral to the spine on the AP view (not available) and represented a kidney stone.

of low back radiographs or other imaging examinations must include careful perusal of the visualized soft tissues. Suspicious findings may require further imaging or special examinations to rule out disease that may be of great significance. It is incumbent upon the doctor of chiropractic as a portal of entry physician to be able to detect such abnormalities and, if unable to adequately diagnose the problems or if the patient needs alternative or complementary care, to refer the patient for such services.

Biomechanical or pathological problems in the hips, lower extremities, especially the feet and ankles, or in other spinal or musculoskeletal structures, as well as systemic or neurological diseases impact on the low back and must be considered in evaluation of low back problems. I remember Dr. Logan in a program on shoulder and upper extremity problems that we were presenting beginning his lecture by saying: "Since we are examining a patient for upper extremity problems, we should begin the examination at the logical location—the feet."

REFERENCES

1. Howard BA, Rowe LJ. Spinal x-rays. In: Haldeman S, ed. *Principles and Practice of Chiropractic* (2nd ed.) Norwalk, Conn: Appleton & Lange; 1992: 361–373.

2. Schultz GD, Phillips RB, Cooley J, et al. Diagnostic imaging of the spine in chiropractic practice: Recommendations for utilization. *Chiro J Austr.* 1992; 22:141.

3. Howe JW. Some considerations in spinal x-ray interpretation. *J Clinical Chiropractic.* 1971; 1:75.

4. Howe JW. Fact & fallacies, myths & misconceptions in spinography. *J Clinical Chiropractic.* Archives Ed 1972; 2:34.

5. Yochum TR, Guebert GM, Kettner NW. The tilt-up view: a closer look at the lumbosacral junction. *Appl Diagn Imag.* 1989; 1:49.

6. Eisenberg RL, Akin JR, Hedgcock MW. Single, well centered lateral view of the lumbosacral spine: Is a coned view necessary? *AJR.* 1979; 133:711.

7. Merrill V. *Atlas of Roentgenographic Positions and Standard Radiologic Procedures* (4th ed) St. Louis, Mo: Mosby; 1975: 1.

8. Jaeger SA. *Atlas of Radiographic Positioning: Normal Anatomy and Developmental Variants.* Norwalk, Conn: Appleton & Lange; 1988.

9. Rowe LJ, Yochum TR. Radiographic positioning and normal anatomy. In: Yochum TR, Rowe LJ, eds. *Essentials of Skeletal Radiology* (2nd ed.) Baltimore, Md: Williams & Wilkins; 1996: 1–138.

10. Howe JW, Foreman SM, Glenn WV Jr. Advanced Imaging Modalities. In: Haldeman S, ed. *Principles and Practice of Chiropractic.* 2nd ed.: Norwalk, Conn: Appleton & Lange; 1992: 361, 371–389.

11. Rothman SLG, Glenn WV Jr. *Multiplanar CT of the Spine.* Baltimore, Md: University Park Press; 1985.

12. Rauschening W. Correlative multiplanar computed tomographic anatomy of the normal spine. In: Post JD, ed. *Computed Tomography of the Spine.* Baltimore, Md: Williams & Wilkins; 1984: 1–57.

13. Shapiro R: Computed tomographic anatomy of the lumbosacral spine. In: Post JD, ed. *Computed Tomography of the Spine.* Baltimore, Md: Williams & Wilkins; 1984: 78–93.

14. Kerber CW, Glenn WV Jr, Rothman SLG. Lumbar computed tomography/Multiplanar reformations, A reading primer. In: Post JD, ed. *Computed Tomography of the Spine.* Baltimore, Md: Williams & Wilkins; 1984: 155–174.

15. Yochum TR, Barry MS. Diagnostic imaging of the musculoskeletal system. In: Yochum TR, Rowe LJ, eds. *Essentials of Skeletal Radiology* (2nd ed). Baltimore, Md: Williams & Wilkins; 1996: 373–545.

16. Modic MT, Masaryk TJ, Ross JS. *Magnetic Resonance Imaging of the Spine.* Chicago, Ill: Year Book; 1989.

17. Edelman RR, Hesselink JR, eds. *Clinical Magnetic Resonance Imaging.* Philadelphia, Pa: Saunders; 1990.

18. Stoller DW, Genant HK. Magnetic resonance imaging of the lumbar spine. In: Weinstein JN, Wiesel SW, eds. *The Lumbar Spine.* Philadelphia: WB Saunders; 1990: 320–336.

19. Ross JS, Masaryk TJ, Modic MT. Gadolinium DTPA–enhanced MR images of the lumbar spine. Time, course, and mechanism of enhancement. *AJNR.* 1989; 10:37.

20. Thrall JH, Ziessman HA. *Nuclear Medicine: The Requisites.* St. Louis, Mo: Mosby; 1995.

21. Lavender JP, Lowe J, Barker JR, et al. Gallium-67 citrate scanning in neoplastic and inflammatory lesions. *Br J Radiol.* 1971; 44:361.

22. Ghelman B. Discography. In: Krikun MR, ed. *Imaging Modalities in Spinal Disorders.* Philadelphia, Pa: Saunders; 1988: 538–556.

23. Aguet L, Lane B. Imaging of degenerative disc of the lumbar spine. *Postgrad Radiol.* 1987; 7:241.

24. Ninomiya M, Mann T. Pathoanatomy of lumbar disc herniation as demonstrated by computed tomography/discography. *Spine.* 1992; 17:1316.

25. Vanharanta H, Sachs BL, Spivey MA, et al. The relationship of pain provocation to lumbar disc deterioration as seen by CT/discography. *Spine.* 1987; 12:295.

26. Weisel SW, Tsourmas N, Feff HL, et al. A study of computer assisted tomography: The incidence of positive CAT scans in an asymptomatic group of patients. *Spine.* 1984; 9:549.

27. Ferguson AB. *Roentgen Diagnosis of Extremities and Spine.* New York, Ny: Hoebner; 1949.

28. Ferguson AB. The clinical and roentgenographic interpretation of lumbosacral anomalies. *Radiology.* 22:934–948.

29. Rowe LJ, Yochum TR. Measurements in skeletal radiology. In: Yochum TR, Rowe LJ, eds. *Essentials of Skeletal Radiology* (2nd ed.) Baltimore, Md: Williams & Wilkins; 1996: 139–196.

30. Banks SD. The use of spinographic parameters in diagnosis of lumbar facet and disc abnormalities. *J Manipulative Physiol Ther.* 1983; 6:113.

31. Hansson T, Bigos S, Beecher P, et al. The lumbar lordosis in acute and chronic low back pain. *Spine.* 1985; 10:154.

32. Hadley LA. Intervertebral joint subluxation, bony impingement, and foraminal encroachment with nerve root changes. *AJR.* 1951; 65:377.

33. Hadley, LA. *Anatomico–Roentgenographic Studies of the Spine* (5th ed.) Springfield, Ill: Charles C Thomas; 1951.

34. Howe JW. Determination of lumbosacral facet subluxations. *Roentgenological Briefs.* Council on Roentgenology, American Chiropractic Assn. Aug 1970.

35. Yochum TR, Rowe LJ. *Essentials of Skeletal Radiology* (2nd ed.) Baltimore, Md: Williams & Wilkins; 1996.

36. Meyerding HW. Spondylolisthesis. *Surg Gynecol Obstet.* 1932; 54:371.

37. *Basic Chiropractic Procedural Manual.* Des Moines, Iowa: American Chiropractic Assn; 1973.

38. Cobb JR. Outline for the study of scoliosis. *Am Acad Orthop Surg.* 1948; 5:261.

39. Risser JC, Ferguson AB. Scoliosis: Its prognosis. *J Bone Joint Surg (Am).* 1936; 18:667.

40. Eisenstein S. Measurements in the lumbar spinal canal in two racial groups. *Clin Orthop Rel Res.* 1976; 115:42.

41. Jones RAC, Thompson JLG. The narrow lumbar canal. *J Bone Joint Surg (Br).* 1968; 50:595.

42. MacGibbon B, Farfan H. A radiologic survey of various configurations of the lumbar spine. *Spine.* 1979; 4:258.

43. Cox JM. *Low Back Pain. Mechanism, Diagnosis, and Treatment* (5th ed.) Baltimore, Md: Williams & Wilkins; 1990.

44. Schmorl G, Junghanns H. *The Human Spine in Health and Disease* (2nd ed.) New York, Ny: Grune & Stratton; 1971.

45. Epstein BS. *The Spine—A Radiological Text and Atlas* (4th ed.) Philadelphia, Pa: Lea & Febiger; 1976.

46. Murray RO, Jacobson HG. *The Radiology of Skeletal Disorders.* New York, Ny: Churchill Livingstone; 1977.

47. Yochum TR, Hartley B, Thomas DP, et al. A radiographic anthology of vertebral names. *J Manipulative Physiol Ther.* 1985; 8:87.

48. Gjorup PA. Dorsal hemivertebrae. *Acta Orthop Scand.* 1964; 35:117.

49. Tini PG, Wieser C, Zinn WM. The transitional vertebra of the lumbosacral spine: Its radiological classification, incidence, prevalence and clinical significance. *Rheumatol Rehabil.* 1977; 16:180.

50. Guebert GM, Yochum TR, Rowe LJ. Congenital anomalies and normal skeletal variants. In: Yochum TR, Rowe LJ, eds. *Essentials of Skeletal Radiology* (2nd ed.) Baltimore, Md: Williams & Wilkins; 1996:197   .

51. Rich EA. *Atlas of Clinical Roentgenology.* Indianapolis, Ind: RAE Publishing Co; 1965.

52. Nachemson A. The lumbar spine–an orthopedic challenge. *Spine.* 1976; 1:59.

53. Magora A, Schwartz A. Relation between the low back pain syndrome and x–ray findings. III. Spina bifida occulta. *Scand J Rehabil Med.* 1980; 12:9.

54. Onitsuka H. Roentgenologic aspects of bone islands. *Radiology.* 1977; 123:67.

55. Greenspan A, Steiner G, Knutzon R. Bone island (enostosis): Clinical significance and radiologic and pathologic considerations. *Skeletal Radiol.* 1991; 20:85.

56. Sickle EA, Gennant HK, Hoffer PB. Increased localization of 99M TE-pyrophosphate in a bone island: Case report. *J Nucl Med.* 1976; 17:113.

57. Davies JA, Hall FM, Goldberg RP, et al. Positive bone scans in bone islands. *J Bone Joint Surg (Am).* 1979; 61:6.

58. Rowe LJ, Yochum TR. Trauma. In: Yochum TR, Rowe LJ, eds. *Essentials of Skeletal Radiology* (2nd ed.) Baltimore, Md: Williams & Wilkins; 1996: 653–   .

59. Krikun M, Krikun R. Fractures of the lumbar spine. *Semin Roentgenol.* 1992; 27:262.

60. Chance GQ. Notes on type of flexion fracture of spine. *Br J Radiol.* 1948; 21:452.

61. Gertzbein SD. Spine update: Classification of thoracic and lumbar fractures. *Spine.* 1994; 19:626.

62. Roaf R. A study of the mechanics of spinal injuries. *J Bone Joint Surg (Br).* 1960; 42:810.

63. Gehweiler JA, Osborne RI, Becker RF. *The Radiology of Vertebral Trauma.* Philadelphia, Pa: Saunders; 1980.

64. Atlas SW, Regenbogen V, Rogers LF, et al. The radiographic characterization of burst fractures of the spine. *AJR.* 1986; 147:575.

65. Jackson H, Kam J, Harris JH. The sacral arcuate lines in upper sacral fractures. *Radiology.* 1982; 145:35.

66. Rogers LF. *The Radiology of Skeletal Trauma* (2nd ed.) New York, Ny: Churchill Livingstone; 1992: 1 & 2.

67. Borkow SE, Kleiger B. Spondylolisthesis in the newborn: A case report. *Clin Orthop.* 1971; 81:73.

68. Turner RH, Bianco AJ. Spondylolysis and spondylolisthesis in children and teen-agers. *J Bone Joint Surg (Am).* 1971; 53:1298.

69. Wiltse LL, Widell EH, Jackson DW. Fatigue fracture: The basic lesion in isthmic spondylolisthesis. *J Bone Joint Surg (Am).* 1975; 57:17.

70. Cyron BM, Hutton WC. The fatigue strength of the lumbar neural arch in spondylolysis. *J Bone Joint Surg (Br).* 1978; 60:462.

71. Yochum TR, Rowe LJ, Barry MS. Natural history of spondylolysis and spondylolisthesis. In: Yochum TR, Rowe LJ, eds. *Essentials of Skeletal Radiology* (2nd ed.) Baltimore, Md: Williams & Wilkins; 1996: 327–372.

72. Frymoyer JW, Newberg A, Pope MH, et al. Spine radiographs in patients with low back pain. *J Bone Joint Surg (Am).* 1984; 66:1048.

73. Waddell G. A new clinical model for the treatment of low back pain. In: Weinstein JM, Wiesel SW, eds. *The Lumbar Spine.* Philadelphia, Pa: Saunders; 1990: 38–56.

74. Wiesel SW, Feffer HL, Rothman RH. A lumbar spine algorithm. In: Weinstein JM, Wiesel SW, eds. *The Lumbar Spine.* Philadelphia, Pa: Saunders; 1990: 358–368.

75. Garfin SR, Herkowitz HN. The intervertebral disc. In: Weinstein JM, Wiesel SW, eds. *The Lumbar Spine.* Philadelphia, Pa: Saunders; 1990: 369–380.

76. Jensen MC, Brant-Zawadsji MW, Obuchowski N, et al. Magnetic resonance imaging of the lumbar spine in people without back pain. *N Eng. J Med.* 1994; 331:69.

77. Giles LGF. *Anatomical Basis of Low Back Pain.* Baltimore, Md: Williams & Wilkins; 1989.

78. Resnick D, Niwayama G. Degenerative diseases of the spine. In: Resnick D, Niwayama G, eds. *Diagnosis of Bone and Joint Disorders.* 2nd ed. Philadelphia, Pa: Saunders; 1988; 3: 1480–1561.

79. Resnick D, Niwayama G, Guerra J, et al. Spinal vacuum phenomena: Anatomical study and review. *Radiology.* 1981; 139:341.

80. Rowe LJ, Yochum TR. Arthritic disorders. In: Yochum TR, Rowe LJ. *Essentials of Skeletal Radiology* (2nd ed.) Baltimore, Md: Williams & Wilkins; 1996: 795–973.

81. Forrester DM, Brown JC. *The Radiology of Joint Disease.* Philadelphia, Pa: Saunders; 1987.

82. Rowe LJ, Yochum TR. Hematological and vascular disorders. In: Yochum TR, Rowe LJ. *Essentials of Skeletal Radiology* (2nd ed.) Baltimore, Md: Williams & Wilkins; 1996: 1243–1326.

83. Bush K, Cowan N, Katz DE, et al. The natural history of sciatica associated with disc pathology. *Spine.* 1992; 17:1205.

84. Rowe LJ, Yochum TR. Infection. In: Yochum TR, Rowe LJ. eds. *Essentials of Skeletal Radiology* (2nd ed.) Baltimore, Md: Williams & Wilkins; 1996: 1193–1241.

85. Resnick D. Neuroarthropathy. In: Resnick D, Niwayama G, eds. *Diagnosis of Bone and Joint Disorders.* 2nd ed. Philadelphia, Pa: Saunders; 1988; 5: 3154–3185.

86. Resnick D, Niwayama G. Osteomyelitis, septic arthritis, and soft tissue infection. The axial skeleton. In: Resnick D, Niwayama G, eds. *Diagnosis of Bone and Joint Disorders* (2nd ed.) Philadelphia, Pa: Saunders; 1988; 4: 2647–2754.

87. Resnick D, Niwayama G. Rheumatoid arthritis: In: Resnick D, Niwayama G, eds. *Diagnosis of Bone and Joint Disorders* (2nd ed.) Philadelphia, Pa: Saunders; 1988; 2: 955–1067.

88. Resnick D, Niwayama G. Rheumatoid arthritis and the seronegative spondyloarthropathies: Radiographic and pathologic concepts. In: Resnick D, Niwayama G, eds. *Diagnosis of Bone and Joint Disorders* (2nd ed.) Philadelphia, Pa: Saunders; 1988; 2: 894–953.

89. Hill HHF, Hill AGS, Bodmer JG. Clinical diagnosis of ankylosing spondylitis in women and relation to the presence of HLA-B-27. *Am Rheum Dis.* 1976; 35:267.

90. Resnick D, Niwayama G. Ankylosing spondylitis. In: Resnick D, Niwayama G, eds. *Diagnosis of Bone and Joint Disorders* (2nd ed.) Philadelphia, Pa: Saunders; 1988; 2: 1103–1170.

91. Resnick D, Niwayama G. Psoriatic arthritis. In: Resnick D, Niwayama G. eds. *Diagnosis of Bone and Joint Disorders* (2nd ed.) Philadelphia, Pa: Saunders; 1988; 2: 1171–1198.

92. Resnick D, Niwayama G. Reiter's syndrome. In: Resnick D, Niwayama G. eds. *Diagnosis of Bone and Joint Disorders* (2nd ed.) Philadelphia, Pa: Saunders; 1988; 2: 1199–1217.

93. Resnick D, Niwayama G. Enteropathic arthropathies. In: Resnick D, Niwayama G. eds. *Diagnosis of Bone and Joint Disorders* (2nd ed.) Philadelphia, Pa: Saunders; 1988; 2:1218–1251.

94. Resnick D, Niwayama G. Gouty arthritis. In: Resnick D, Niwayama G. eds. *Diagnosis of Bone and Joint Disorders* (2nd ed.) Philadelphia, Pa: Saunders; 1988; 3: 1618–1671.

95. Resnick D, Niwayama G. Calcium hydroxyapatite crystal deposition disease. In: Resnick D, Niwayama G, eds. *Diagnosis of Bone and Joint Disorders* (2nd ed.) Philadelphia, Pa: Saunders; 1988; 3: 1733–1764.

96. Resnick D, Niwayama G. Calcium pyrophosphate dihydrate (CPPD) crystal deposition disease. In: Resnick D, Niwayama G, eds. *Diagnosis of Bone and Joint Disorders* (2nd ed.) Philadelphia, Pa: Saunders; 1988; 1673–1764.

97. Resnick D, Niwayama G. Alkaptonuria. In: Resnick D, Niwayama G. eds. *Diagnosis of Bone and Joint Disorders* (2nd ed.) Philadelphia, Pa: Saunders; 1988; 3: 1787–1803.

98. Rowe LJ, Yochum TR. Nutritional, metabolic and endocrine disorders. In: Yochum TR, Rowe LJ, eds. *Essentials of Skeletal Radiology* (2nd ed.) Baltimore, Md: Williams & Wilkins; 1996; 1327–1370.

99. Resnick D, Niwayama G. Osteoporosis. In: Resnick D, Niwayama G, eds. *Diagnosis of Bone and Joint Disorders* (2nd ed.) Philadelphia, Pa: Saunders; 1988; 4: 2022–2085.

100. Resnick D. Hemoglobinopathies and other anemias. In: Resnick D, Niwayama G, eds. *Diagnosis of Bone and Joint Disorders* (2nd ed.) Philadelphia, Pa: Saunders; 1988; 4: 2321–2357.

101. Rowe LJ, Yochum TR. Hematologic and vascular disorders. In: Yochum TR, Rowe LJ. eds. *Essentials of Skeletal Radiology.* 2nd ed. Baltimore MD: Williams & Wilkins; 1996; 1243–1326.

102. Resnick D. Disorders of other endocrine glands and of pregnancy. In: Resnick D, Niwayama G, eds. *Diagnosis of Bone and Joint Disorders* (2nd ed.) Philadelphia, Pa: Saunders; 1988; 4: 2287–2317.

103. Pitt MJ. Rickets and osteomalacia. In: Resnick D, Niwayama G. eds. *Diagnosis of Bone and Joint Disorders* (2nd ed.) Philadelphia, Pa: Saunders; 1988; 4: 2087–2126.

104. Resnick D, Niwayama G. Parathyroid disorders and renal osteodystrophy. In: Resnick D, Niwayama G, eds. *Diagnosis of Bone and Joint Disorders* (2nd ed.) Philadelphia, Pa: Saunders; 1988; 4: 2219–2285.

105. Yochum TR, Rowe LJ. Tumors and tumorlike processes. In: Yochum TR, Rowe LJ. eds. *Essentials of Skeletal Radiology* (2nd ed.) Baltimore, Md: Williams & Wilkins; 1996; 975–1191.

106. Resnick D, Niwayama G. Skeletal metastasis. In: Resnick D, Niwayama G, eds. *Diagnosis of Bone and Joint Disorders* (2nd ed.) Philadelphia, Pa: Saunders; 1988; 6: 3945–4010.

107. Resnick D, Kyriakis M, Greenway GD. Tumors and tumor-like lesions of bone: Imaging and pathology of specific lesions. In: Resnick D, Niwayama G, eds. *Diagnosis of Bone and Joint Disorders* (2nd ed.) Philadelphia, Pa: Saunders; 1988; 6: 3617–3888.

108. Wilner D. Ewing's sarcoma. In: Wilner D. ed. *Radiology of Bone Tumors and Allied Disorders*. Philadelphia, Pa: Saunders; 1982; 3: 2462–2573.

109. Wilner D. Osteogenic sarcoma (osteosarcoma). In: Wilner D, ed. *Radiology of Bone Tumors and Allied Disorders*. Philadelphia, Pa: Saunders; 1982; 3: 1897–2095.

110. Deutch A, Resnick D. Eccentric cortical metastases to the skeleton form bronchogenic carcinoma. *Radiology*. 1980; 137:49.

111. Hendrix RW, Rogers LF, Davis TM Jr. Cortical bone metastasis. *Radiology*. 1991; 181:409.

112. McDougal IR. Skeletal scintigraphy. *Western J Med*. 1979; 130:503.

113. Litterer WE. Nuclear bone scanning—Skeletal imaging. *J Clin Chiro*. 1980; 3:7.

114. Lodwick, GW. The bones and joints. In: Hodes PJ, ed. *An Atlas of Tumor Radiology*. Chicago, Ill: Year Book; 1973.

115. Resnick D. Tumors and tumor-like lesions of bone: Radiographic principles. In: Resnick D, Niwayama G, eds. *Diagnosis of Bone and Joint Disorders* (2nd ed.) Philadelphia, Pa: Saunders; 1988; 6: 3603–3615.

116. Resnick D, Niwayama G. Paget's disease. In: Resnick D, Niwayama G, eds. *Diagnosis of Bone and Joint Disorders*. Philadelphia, Pa: Saunders; 1988; 4: 2127–2170.

117. Resnick D, Haghighi P. Myeloproliferative disorders. In: Resnick D, Niwayama G, eds. *Diagnosis of Bone and Joint Disorders* (2nd ed.) Philadelphia, Pa: Saunders; 1988; 4: 2459–2496.

118. Feldman F Tuberous sclerosis, neurofibromatosis, and fibrous dysplasia. In: Resnick D, Niwayama G, eds. *Diagnosis of Bone and Joint Disorders* (2nd ed.) Philadelphia, Pa: Saunders; 1988; 6: 4033–4072.

119. Resnick D. Plasma cell dyscrasias and dysgammaglobulinemias. In Resnick D, Niwayama G, eds. *Diagnosis of Bone and Joint Disorders* (2nd ed.) Philadelphia, Pa: Saunders; 1988; 4: 2358–2403.

120. Wilner D. Myeloma. In: Wilner D, ed. *Radiology of Bone Tumors and Allied Disorders*. Philadelphia, Pa: Saunders; 1982; 3: 2039–2765.

121. Mirra JM. *Bone Tumors*. Philadelphia, Pa: Lippincott; 1980.

122. Ludwig H, Kumpan W, Sinzinger H. Radiography and bone scintigraphy in multiple myeloma: A comparative analysis. *Br J Radiol*. 1982; 55:173.

123. Wilner D. Chondrosarcoma. In: Wilner D, ed. *Radiology of Bone Tumors and Allied Disorders*. Philadelphia, Pa: Saunders; 1982; 3: 2170–2280.

124. Wilner D. Fibrosarcoma. In: Wilner D, ed. *Radiology of Bone Tumors and Allied Disorders*. Philadelphia, Pa: Saunders; 1982; 3: 2281–2326.

125. Wilner D. Chordoma. In: Wilner D, ed. *Radiology of Bone Tumors and Allied Disorders*. Philadelphia, Pa: Saunders; 1982; 3: 2807–2856.

126. Wilner D. Malignant hematologic and lymphoid disorders of bone. In: Wilner D, ed. *Radiology of Bone Tumors and Allied Disorders*. Philadelphia, Pa: Saunders; 1982; 3: 2859–2945.

127. Wilner D. Malignant giant cell tumor. In: Wilner D, ed. *Radiology of Bone Tumors and Allied Disorders*. Philadelphia, Pa: Saunders; 1982; 3: 2356–2386.

128. Wilner D. Benign vascular tumors and allied disorders of bone. In: Wilner D, ed. *Radiology of Bone Tumors and Allied Disorders*. Philadelphia, Pa: Saunders; 1982; 1: 660–782.

129. Wilner D. Osteochondroma. In: Wilner D, ed. *Radiology of Bone Tumors and Allied Disorders*. Philadelphia, Pa: Saunders; 1982; 1: 271–386.

130. Wilner D. Osteoid osteoma. In: Wilner D, ed. *Radiology of Bone Tumors and Allied Disorders*. Philadelphia, Pa: Saunders; 1982; 1: 144–216.

131. Wilner D. Benign osteoblastoma. In: Wilner D, ed. *Radiology of Bone Tumors and Allied Disorders*. Philadelphia, Pa: Saunders; 1982; 1: 217–270.

132. Wilner D. Enchondroma. In: Wilner D, ed. *Radiology of Bone Tumors and Allied Disorders*. Philadelphia, Pa: Saunders; 1982; 1: 387–437.

133. Wilner D. Aneurysmal bone cyst. In: Wilner D, ed. *Radiology of Bone Tumors and Allied Disorders*. Philadelphia, Pa: Saunders; 1982; 1: 1003–1103.

134. Wilner D. Paget's disease of bone (Osteitis deformans). In: Wilner D, ed. *Radiology of Bone Tumors and Allied Disorders*. Philadelphia, Pa: Saunders; 1982; 2: 1646–1750.

135. Wilner D. Fibrous dysplasia of bone. In: Wilner D, ed. *Radiology of Bone Tumors and Allied Disorders*. Philadelphia, Pa: Saunders; 1982; 2: 1443–1580.

136. Wilner D. Neurofibromatosis. In: Wilner D, ed. *Radiology of Bone Tumors and Allied Disorders*. Philadelphia, Pa: Saunders; 1982; 2: 1551–1645.

Muscle testing is essential in the examination of all musculoskeletal problems. A muscle imbalance becomes an important objective finding when it verifies subjective complaints, the observation of functional tests, and palpation findings. If muscle weakness is found to be a causative factor, it becomes an important part of the treatment protocol.

Testing of an individual muscle is difficult, if not impossible. When isolating a primary muscle, evaluating it will include the secondary support muscles and stabilizers of the part being tested. The most definitive text on testing is *Muscles: Testing and Function* by Kendall.[1]

Muscle testing is the continuation of an active movement by the patient while the examiner uses his or her skill to provide resistance. That resistance should be from a direction where the part being tested is in a position that elicits the greatest response from the primary muscle. The skilled examiner has a clear understanding of the muscles, their origins, insertions, and function. It is important to observe the patient's effort and the body reaction during the test.

The movement of an articulation requires primary and secondary movers and joint stabilizers. Secondary support muscles stabilize the structures upon which the movers originate. A lack of normal strength in muscles other than the primary mover may result in compensation, adaptation, or abnormal recruitment for stabilization by the affected person.

Testing of the primary mover may seem normal yet be accompanied by obvious shifting of the body to give the secondary muscles greater advantage. An abnormal muscle reaction, such as shaking of the primary muscle during the test, may be observed. Often, in the presence of a weak primary muscle, there will be an exaggerated attempt to secure the rest of the body during the test. The prime mover may test weak in the presence of a weak secondary muscle that fails to secure the primary's origin. For example, testing the hip flexors (psoas and iliacus) with a weak iliocostalis lumborum on the opposite side will result in an apparent weakness. Observation of the patient will show abnormal abdominal movement during the test.

To effectively test a muscle, the patient must understand what is being done and what is expected of him or her. Place the patient in a position that gives the muscle being tested the greatest advantage. Have the patient hold that position. By using an open hand (if possible) to apply resistance, the patient is better able to discern the direction of the applied force. Grasping the area to be tested can confuse the patient as to the direction in which to resist.

Apply light pressure, instructing the patient to resist, and determine if any pain is elicited. Pain will negate the test. To determine the relative strength of the muscle, apply force in a gradual manner until you have satisfied yourself that the muscle has sufficient strength, or gives way. It is best to test the muscle several times and compare bilaterally or with its antagonist or both where possible. Comparing both sides for signs of weakness or imbalance is essential to a correct diagnosis. Muscle balance, not strength, is the key to comfort and normal function. By testing the muscle several times in a row, a more accurate assessment can be made. If the muscle tests within normal limits the first time but weakens on subsequent attempts, it can be assumed to be dysfunctional.

The object of muscle testing is not to overpower the muscle, but to determine whether the muscle responds in a manner that appears normal for the patient. Age, sex, and general body type of the patient must be considered. Even a strong athlete can be assessed with proper technique. Testing muscles in this fashion can be reasonably objective as long as the examiner is careful to keep an open mind, not allowing other evaluation findings to prejudice his or her expectations. Experience and practice, being careful to use a consistent pressure and test setup, give the examiner the ability to objectify the procedure.

As stated previously, pain negates the test. It is important to observe the patient for signs of bodily pain as well as facial expression in response to the test. Patients are often reluctant to report pain, and they should be informed to relate any symptoms to the examiner. It is important to know the point in the test where the pain is noted. The location and functional point of pain will be important information in the diagnosis, helping locate a muscle tear, tendonitis, or bursitis. Pain away from the area being tested may indicate a problem with the support structures.

Recruitment of other muscles may be necessary for the patient to perform the test. Most movements of the body are carried out smoothly with ease and strength against varying degrees of resistance. In the presence of pain, joint dysfunction, or weakness, the body cannot perform normally and is forced to use alternative methods to achieve the desired function.

The normally smooth action gives way to an obviously adaptive action. The body may shift to establish a new point of stability. Unusual movement of other muscles may occur to provide better support. There may be a deviation in the direction of resistance away from the expected direction of the test. The body "cheats" in order to achieve the desired action or response. The cheating is quite individualized and can be subtle. The experienced examiner knows what to expect from normal, functioning anatomy and should be able to read these attempts to cheat.

To determine whether a secondary muscle is at fault, apply manual assistance to the suspected muscle, or do its job by stabilizing the structure while retesting the primary muscle.

When a muscle tests weak, goad the origin and insertion. Goading is a rapid, deep oscillating pressure using the finger or thumb pad, without allowing the contact to slide over the skin. If the muscle has had a mild stretch, it may not be weak and will respond to goading that will stimulate the Golgi tendon organs and "reset" the muscle. Retest several times. If the muscle is truly weak, it may seem normal on the first test but weaken quickly.

When a true weakness is found there are a number of possible causes to consider. A muscle can be weak from lack of use in a lazy patient. A muscle may be stretched as a result of a loss of use and normal habit patterns. For example, the abdominals during pregnancy are stretched and are out of use. If they are not deliberately restored by consistent exercise postpartum, they may remain chronically weak. This is a common finding in women. Another common situation is an overstretching of the popliteus muscle with excessive hyperexten-

sion of the knee, as in sitting with the heels on a footstool and the knees unsupported in hyperextension.[2]

A muscle may be weak from a loss of normal joint alignment that can alter the fulcrum of action. Hypertonic muscles will often test weak. Spinal subluxation may weaken the nerve supply to a muscle. Fixations can inhibit muscle function (see Appendix A). Fixations are spinal articulations that have no movement but are not necessarily out of alignment.

Dr. Logan found in his clinical research two fixation patterns that consistently cause specific muscle reactions. One is an anterior fixation of the atlas with the occiput causing a weakness of the dorsiflexors of the foot. The other is a fixation of L5 causing a weakness of the gluteus maximus. Fixation theory has proven consistent in the clinical setting. It may elude explanation from a purely anatomical perspective, but is worth considering for further research. Organic problems can affect muscle function (see Appendix A).

Injury to a muscle can affect strength. A minor strain without fiber damage can cause prolonged underfunctioning and may respond to mild exercise. A mild strain with minimal fiber damage may test at 80% of normal without significant pain. A moderate strain will test weak or show little function and demonstrate palpable pain. Severe injuries can cause disruption of the muscle or tendon and require surgical repair. Muscle injury can be tears in the belly of the muscle, at the muscle/tendon interface, or at the tendon/bone interface. In examining the muscles, abnormal function will lead to an investigation of all the factors affecting their function and to a diagnosis.

MUSCLE EXAMINATION

Gluteus Maximus

The gluteus maximus (Fig. 4–1) is the primary extensor of the thigh and is tested while the patient is prone. Grasp the ankle and flex the knee to 90°, then lift the thigh off the table (Fig. 4–2). The examiner's other hand should stabilize the lumbosacral area. The patient should be relaxed and encouraged not to help. Ascertain if there is any discomfort, and ask the patient to attempt to hold the leg in the elevated position. When the patient is secure, test the muscle by applying pressure against the posterior thigh just above the knee. The pressure is in the direction of flexion.

When lifting the thigh from the table, note any lateral deviation. An immediate "popping out" of the knee laterally indicates a probable piriformis hypertonicity (Fig. 4–3). A more gradual lateral deviation as the end point of lift is reached suggests the maximus itself may be hypertonic. Weakness of the contralateral quadratus lumborum (Q-L) will reduce the support needed to stabilize the low back and pelvis, allowing the maximus to function. Grasp the Q-L and assist it while testing

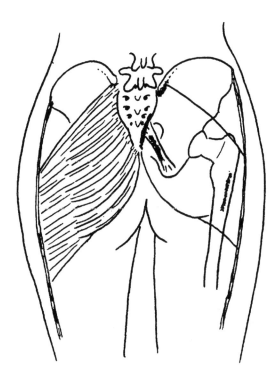

Fig. 4–1 Gluteus maximus: left superficial, right deep attachments.

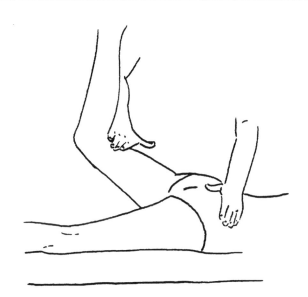

Fig. 4–2 Gluteus maximus test.

the maximus. If there is a better response, correct the Q-L.

The gluteus maximus is innervated by fibers from L5, S1, and S2 via the inferior gluteal nerve. Fixation theory finds a bilateral weakness associated with an upper cervical fixation (see Appendix A). A unilateral weakness can be affected by a

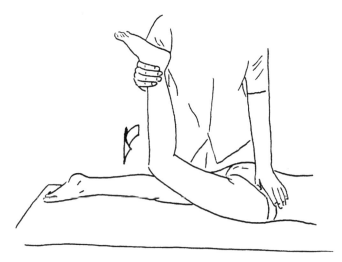

Fig. 4–3 Passive hip extension—lateral flare of knee indicates piriformis or gluteus maximus hypertonicity.

posterior rotation fixation of L5 on the opposite side. Weakness can also be found with prostate or menstrual problems (see Appendix A).

Gluteus Medius

The medius (Fig. 4–4) is a major abductor. The anterior fibers assist in medial rotation, and the posterior fibers assist in lateral rotation. The best way to isolate this muscle is with the patient lying on his or her side. Have the patient bend the under leg. The examiner should stabilize the pelvis with the free hand. Test the side that is up by abducting the leg with slight

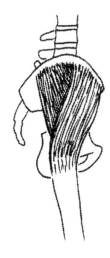

Fig. 4–4 Gluteus medius.

extension and lateral rotation. Apply pressure near the ankle in the direction of adduction and flexion (Fig. 4–5). This is the primary lateral stabilizer of the pelvis and should be strong in order to function normally.

Gluteus Minimus

The minimus (Fig. 4–6) is the primary abductor of the leg. The test is done with the patient in the same position as for the medius test. The upper leg is placed in neutral abduction (no extension or rotation). Pressure is directed into adduction with slight extension.

A second method of testing is with the patient supine. The leg is abducted and resistance is applied against adduction pressure (Fig. 4–7).

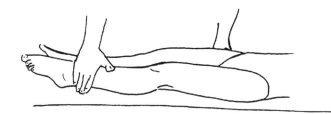

Fig. 4–7 Gluteus minimus test—patient supine.

Piriformis and Lateral Rotators

The piriformis (Fig. 4–8) is the major lateral rotator. It is impossible to isolate it from the other muscles in the group, the quadratus femoris, obturators, and gemelli. Fine-tuning a diagnosis of these muscles can be done with careful palpation, isolating origins and insertions that are reactive.

The patient is prone. Flex the knee to 90°. Use the open hand against the medial ankle (Fig. 4–9). Grasping the ankle can confuse the patient. Make sure the patient understands the direction of force that is lateral. The lateral movement is actually medially rotating the thigh.

Kendall[1] demonstrates this test with the patient in the sitting position; however, Kendall tests the rotational aspect when the muscle is acting more as an abductor. It is more accurate to test its abduction action in the sitting position (Fig. 4–10). Testing rotation in this position may remove the piriformis to an extent that brings out more of the other lateral rotatores' function.

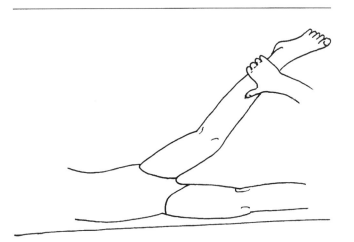

Fig. 4–5 Gluteus medius test.

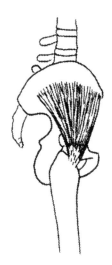

Fig. 4–6 Gluteus minimus.

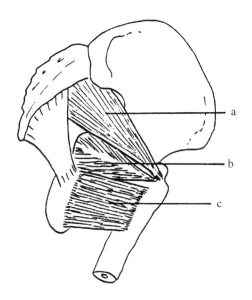

Fig. 4–8 Lateral rotatores, a. piriformis, b. gemelli, c. quadratus femoris.

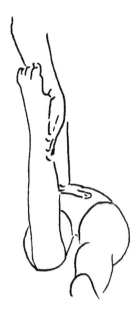

Fig. 4–9 Piriformis test—patient prone.

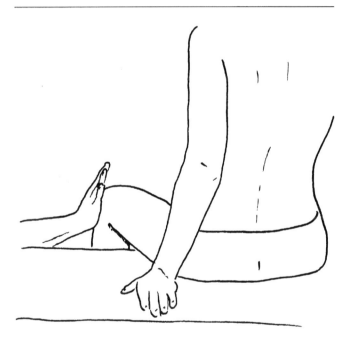

Fig. 4–10 Sitting piriformis test.

The piriformis is innervated by branches from the first and second sacral nerves and is associated with bladder problems (see Appendix A).

Medial Rotators

There is no way to isolate individual muscles. The adductors, pectineus, iliacus, and fibers from the gluteus medius and minimus are involved. The test is the opposite of the prone piriformis test with resistance pressure directed medially against the lateral ankle (Fig. 4–11). The nerve supply to these muscles comes from L2–5 and S1. There is an organ association with the ileocecal valve (see Appendix A). Adjusting T12–L1 affects the ileocecal valve and appendix.

Sartorius and Gracilis

The sartorius (Fig. 4–12) is involved in flexing the hip and knee, can medially rotate the thigh, and with the knee in flexion assists in further medial rotation of the knee. It is also responsible for influencing the ilia anteriorly in the erect position.

The gracilis (Fig. 4–12) is the most superficial muscle medially on the thigh. It is a weak adductor and assists the hamstrings in knee flexion, as well as stabilizing the knee when the body is erect. It also works with the sartorius in medial rotation of the knee.

Testing either muscle alone is difficult. With the patient in the supine position, place the heel above the opposite knee and abduct the thigh approximately 40°. Have the patient hold this position. Place an open hand on the medial aspect of the knee, signaling to the patient that an abduction and slight extension force will be applied. Place the other open hand against the heel and ankle, signaling that a pressure to extend the leg with slight abduction will be made.

As the patient resists, apply pressure simultaneously at both contacts (Fig. 4–13). The knee contact will gauge the gracilis, and the ankle contact will gauge the sartorius. Watch for support muscle dysfunction. The hip may extend to support the gracilis with the adductors, or the ilia may rotate posterior to support the sartorius.

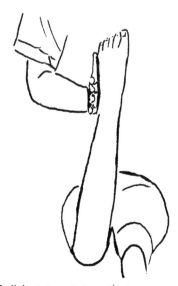

Fig. 4–11 Medial rotatores test—patient prone.

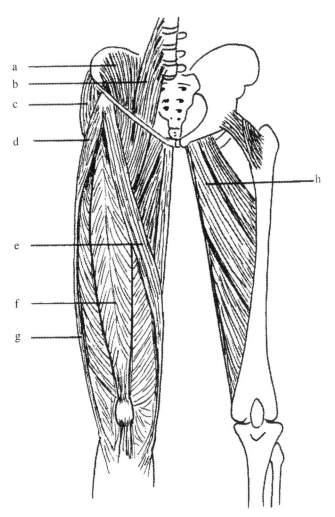

Fig. 4–12 Anterior view pelvic and thigh muscles. a. iliacus, b. psoas, c. gluteus medius, d. tensor fascia lata, e. sartorius, f. rectus femoris, g. iliotibial tract, h. adductor group.

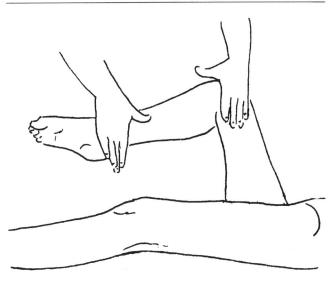

Fig. 4–13 Sartorius and gracilis test.

A weakened sartorius must be considered in persistent posterior rotation fixations of the ilia. It may also be a sign of adrenal problems (see Appendix A). If adrenal weakness is suspected, the specific area to adjust is T9. The nerve supply for both muscles is L2 and L3, the femoral nerve.

Tensor Fascia Lata (TFL)

This muscle (Fig. 4–14) stabilizes the iliotibial tract and assists in flexion, medial rotation, and abduction of the thigh. This muscle is tested with the patient supine. Raise and slightly abduct the leg to approximately 50° with slight medial rotation of the thigh. Pressure is applied with the open hand at the ankle in the direction of extension and adduction (Fig. 4–15). Support the pelvis on the same side. Support muscles

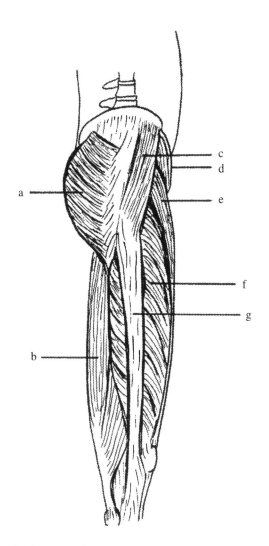

Fig. 4–14 Lateral view pelvic and thigh muscles. a. gluteus maximus, b. biceps femoris, c. TFL, d. sartorius, e. rectus femoris, f. vastus lateralis, g. iliotibial tract.

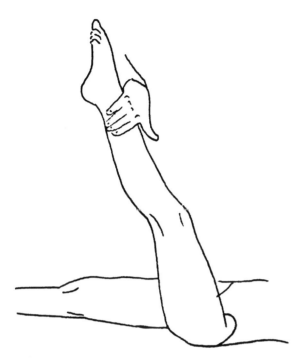

Fig. 4–15 TFL test.

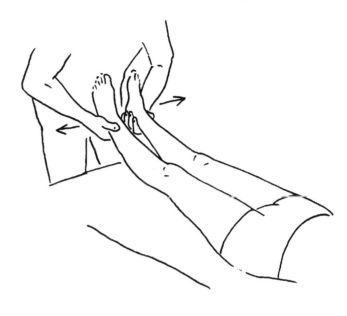

Fig. 4–16 Adductor test—supine.

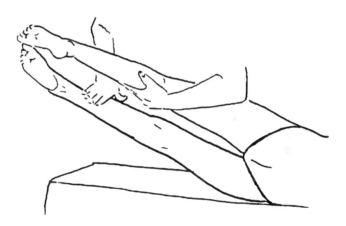

Fig. 4–17 Adductor test—side position.

include the quadriceps to keep the knee extended, the abdominals to keep the pelvis from tilting anteriorly, and the Q-L and other lumbar paravertebral muscles to stabilize the spine.

The nerve supply is from the superior gluteal nerve, L4, L5, and S1. Organic relationship is with the large intestine. L1 is often subluxated in colon problems.

Adductors

The adductors (Fig. 4–12) are a large and powerful group of muscles composed of the pectineus, adductors magnus, longus and brevis, and the gracilis. These can be tested in the supine position. Pull laterally on the ankles in the direction of abduction. There should be no movement (Fig. 4–16).

A more specific test is demonstrated in Kendall.[1] The patient is placed on his or her side. The under leg is adducted, up off the table, with the examiner supporting the upper leg and applying pressure against the inner aspect of the under leg toward abduction (Fig. 4–17). The innervation is via the obturator nerve, L3 and L4. Its organic association is with the ileocecal valve. Specific adjusting should be directed toward L1.

Transversus Perineus

These muscles (Fig. 4–18) are difficult to isolate. Their action is most primary in initiating adduction from an abducted position. The most specific test is done in a similar manner to

the adductor test. The legs are abducted approximately 15° and the patient resists an attempt to further abduct the legs (Fig. 4–19). The transversus perinei must contract first to stabilize the ischial tuberosities. This contraction allows a better support for the adductors. The nerve supply is via the perineal branch of the pudendal nerve.

Hamstrings

The hamstrings (Fig. 4–20) arise from the ischial tuberosity with the biceps long head also accepting fibers from the sacrotuberous ligaments. The short head of the biceps originates on

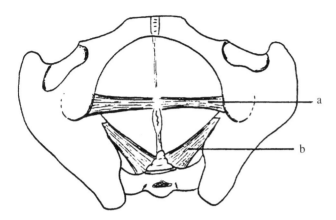

Fig. 4–18 Inferior view of pelvic basin a. transversus perineus, b. coccygeus.

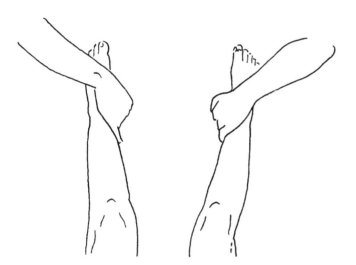

Fig. 4–19 Transversus perineus test.

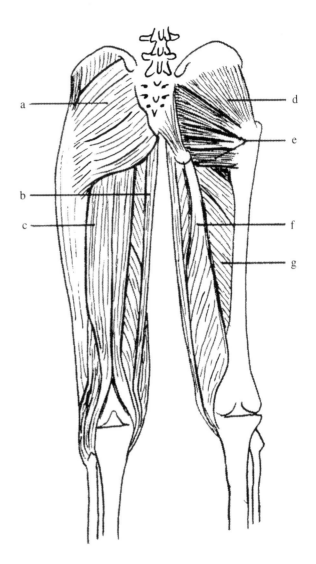

Fig. 4–20 Posterior view pelvic and thigh muscles. a. gluteus maximus, b. gracilis, c. hamstrings, d. gluteus medius, e. lateral rotatores, f. semimembranosus, g. adductors.

the posterior femur beginning at the lowest insertion of the gluteus maximus.

The semitendinosus forms the medial border of the popliteal fossa and inserts on the anteromedial tibia in the area known as the pes anserinus. The semimembranosus lies deep to the semitendinosus. The biceps forms the lateral border of the popliteal fossa and inserts generally on the fibula.

Acting together, the hamstrings flex the knee and extend the hip. With the knee flexed, the biceps is a lateral rotator of the tibia, and the medial hamstrings are medial rotators.

The hamstrings become posterior rotators of the pelvis only if it is flexed forward, assisting in returning the pelvis to neutral. In the erect posture, the hamstrings' effect on pelvic rotation is minimal. If it were significant, there would be a large number of the shortened hamstrings found clinically, which would produce a predominance of posteriorly rotated pelves.

If anything, the opposite is the case. Many cases of hamstring contracture are seen clinically with anterior pelvic rotations.

The hamstrings act as lateral stabilizers of the pelvis in the erect stance, and assist in shifting the pelvis from side to side. The biceps can affect the fibula and consequently plays a role in knee, foot, and ankle problems.[2] To test the hamstrings, have the patient in the prone position. Flex the knee to 90°. The support hand should cover the belly of the muscle. Apply extension pressure with the back of the wrist or hand (Fig. 4–21).

If a spasm should occur, immediately extend the leg and apply steady pressure laterally across the belly of the muscle. Do not attempt to retest. Testing the muscles with the leg at varying angles of flexion, from 45° to 90°, can elicit problems with various structures at the knee.[2]

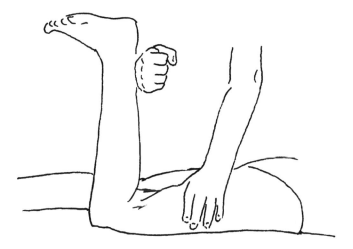

Fig. 4–21 Hamstring test.

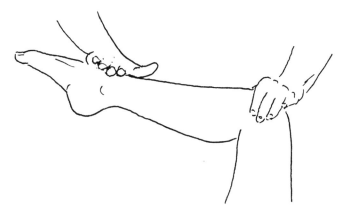

Fig. 4–22 General test for quadriceps femoris.

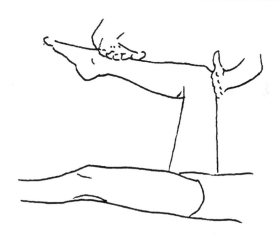

Fig. 4–23 Quad test emphasizing rectus femoris.

To emphasize the medial hamstrings, rotate the thigh medially (move the foot laterally). This brings the medial muscles into prominence and reduces the biceps effectiveness. The lateral hamstrings can be brought to prominence by rotating the thigh laterally.

The nerve supply comes from the sciatic nerve, L5, S1, and S2. The hamstrings are associated with the rectum and can be weakened by sacral fixations.

Quadriceps Femoris

The quads (Fig. 4–12) are the primary extensors of the leg. The rectus crosses two joints, the hip, and knee and has the added role of flexing the hip. The quads as a group can be tested, and the rectus can be somewhat isolated from the vastus group as well as from the flexor group (psoas and iliacus).

To test the quads, flex the hip and knee both to 90° (patient supine). Test the hip flexors first by pushing inferiorly on the knee in the direction of hip extension before applying flexion pressure at the ankle (Fig. 4–22). This will give the examiner a basic idea of the strength of the hip flexors. If they appear weak, it will be difficult to determine the status of the rectus, and interfere with stabilizing the body for testing of the quads.

To further isolate the rectus, apply inferior extension pressure at the knee at the same time as flexion pressure is applied at the ankle (Fig. 4–23). If the hip flexors are functioning normally, this will put the rectus to work. Usually, if the hip flexors are normal and the rectus is weak, there will be noticeable movement of the pelvis and exaggerated abdominal effort to compensate.[2]

The vastus lateralis can be emphasized by medially rotating the foot and applying a slightly medial downward pressure on the ankle. The vastus medialis can be emphasized with lateral rotation and lateral downward pressure. The oblique fibers of the vastus medialis (VMO) are the most inferior fibers running almost laterally from the femur to the patella.

Any weakness of the quadriceps should cause the examiner to suspect the VMO first as it is the more commonly dysfunctional part of the vastus group and plays an important part in knee problems.[2] To test for the VMO, hook the thumb of the support hand around the patella influencing it medially and slightly superior while retesting the quads. If improvement is noted, the VMO is weak and in need of treatment or exercise or both.

The nerve supply to the quads is L2–L4. The quads are used as an indicator for nerve root compromise, especially of L4. Adjusting T10–12 and L1 has more often affected quad tone in clinical experience.[2] It is theorized that spinal fixations can affect the segments and somatic innervations above or below the site of fixations. Another theory is that the actual origin of the nerve roots from the spinal cord occur higher up than their site of exit through the intervertebral foramen (IVF; recall that the cord ends at L2 in the filum terminale). Adjusting higher up the spine can affect the nerve root at its origin.

The quads are associated with the small intestine, especially the duodenum (see Appendix A). Any weakness in the presence of digestive disturbance can be helped by adjusting the lower six thoracics.

Psoas

The psoas (Fig. 4–24) originates from the transverse processes' bodies, and disks of the five lumbar vertebrae. It can be seen as five distinct muscle slips that join with the iliacus to form a common tendon inserting on the lesser trochanter of the femur. It is often necessary to consider the slips separately as it is common to find them doing different things. For instance the L4–L5 slips are more likely to be hypertonic, but the upper slips may be normal or weak.

The psoas figures significantly in low back problems. It is the principal flexor of the hip with its origin fixed. It is also involved in abduction as well as lateral and medial rotation, depending on the position of the hip. With the insertion fixed, it flexes the lumbar spine, and acting unilaterally it can laterally bend the spine. Acting segmentally, it supports the individual vertebra in its movements. As mentioned in Chapter 1, the psoas can increase the lordosis by a compressive action.

The psoas is often hypertonic, and palpation of the insertion is often painful. In the supine position, a hypertonic psoas muscle will exaggerate the lordosis, arching the back and producing a gap between the back and examination table.

To test the psoas, the patient should be supine. The test will tell the general tone of the iliacus and psoas. Raise the leg with the knee straight to approximately 55°, and place it in slight abduction and lateral rotation. Stabilize the pelvis on the opposite side and apply pressure, at the ankle or knee (either is appropriate, but contact should be consistent), in the direction of extension with slight abduction (Fig. 4–25). Test several times, and watch for weakening.

The psoas is innervated by the second and third lumbar nerves via the lumbar plexus. Adjusting the T9–10–11 segments often affects the nerve roots. The psoas is also weakened by lateral rotation of the femur and lateral tarsal fixations of the foot. The psoas is related to the kidneys (see Appendix A).

The psoas and iliacus can be tested with the patient in the sitting position. Have the patient flex the hip and resist a downward pressure on the knee (Fig. 4–26). The L5 slip and iliacus can be isolated by leaning forward, which reduces the upper lumbar slips' influence.

Iliacus

The iliacus originates on the inside of the ilia, a broad attachment from the anterior superior iliac spine (ASIS) to the sacroiliac (SI) joint. It joins the psoas to attach to the lesser trochanter. It is not readily tested and contributes to the general actions associated with the psoas. Its anterior fibers also pull the ilium medially. The middle and posterior fibers pull the ilium anteriorly. The sacral fibers can influence the sacrum anteriorly.

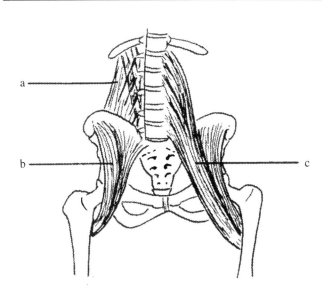

Fig. 4–24 Anterior view: deep muscles. a. quadratus lumborum, b., iliacus, c. psoas.

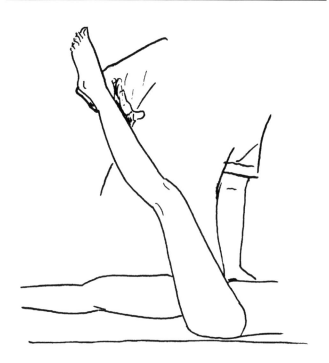

Fig. 4–25 Psoas test.

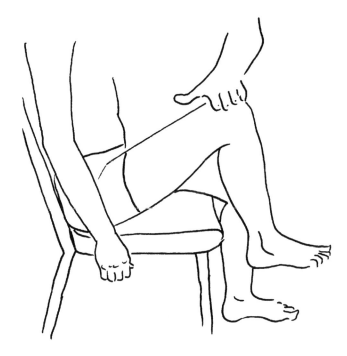

Fig. 4–26 Sitting psoas test.

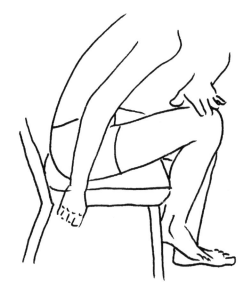

Fig. 4–27 Isolating iliacus and lower psoas fibers.

The L4 and L5 psoas slips and the iliacus can be isolated by testing in the sitting position and having the patient lean forward eliminating the upper psoas slips (Fig. 4–27).

Quadratus Lumborum

The Q-L (Fig. 4–24) originates on the iliac crest and iliolumbar ligament and inserts on the twelfth rib, with another layer inserting into the upper four lumbar transverse processes. Another layer often arises from the first four lumbars and inserts into the last rib. Its basic function is considered to be pulling down on the last rib and laterally flexing the lumbar spine. It has important functions in stabilizing the lumbar vertebrae, controlling anterior and rotational influences.

The Q-L is not accurately tested. The most common test is to have the patient prone, traction the leg inferiorly, and have the patient attempt to pull the pelvis cephalad. There are too many support muscles that can mask a weakness. The Q-L is often weakened in low back dysfunctions. Weakness is detected in its basic tone. The most accurate way to access weakness is to test for tone.

If the pelvis is level and free of fixation or rotations or both, grasp the supine patient's ankles and traction caudad with enough force to rock the pelvis and almost pull the patient from the table. Pull with equal force on both legs (Fig. 4–28). If there is a unilateral weakness, the weak side will demonstrate an elongation of the leg and an inferior ilium. The weak

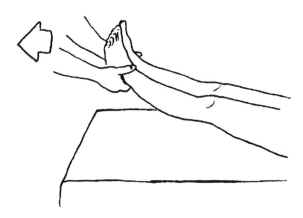

Fig. 4–28 Tug inferiorly for Q-L imbalance.

side will be pulled down due to the lack of tone. Push the legs cephalad and recheck for level iliac crests and legs. Retest several times to confirm.

If the weakness is due to subluxation, adjusting the lower thoracics will eliminate the inferior shift upon testing. Goading the insertion on the twelfth rib can improve function, but only temporarily if the muscle is in need of exercise.

The Q-L is associated with the appendix. It is innervated by the T12 and L1.

Abdominals

The abdominals are often observed to be weak in men due to a lack of exercise and ever-increasing abdominal fat layers

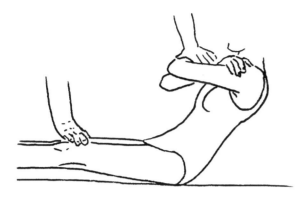

Fig. 4–29 Abdominal muscle test emphasizing the rectus.

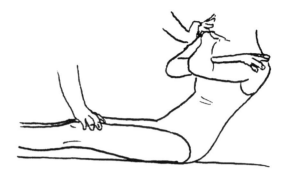

Fig. 4–30 Abdominal test emphasizing oblique and transverse groups.

and in women due to the overstretching of pregnancy and lack of exercise postpartum. The rectus, obliques, and transverse are necessary to maintain a stable low back and support the viscera.

Test the abdominals with the patient sitting up with legs extended and arms crossed over the chest. Have the patient lean back slightly. Stabilize the legs and contact the crossed arms. Attempt to push the patient down (Fig. 4–29). A normal response should be no movement. Test the obliques and transverse fibers by turning the patient to one side and then the other and repeat the test (Fig. 4–30). No movement should be noted.

The abdominals are innervated by the T8–T12 intercostals and the ilioinguinal and iliohypogastric nerves. This muscle group is associated with the duodenum.

CONCLUSION

The muscles discussed in this chapter are those most directly and most commonly involved in low back and pelvic conditions. It should be recognized that muscles in the neck, upper back and shoulder girdle or below the knee and into the foot can be a factor in low back and pelvic problems.

When evaluation fails to reveal significant findings in the immediate area, the investigation should move to structures above or below to rule out causal factors. For instance, the psoas muscles can be affected by diaphragmatic dysfunction. The latissimus dorsi can affect the third lumbar, its distal insertion, and thereby affect the lower erector spinae muscles inserting at L3 from below. Foot imbalances due to tibialis anterior or peroneus muscles can upset lumbopelvic function.

REFERENCES

1. Kendall H. *Muscles: Testing and Function* (2nd ed). Baltimore, Md: Williams & Wilkins; 1971.

2. Logan A. *The Knee: Clinical Aspects.* Gaithersburg, Md: Aspen; 1994.

Chapter 5

Adjustive Techniques

The manipulation of the human body for the express purpose of restoring health is documented in the earliest of recorded history. Forms of manipulation were used in ancient Egypt and Greece and the healing arts of the Orient still include manipulative procedures.

In the United States, in modern history, Andrew Still linked manipulation to the principles of osteopathy. He founded the first school in 1874. In 1895, D.D. Palmer founded the principles of chiropractic. He did not claim to have discovered manipulation, but did claim to be the first to use the vertebral processes as levers to adjust specific segments. He referred to adjusting all 300 articulations of the body including the spine, pelvis, and extremities.

Over the last one hundred years, the chiropractic profession has evolved a varied philosophy and methodology, yet Palmer's basic concept—the idea that articular dysfunction especially of the spine can interfere with the flow of nervous energy, compromising health—remains. Specific manipulation to restore normal function can free the innate mechanisms allowing the body to be as healthy as possible.

The history of chiropractic is a lively subject, full of large egos, and strong differences of opinion as to the best way to explain and implement treatment. The controversy began with some of the first students to pass through the Palmer College. Willard Carver was a constant critic of Palmer's methods and went on to found four other chiropractic institutions. Much of the early controversy has left the profession divided and even fractionated by philosophical and technical differences.

In spite of these differences, chiropractic has persevered as a vital alternative to traditional medicine. Despite the efforts of its detractors to eradicate chiropractic, it continues to see growing popular support and a growing body of valid research that supports its hypotheses. As we enter a new era, that of managed care, chiropractic needs to continue its efforts to validate and standardize its evaluation and treatment protocols in order to participate as equals. My hope is that chiropractic will develop its own protocols instead of being forced into, or accepting, medical models.

The list of notable contributors to chiropractic technique is large. From D.D. and B.J. Palmer, through Joseph Janse, Major DeJarnette and D.J. Metzinger to George Goodheart and Alan Fuher, the art and science of manipulation has grown. Many of the techniques are touted by their supporters as the only valid methods of analysis and correction. Without valid research, such a claim is little more than bombast.

In studying the various techniques, one is much more likely to find valid bits and pieces that seem to make sense and appear to be clinically consistent. Out of such research, the concept of diversified technique has developed. This loosely defined amalgam of adjustive techniques was named diversified technique by D. J. Metzinger. He believed in learning from anyone and everyone, testing for himself, and collecting the procedures that worked for him. The distilled essence of his work, and the continued contributions of many, is the diversified approach.

Dr. Metzinger taught at what is now the Los Angeles College of Chiropractic in the 1940s and is remembered for his common sense approach to adjusting, based on a thorough command of anatomy and what we now call biomechanics. He developed many new adjustive techniques for the spine and is credited with pioneering manipulation of the ribs and extremities.

Dr. A.L. Logan was a student and protegé of Dr. Metzinger. The concepts described in this text are the result of a continuum from those who taught Dr. Metzinger through those who have learned from Dr. Logan, who continued to refine and add to the body of knowledge known as diversified technique throughout his career.

There is no one way to move a bone. Many of the techniques taught today have excellent ways to correct osseous disrelationships. They range in application from "nonforce," or more appropriately, low force, to an aggressive dynamic thrust. The adjustive procedures included in this text are those we have found to be the most effective. Where possible, alternative methods are described. In using this text, any method of manipulation that the reader feels will effectively correct the subluxations described is likely to be as valid as those included.

However, I am of the opinion that the more aggressive (not necessarily forceful) the adjustment, the more effective and rapid the improvement in the patient. Dr. Warren Hammer,[1] who has written extensively on chiropractic adjusting, said:

> The so-called 'painless,' gentle, nonforce techniques used by practitioners who deride the spinal adjustment can never be as effective as the chiropractic thrust. I also doubt that the use of the activator instruments could stimulate the amount of mechanoreceptors that a good old fashioned adjustment is capable of stimulating. The chiropractic adjustment by hand is the mainstay of our art and science. I fear that the lack of proficiency and confidence present in many chiropractors causes them to seek alternative methods of spinal care.

In studying the intricacies of the neurophysiological system and how the body learns, it may be that the so-called nonforce techniques may show greater results in correcting long-term proprioceptive irregularities due to chronic subluxation patterns. Rywerant,[2] writing on the Feldenkrais method of functional integration, alludes to the greater informational input from gentle manipulation than from forceful approaches.

It is my experience that aggressive manipulation, the core of "classic" chiropractic, is effective in restoring normal function when there is significant fixation or contracture of tissue around the joint in question. However, I have had success in using low-force techniques. It may be that low-force adjusting may be more effective in reestablishing normal neurophysiological function, which involves relearning processes. At this time, I am of the opinion that a combination of aggressive and gentle techniques may be the most effective. These are areas for future research.

It is likely that the paranoia over cervical manipulation, based on the erroneous assumption that there is valid evidence of possible harm, has led some educators and schools to discontinue the teaching of effective cervical manipulation, and to substitute cautious approaches that may be less effective. This caution, in my opinion, speaks to an element in chiropractic that wishes to have the sanction of the established medical powers, with no courage to stand up for chiropractic as an alternative choice in health care.

Most practitioners today have developed their own style of manipulation based on their undergraduate training and what they have picked up in postgraduate education. A diversified approach to adjustive procedures should give the practitioner a variety of ways to correct a subluxation. Different patients will respond better to different techniques.

An elderly patient with advanced osteoporosis should not be adjusted with a dynamic thrust. A lower force approach would obviously be more judicious. I often use the same basic approach as with more aggressive techniques but reduce the force. On some occasions, I have used an impact tool (often referred to as an activator), again with the basic setup, substituting the impactor instead of a thrust.

Learning adjustive techniques out of a textbook is incomplete. Throughout the history of manipulative healing, culminating in chiropractic, the methods were handed down by one-on-one instruction. This is obviously the best method. Most of the technique texts I have consulted have seemed static, listing contact and stabilization points, with little else to give a feeling of the dynamics of physician and patient interaction. In attempting to describe adjustive techniques in this text, I will list the basics of setup and points of contact. I will also attempt to describe the flow of movement as I learned it. This may seem wordy, but should help to more fully convey the sensation of executing these moves.

DIVERSIFIED TECHNIQUE

The basic concepts of diversified technique are as follows:

1. All articulations of the body are subject to subluxation or dysfunction. It is necessary to be able to adjust all of them, from the cranium to the toes, with the spine obviously the most important.

2. The application of carefully controlled force with the utmost speed, when executing the adjustment is a fundamental aspect of effective manipulation. This requires quick reflexes and a keen hand/eye coordination. This does not imply the use of great force, but the rapid split-second application of a controlled amplitude, specifically directed force, a force that is determined by the situation, the area adjusted, the age of the patient, and the degree of injury or degeneration.

3. Hands-on palpation, touching one's patients, feeling for hyper- and hyopmobility, muscle tone, and altered sensation is the principal analytic tool. Your palpatory and clinical experience should leave little room for surprise when reviewing radiographs.

4. The reason for giving an adjustment must have an explanation that is compatible with the anatomy and function of the area being treated and to the overall function of the body.
5. The importance of muscles and their effects on joint dysfunction is fundamental to effective, lasting correction.
6. The technique must demonstrate clinical consistency from physician to physician.
7. The technique should be adaptable and allow for creativity. It should be open-ended.

An important factor in successful adjusting is the comfort and confidence the patient has in the physician. When positioning the patient for an adjustment, the practitioner will place the body into a position that allows access to the part being adjusted. Tension or traction is applied to the tissues to take up the slack in the articulation and the adjustment is made. If the physician is confident and assertive in setting up for an adjustment, it is far more likely the patient will relax. A relaxed, comfortable patient makes for an easy, comfortable adjustment. It is obvious to the experienced practitioners of hands-on therapeutics, such as massage, chiropractic, osteopathy, and physical therapy, that the patient can read the practitioner. Uncertain hands tell the patient to resist and protect themselves.

If the patient cannot relax, any attempt to adjust is met with instinctual and often conscious resistance that means the physician is fighting tight muscles that counter the adjustment. In this case, the adjustment will likely be painful and far less effective. A tense patient can often be "tricked" into relaxing by distracting their attention, sometimes only for a split second. The skilled adjuster should be able to sense that moment of broken concentration and execute, with speed, an adjustment that is quick and comfortable. Once a patient is confident in the chiropractor's handling, he or she becomes easier to adjust. Those that are difficult to get to relax are candidates for low-force adjusting.

PRINCIPLES OF EFFECTIVE ADJUSTMENT

The principles of an effective adjustment are as follows:

1. Positioning. Careful and confident handling of the patient is fundamental. Place the patient into the desired position, explaining what is expected of him or her and what is going to be done.
2. Traction. Take up the "slack" in the tissue and surrounding structures. Make sure the patient is comfortable. Any pain noted should warn the physician that another approach may be necessary, or that it is too soon to attempt that particular correction.
3. Contact point/line of drive. Accurate palpation and a keen sense of anatomy are vital in order to make the contact point as precise as possible. In lumbar and pelvic adjusting, the pisiform contact is most effective. With a "pull" technique, finger tip contact will be used.

Care in establishing the line of drive so that it coincides with the plane of articulation and natural range of motion is also important. The line of drive is established in diversified technique by the positioning of the forearm. The physician's body should drop into a position that lines up the forearm behind the pisiform and in line with the articular plane. This gives a solid drive to the adjustment.

In diversified techniques, all adjustments should be made with respect to the natural joint play and range of motion. In my opinion, adjustive techniques that "go against the grain" are likely to produce irritation and possibly cause ligament damage. As an example, the cervical break is a thrust perpendicular to the spine with no respect to the plane of articulation of the cervical apophyseal joints. This approach is likely to overstretch the ligaments and lead to joint instability.

4. Stabilization. Stabilizing is based around balancing the body so that traction can remove all slack in the tissues that support the joint and an end point in joint play can be reached. In handling patients, it is best to utilize the patient's body weight for leverage whenever possible. An effective adjustment can be delivered with less effort and force if the patient is relaxed, balanced, and placed in the most advantageous position. If the patient is set up properly, the physician can better use his or her own body more economically, reducing the stress on the physician's own body.
5. The impulse. Executing the adjustment at the culmination of the setup should be fast. The depth of the thrust is determined by the area being adjusted, the body type, and age of the patient. As a rule, the depth of thrust should always be minimized. If the setup is correct and the patient is relaxed, the need for a deep thrust is unwarranted. Speed is the key. There is an instinctual tightening of the body in response to stretching forces like those in making an adjustment. The speed of the impulse can beat this built-in contraction response. The adjustment is over before the body can respond. I have found that a recoil method works to increase the speed. The idea is to back off as fast or faster than the thrust.
6. Repalpate. After making an adjustment, recheck your findings to ascertain if a correction has been made. An audible release or pop is not always a clear indicator of correction. Not all patients will make audible releases, and some pops may be incidental fixations other than the joint being adjusted. In cases of chronic subluxation, where trophic changes have progressed toward ankylosis, it may take a series of adjustments to reduce

the adhesions and restore normal movement. Attempting to break down a chronic fixation too quickly can create inflammation and increased symptoms that can complicate a patient's recovery.

These steps in setting up and making an adjustment are at first awkward, and the student of diversified adjusting needs to spend time perfecting a smooth, quick, and confident execution. The idea is to flow from positioning, to tractioning, to thrusting quickly. In teaching technique, I have noticed that the longer one fools around setting up an adjustment, the more tense the patient becomes. The adjustment will then be diminished by resistance, may be painful, and will likely be ineffective.

Most diversified adjusting of the low back and pelvis is done with the patient in the side posture position (Fig. 5–1). When properly positioned, the upside knee and hip are flexed, and the downside hip and knee are extended. Tuck the upside foot into the popliteal fossa of the downside knee and instruct the patient to keep it there. The pelvis is rotated, and the shoulders should remain relatively flat on the table. Make sure that the patient is not hunched up or flexed, but relaxed and extended, as if erect. Many patients will curl up approaching the fetal position if you let them. Have the patient firmly interlace their fingers and rest them on the lower part of the upside rib cage.

When properly positioned, the patient will be balanced. The physician should stand to the side, facing the patient with the cephalad leg against the table and bracing the patient. This gives the patient the feeling of being secured on the table as they are rolled further to take up slack (Fig. 5–2). The caudad leg is used to contact the upside flexed hip and knee. The physician's knee is placed at approximately the ischial tuberosity and his or her ankle at the patient's knee. This stabilization contact is used to complete traction and, in certain adjustments, a slight leg kick (a rapid shallow extension of the physician's leg) is used to "gap the articulation."

The support hand should comfortably contact the upside shoulder with a broad contact. If the patient is large or has shoulder pathology, grasp the upside arm just above the elbow (remember to instruct the patient to keep the fingers firmly interlaced). Stabilize the shoulder and upper torso, keeping it as flat against the table as possible.

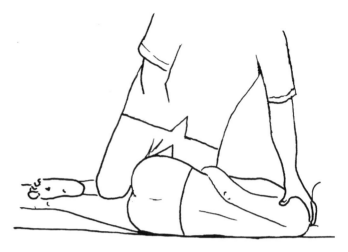

Fig. 5–2 Side posture—contact and traction points.

The physician's caudad leg is used to further rotate the low back and pelvis by extending the (physician's) leg (Fig. 5–3). The combination of upper torso stabilization and torquing of the pelvis will take up all slack in the patient's low back and pelvis. Both physician and patient should be balanced and relaxed.

The adjusting hand is free to make the appropriate contact. This position can be used to adjust the sacrum, ilia, and all the lumbars. With one exception, the upside is the side that is to be adjusted. The exception will be discussed in the section on lumbar adjusting.

To complete the removal of slack and make the adjustment more specific, further flexion or extension of the patient's upside hip can be effectively done by moving the patient's thigh with the adjuster's caudad leg contact. Use the adjusting hand

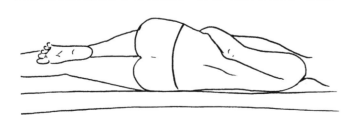

Fig. 5–1 Side posture.

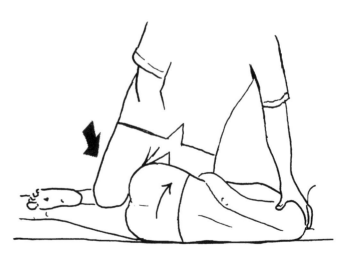

Fig. 5–3 Physician's leg extension causes further pelvic rotation.

to palpate the paravertebral muscles at the level being adjusted, by flexing the upside hip until tension is noted in the paravertebral muscles at the desired level (Fig. 5–4). All slack is removed up to one level below the segment to be moved. For example, adjusting L3 would be more effective if the upside hip is flexed until the paravertebral muscles at L4 become taut. To adjust below L5, the hip is extended until no tension is noted at the L5 level. To adjust L5, flex the hip until tension is felt at the L5–S1 level.

When executing a lumbopelvic adjustment, the flow from rolling the patient into the side posture, taking stabilizing and adjustive contacts, to firing the impulse, should be a smooth maneuver. The "force" of the adjustment is originated not from the shoulder, but from a drop of the physician's torso. This is a more economical use of the physician's body, less likely to lead to shoulder injury or problems from repetitive trauma.

The way this works is to set up the patient and test the point of tension (remove all slack). Bring the paravertebral muscles up tight (hip flexion). Take the adjustive contact. Drop your body down quickly, over the patient (Fig. 5–5a). When you reach the correct line of drive, that is, your forearm is in line with the specific plane and angle of articulation, fire your impulse (Fig. 5–5b). When indicated, a simultaneous leg kick gaps the joint and the adjustment is made. This body drop transfers the weight and momentum from your torso through the shoulder into the pisiform.

There is no question that diversified technique is a physical technique that requires some strength and agility. Women in chiropractic are every bit as capable of practicing diversified technique. They often have a greater need to strengthen their upper bodies in order to avoid injuring themselves. We have always stressed to our students that conditioning is important.

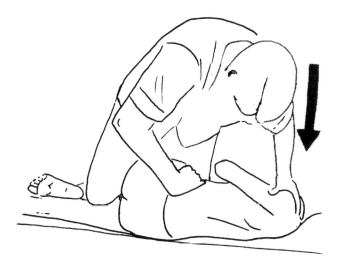

Fig. 5–5a Taking up slack and beginning body drop.

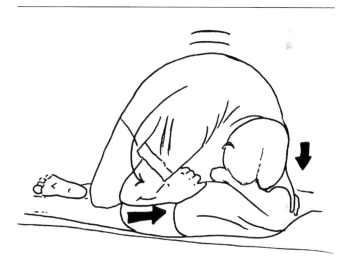

Fig. 5–5b Completion of body drop and transfer of momentum into adjusting arm.

Many physicians will opt for less strenuous techniques rather than train for what could offer the practitioner a more complete chiropractic regimen.

PI Ilium

Patient Position:	side posture
Stabilization:	upside shoulder or arm, and thigh
Contact Point:	pisiform at the posterior superior iliac spine
Line of Drive:	anterolateral

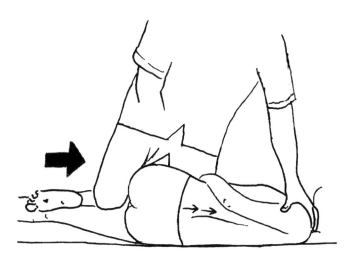

Fig. 5–4 Moving upside hip into further flexion tenses lumbar paravertebral muscles higher up the spine.

A posterior rotation subluxation of the ilium is noted when the supine patient has a superior anterior superior iliac spine (ASIS; Fig. 5–6) and passive motion palpation (PMP) shows no anterior movement. The sacroiliac (SI) plane of articulation is anterolateral/posteromedial. Adjusting a PI ilium, will require an anterolateral line of drive. The forearm should be aligned with the SI joint plane. As the adjuster's body drops into the adjustment the forearm should be lowered past the posterior superior iliac spine (PSIS) contact so that the impulse is directed anterolaterally (Fig. 5–7). Use a leg kick.

AS Ilium

Patient Position:	side posture
Stabilization Point:	upside shoulder and thigh
Contact Point:	ischial tuberosity
Line of Drive:	anteromedial

An AS ilium is indicated by an inferior ASIS (Fig. 5–6). PMP shows a lack of posterior movement. When the ilium is anteriorly rotated, the ischial tuberosity is moved posterior and slightly lateral. The line of drive needs to be anterior and slightly medial. To do this, the adjuster's shoulder must be internally rotated to bring the pisiform into contact with the ischial tuberosity. The elbow will be pointed toward the opposite side of the patient and slightly cephalad (Fig. 5–8). This is easier to do if the patient is rolled further over than for the PI adjustment. No leg kick is used.

An alternative technique that is sometimes effective is the use of blocks. First used by Willard Carver, who started correcting pelvic rotations with the patient's shoes, it was popularized by Major DeJarnette in his sacro-occipital technique (SOT).

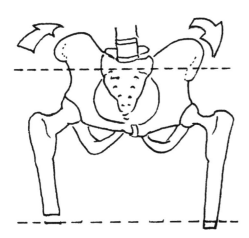

Fig. 5–6 Right PI ilium, left AS ilium.

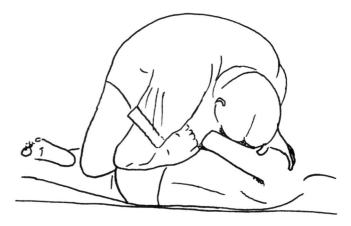

Fig. 5–7 PI ilium adjustment.

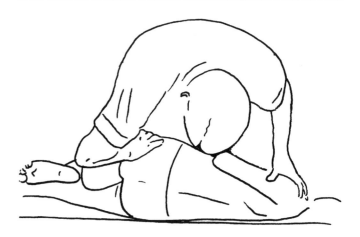

Fig. 5–8 AS ilium adjustment.

I have found the blocks effective in acute cases where the side posture was contraindicated and as a low-force method in very frail patients. I have found that a precise setup and a relaxed patient make the side posture adjustment easy with very light force. The blocks are not always effective if the fixation is set too hard. I do not follow the SOT criterion.

I place the blocks under the supine patient. The PI ilium is blocked under the posterior iliac crest in line with the SI joint space. The AS ilium is blocked under the greater trochanter (Fig. 5–9). It should take less than a minute to see results. If no change is noted, the fixation will require a more direct adjustment. Blocking is more effective when there is little or no fixation and the rotation involves muscle imbalance. The blocks are often effective in acute cases as they more often involve widespread muscle reaction.

In all cases, the muscles that produce and allow AS and PI ilia should be evaluated (see Chapter 1 on Anatomy). The gluteus maximus, hamstrings, and posterior abdominal and quadratus lumborum can produce a PI and will allow an AS

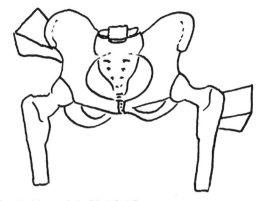

Fig. 5–9 Blocking a right PI, left AS.

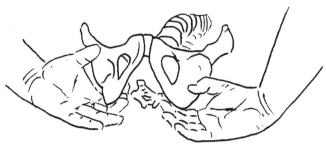

Fig. 5–11 Motion palpation of ischia.

ilium. The iliacus and to a lesser extent the sartorius, rectus femoris, and tensor fascia lata can produce an AS and allow a PI ilium. The chapter on conditions and treatment will discuss this further.

Medial Ischium

A medial ischium (MI) is often described as a flaring of the iliac crest (Fig. 5–10). It is readily found with PMP of the ischial tuberosities. By grasping the medial aspect of the tuberosities and attempting to pull them laterally, there should be a noticeable joint play (Fig. 5–11). Often there is palpable pain in the SI joint due to the flaring of the ilia and a straining of the SI ligaments.

The muscles involved are the transversus peronei, originating on the medial ischial tuberosities and inserting into a central tendinous speta. The muscles are a major support for the rectum and floor of the pelvis. The lateral-most iliacus fibers act to pull the iliac crest medially countering the lateral flare.

A hypertonic transversus peroneus can pull the ischial tuberosity medially. When weak, they can allow excessive lateral play.

Patient Position:	side posture
Stabilization Point:	upside shoulder or arm
Contact Point:	pisiform on medial ischial tuberosity
Line of Drive:	lateral

This adjustment requires the deepest body drop in order to bring the forearm into a correct line of drive. The elbow should be pointed almost toward the floor so that a true lateral thrust can be delivered. The thrust will be practically toward the ceiling, depending on how far the patient can be rolled (Fig. 5–12a,b,c).

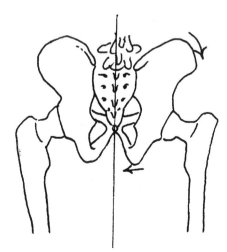

Fig. 5–10 Right medial ischium.

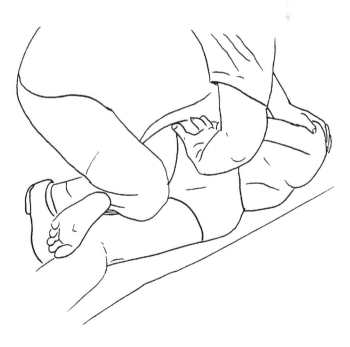

Fig. 5–12a MI adjustment—beginning body drop.

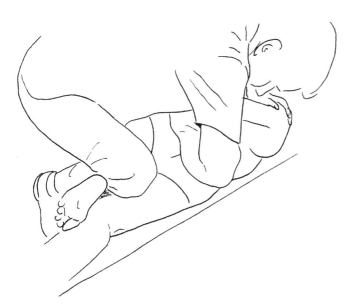

Fig. 5–12b MI adjustment—midway in body drop.

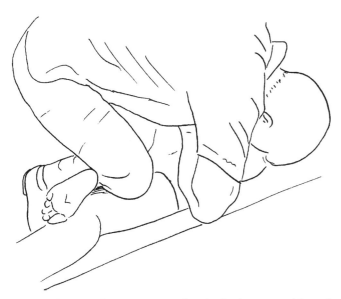

Fig. 5–12c MI adjustment—complete body drop to position of thrust.

The PI, AS, and MI ilia are the most common pelvic subluxations.

Inferior Ilium

An inferior ilium (Fig. 5–13) is indicated by a low iliac crest, usually accompanied by an ipsilateral long leg and often associated with a weak quadratus lumborum (Q-L). It is detected by finding a persistent low iliac crest, even after weight-bearing simulation. The ASIS findings will be consistent as

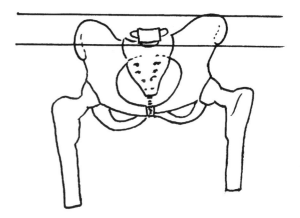

Fig. 5–13 Inferior right ilium.

well, except if there are AS or PI rotations. Adjust the inferiority first and recheck the crest and ASIS listings. After setting the supine patient, with cephalad force, into simulated weight bearing, if the iliac crest remains inferior, an adjustment for an inferior ilium is indicated.

The adjustment of inferior segments in the pelvis and lumbar spine requires a modified side posture. With the patient rolled to the side, place the upside arm over the patient's head and the downside hand in the upside axillary area. The knee stabilization is set with tension below the SI joint. This position accentuates the line of drive, which is cephalad.

Patient Position:	modified side posture
Stabilization Point:	upside axilla over patient's hand
Contact Point:	pisiform on inferior ischial tuberosity
Line of Drive:	cephalad

The adjuster's forearm should be parallel to the table with the elbow pointed caudad. The thrust is a superior thrust on the ischial tuberosity. Traction on the spine is accomplished by the adjuster's body shifting from caudad to cephalad, with a rigid "stiff arm" contact on the shoulder. By the adjuster's shifting headward, with firm contact and stabilization points, the force of body momentum can be transferred to the patient. A final impulse, at the ischial contact, at the peak of superior movement makes the adjustment. This should be a smooth, fast, shallow adjustment (Fig. 5–14).

Lateral Rotation Subluxation of the Femur

The hip joint is commonly subluxated. If not detected and corrected, the subluxation can confuse the findings in a diagnosis of low back and pelvic conditions. The lateralp femoral rotation (LRF) subluxation is an incomplete seating of the

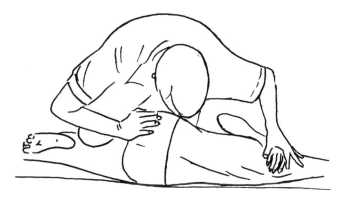

Fig. 5–14 Inferior ilium adjustment.

head of the femur in the acetabulum. The wraparound design of the capsular ligaments "screws home" the head into the acetabulum when the hip is extended as in the standing position. Apparently the intercapsular fat pad can become trapped between the head and rim of the socket preventing complete seating. The femur remains laterally rotated and longer.

There are common postural faults that cause this subluxation. They include sitting cross-legged, sitting with one ankle resting on the opposite thigh, and sleeping on one's stomach. The femur can also subluxate in compensation for other low back and pelvic distortions (see Chapter 6 on Conditions and Treatment).

The detection of an LRF can be made by first noting any leg length discrepancy. The LRF will cause the leg to appear longer. This is often an unreliable primary indicator unless all other causes of a leg length inequality are ruled out including an anatomical difference. A better indicator is to compare internal rotation of both legs. Grasp the supine patient's ankles and internally rotate them (Fig. 5–15). If there is a noticeable

loss of movement, there may be an LRF or only hypertonicity of the lateral rotator muscles, primarily the piriformis.

Another confirmatory check is to flex the knee and then the thigh as fully as possible. With an LRF, there will be a significant medial deviation of the foot as the thigh is flexed, which is due to lateral rotation of the femur. A normal hip will flex with the foot remaining in line with the thigh.

A lateral rotation of the femur will often cause hip pain, most often across the buttock, or radiating down the anterior thigh.

Patient Position:	supine with hip and knee flexed
Stabilization Point:	none
Contact Point:	interlocked fingers over the knee
Line of Drive:	inferior (toward the floor)

This adjustment is done with a body drop. The adjuster stands next to the hip to be adjusted, facing cephalad. The back should be straight. A partial crouch is done to contact the knee. Interlace your fingers over the knee and clamp the leg to your body with your caudad arm. You should be crouched so that your hands are at shoulder level and your shoulder should be level with the patient's raised knee. Use the leg to rotate the thigh medially (pull it laterally by rotating your body). Pull it to tension, removing all slack. At this point a short amplitude body drop makes the adjustment. Keep your interlaced hands, arms, and shoulders rigid. Your body should drop as if it were a solid unit (Fig. 5–16).

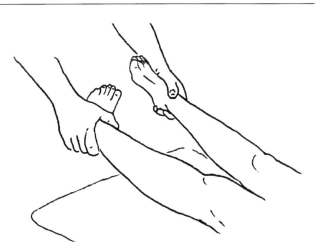

Fig. 5–15 Decreased internal rotation of right leg—suggests lateral femoral rotation subluxation.

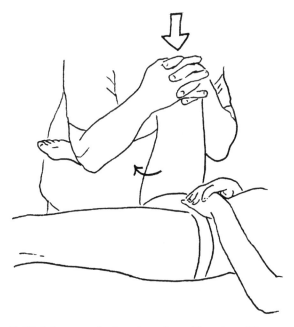

Fig. 5–16 Adjustment for lateral rotation subluxation of femur.

There is often a loud audible release, rarely uncomfortable. It should be used with caution in patients you suspect of having osteoporosis, acute arthritic inflammation, or fracture. An alternative adjustment can be done if this adjustment is contraindicated. The patient is supine. Grasp the ankle and traction the leg caudad making sure the patient relaxes the hip and low back. When you are certain of relaxation and all slack is tractioned out, a rapid caudad tug of short amplitude will gap the joint and seat the hip. With LRF subluxation, the lateral rotator muscles are often hypertonic and may need to be stretched.

The second method is safer if hip pathology is evident but could aggravate any low back pathology. I have used the first adjustment in many questionable circumstances. Often a gentle stretch and mild drop, or a rapid series of gentle drops will achieve a correction with no discomfort or further harm to the patient.

Posterior Sacrum

A posterior sacrum subluxation will palpate as a decreased space between the PSIS and lateral border of the sacrum (Fig. 5–17). PMP will show the subluxated SI to have no anterior joint play. The sacrum may even feel as if it is in a relatively normal position, but if PMP reveals a loss of anterior movement, it is likely to be fixed.

Patient Position:	side posture
Stabilization Point:	upside shoulder or arm
Contact Point:	pisiform on upside lateral border S1–2
Line of Drive:	anterolateral (in line with joint space)

This adjustment is similar in all respects to the PI and lumbar adjustment, with the exception of the contact and line of drive being consistent with the plane of the articulation being adjusted. The sacrum has a line of drive that is more anterior to posterior (A-to-P) than the PI ilium (Fig. 5–18).

Anterior Sacrum

An anterior sacrum will palpate as a deeper space between the PSIS and the lateral border of the sacrum (Fig. 5–17). It is not possible to motion palpate for a lack of posterior joint play. Comparison of the opposite SI can aid in confirming the anterior fixation. If the opposite SI joint is in a normal position and has normal joint play, the likelihood of anterior fixation is great.

Adjusting anterior fixations in the sacrum and lumbar spine is done with the patient in the side posture. There is a reversal of stabilization and contact points. The idea is to influence an anteriorly fixed segment posteriorly. The concept of adjusting anteriorities is to bring tension in the paravertebral muscles up to the level below the segment to be adjusted, and by thrusting posteriorly the segments above the anterior segment, release it from its fixation.

Patient Position:	side posture
Stabilization Point:	upside ilium adjacent to SI joint
Contact Point:	upside shoulder or arm
Line of Drive:	posterior rotation of the spine

The stabilization of the ilium is done with pisiform or index contact on the ilium at the SI joint with the forearm establishing the same position as if adjusting a PI. Contact at the shoulder or arm is where the thrust will be made. Bring the patient to tension by rotating the pelvis toward you with leg extension and a firm hold on the ilia. Roll the shoulder away. When all slack is removed, a rapid thrust is made at the shoulder or arm, while the pelvis is held firm. This will pull the sacrum poste-

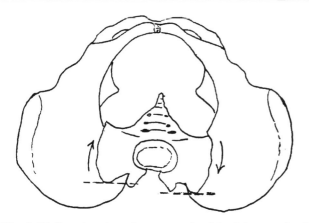

Fig. 5–17 Superior view of sacrum and pelvis, right posterior, left anterior sacral subluxation.

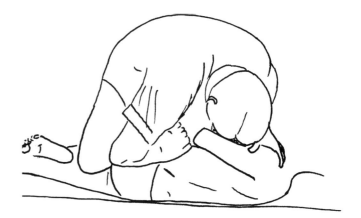

Fig. 5–18 Posterior sacrum adjustment.

rior along with the rest of the spine. This adjustment is rapid and of short amplitude (Fig. 5–19). The key to a comfortable anterior adjustment is patient relaxation and precise tension levels set with the flexion/extension mechanism of the patient's upside leg. Care should be taken to avoid adjusting if significant muscle hypertonicity or spasm or acute injury to spinal segments is present.

Inferior or Oblique Sacrum

An inferior or oblique sacrum (Fig. 5–20) is detected by bringing the thumbs up against the lower borders of the sacrum above the sacrococcygeal joint with the patient prone. It is easy to spot any unleveling of the sacrum. An inferior sacrum is often found along with an inferior ilium on the same side. In some cases, correcting one corrects the other. If both are present, I will usually adjust the ilium first and repalpate before adjusting the sacrum.

Patient Position:	side posture, inferior side up
Stabilization Point:	axillary, patient's arm overhead
Contact Point:	pisiform on lateral border of sacrum
Line of Drive:	cephalad

The setup and adjustment are the same as for the inferior ilium (Fig. 5–14). The contact is on the inferolateral aspect of the sacrum, with a cephalad line of drive.

An alternative method is to reverse the side posture so that the inferior side is down and patient is positioned as for a posterior fixation. The pisiform contact is on the downside lateral sacral border. The line of drive is lateral and slightly superior, which means a deep body drop with the forearm lined up as in the MI adjustment (Fig. 5–12c).

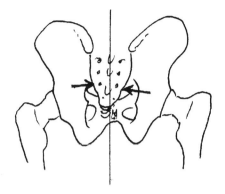

Fig. 5–20 Right inferior or oblique sacrum.

Posterior L1–L5

A posterior subluxation of a lumbar vertebra will palpate (Fig. 5–21) as a lack of anterior joint play when pressing anteriorly on the mamillary process, with supine PMP. It will usually feel closer to the surface (Fig. 5–22).

Patient Position:	side posture, subluxation side up
Stabilization Point:	upside shoulder or arm
Contact Point:	pisiform on upside mamillary process
Line of Drive:	anterolateral

The line of drive can vary according to the plane of facetal articulation. If PMP or radiological evidence or both show facetal asymmetry, correct the line of drive as necessary. Use a leg kick.

An effective alternative for adjusting a posterior subluxation that is often effective with less force and less torquing of

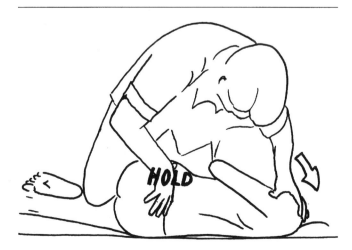

Fig. 5–19 Anterior sacrum adjustment.

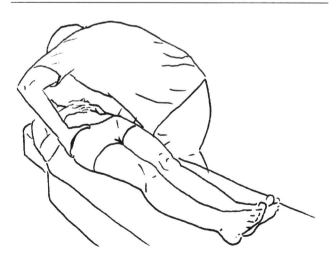

Fig. 5–21 Basic position for palpation of low back and pelvis.

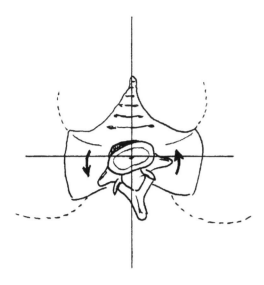

Fig. 5–22 L5–S1 superior view: L5 is anterior on right, posterior on left.

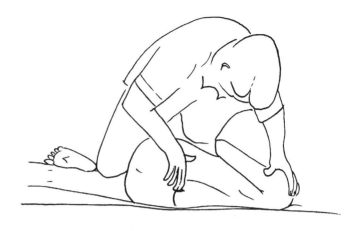

Fig. 5–23 Pull adjustment on lumbars.

the body is a pull adjustment. When setting up for a pull adjustment, use the side posture and put the posteriority on the downside. The stabilization and upside leg positions are the same. The contact point is with the tips of the first two fingers on the downside mamillary process (Fig. 5–23). Take tension in the same fashion but note that less is necessary. When the end point is reached, pull your rigid hand, fingers, and arm toward you. This is not a spinous pull. Another way of considering how to make this move is to think that you are "poking" the mamillary to move it anteriorly. A patient that is in too much pain to take much rotation may be easily adjusted with a pull technique.

Anterior L1–L5

An anterior subluxation will palpate deeper before contacting the mamillary process (Fig. 5–22). The opposite side may feel posterior in comparison.

Patient Position:	side posture, subluxation side up
Stabilization Point:	segment below subluxated segment
Contact Point:	upside shoulder or arm
Line of Drive:	posterior thrust on upside shoulder/arm

Adjusting lumbar anteriorities is the same as for the sacrum (Fig. 5–19). The concept is to bring the subluxated segment posterior. Bring the tension up to the next lowest segment by flexing the patient's upside leg. Stabilize that segment and make the adjustment, thrusting on the upside shoulder or arm.

Inferior L1–L5

A vertebra that is subluxated inferiorly will not have any superior joint play with PMP. The setup is the same as for an inferior ilium or sacrum (Fig. 5–14). Flex the upside leg to bring tension up to the segment below the subluxated segment.

Patient Position:	side posture, inferior side up
Stabilization Point:	axillary, upside arm overhead
Contact Point:	pisiform—underside of mamillary
Line of Drive:	superior

Combination Subluxations

It is rare to have a solitary subluxation. Most often you will find various combinations of subluxations. Any segment can be bilaterally subluxated, posterior on both sides or posterior on one and anterior on the other side. There is not a set way to discern which one to adjust first. The most confusing combination is an anterior and posterior combination at the same level. Palpation will tell you that you have a posterior fixation, but until you adjust and recheck you cannot be sure of the anteriority. The best way to approach correcting lumbopelvic subluxations is to start in, adjust, recheck, and adjust the next finding. In some cases, the first adjustment will correct other listings.

As a rule, I usually adjust L5 first, as L5 subluxations have the ability to mask or alter other subluxations. From there, use your own method or intuition.

A combination of a posteroinferior subluxation on the same side can be adjusted separately or by putting a "spin" on the pisiform, a combination of anterior thrust with a superior torque can be applied at the same time, often correcting both subluxations.

There are often several overlapping subluxations that need to be unraveled. For instance, initial findings at the iliac crest show a right inferior ilium with equal leg lengths, which may be a lateral rotation of the left femur. Testing for lateral rotation of the femur is negative. Checking the ASIS levels shows them to be level. If the right ilium is inferior, the ASIS should be as well. Checking for PI fixation on the right is positive. The PI rotation has leveled out the ASISs and leveled out the legs. By correcting the PI fixation, there will be a more logical finding of a long leg on the right, and correction of the inferior right ilium will balance out the pelvis. There are many variations of combined fixation/subluxation patterns that can be found. By eliminating one, others self-correct or become more apparent.

Pubic Symphysis

The pubic symphysis has little movement, but can shift superiorly on one side (Fig. 5–24). The pubis will often be painful when palpated. Sight down over the pubic symphysis while pressing evenly with the thumbs on the superior aspect of the pubes. It is easy to determine if one is riding higher. The adjustment is best done with a light force. A reinforced pisiform (the web of the other hand over the wrist of the contact hand) is best with a rapid shallow thrust. This can be uncomfortable to the patient. The area is usually sensitive. I find the impact tool used in Activator technique effective.

Coccyx

The coccyx can subluxate anteriorly. The coccygeus muscle can become hypertonic, pulling the coccyx forward. Prat falls can jam it forward. Weakness of the coccygeal fibers of the gluteus maximus can allow the coccyx to shift anteriorly. Unilateral weakness can allow it to deviate to the opposite side.

The first thing to do is to goad the coccygeal fibers of the gluteus maximus. Often this stimulation is enough to correct the problem. Adjusting the coccyx can be done with relative comfort. It is adjusted by rectally contacting the anterior tip of the coccyx and gently pulling with a steady comfortable force for a period up to one minute (Fig. 5–25). A release is often felt as the coccygeus relaxes and moves posteriorly. Some techniques for the coccyx teach a rapid forceful pull that can be very painful and is not necessary. The ganglion of impar is situated at the upper levels of the coccyx. Be sure to contact only the lower segment.

While contacting the coccyx, note if it is deviated to one side. This indicates that the gluteus maximus fibers may be weak on the side opposite the deviation. Varying the direction of pull toward the midline and goading the weak gluteal fibers at their insertion on the femur, will bring the area into balance.

CONCLUSION

It is wise to consider the importance of knowing when and when not to adjust. It is reasonable to consider adjusting when there is a complete understanding of the factors that warrant adjustive intervention and there is a reasonable likelihood of a favorable outcome based on clinical experience. It is wise not to adjust if this understanding is not clear, if a fracture or other pathology is suspected, or if there is significant instability of the articulation.

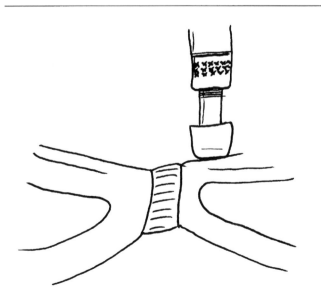

Fig. 5–24 Left superior pubis—adjusting with impactor.

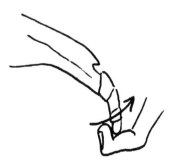

Fig. 5–25 Adjusting the coccyx.

REFERENCES

1. Hammer W. Adjustment by hand only. *Motion Palpation Institute's Dynamic Chiropractic* 1994;12:24.

2. Rywerant Y. *The Feldenkrais Method: Teaching by Handling.* New York, NY: Gininger; 1983.

Chapter 6

Conditions and Treatment

The treatment of various conditions of the somatic (neuro-musculoskeletal) system should, in my opinion, follow a protocol of:

1. assessing and controlling inflammation, acute or chronic.
2. assessing and correcting muscle imbalances, hyper- or hypotonic.
3. determining articular dysfunction and correcting by manipulation.
4. rehabilitating the damaged articulations and their surrounding connective tissue components by corrective manipulation, physical therapy modalities and exercise of involved structures. Corrective manipulation is an adjustive program designed to increase and normalize range of motion (ROM) and reduce connective tissue restrictions related to chronic dysfunction.

Conservative management of somatic pathophysiology begins at varying stages. Some patients present within hours of being injured, some will come in after several days, weeks, or some even months later. Some will have attempted self-treatment with over-the-counter (OTC) pain and anti-inflammatory drugs, heat, liniments, and probably little rest.

Others have seen traditional medical physicians and have been prescribed relaxants and more powerful NSAIDs (nonsteroidal anti-inflammatory drugs) or aggressive physical therapy (PT) that can actually aggravate the condition, and have had no rest. Those with a more chronic inflammatory process will likely have degenerative changes in the surrounding, related structures. Many patients present with significant degenerative joint disease, related to an old injury, poor healing, multiple injuries, and a history of various multidisciplinary attempts to stop the pain.

The most common causes of chronic low back problems are undiagnosed anatomical and functional leg length inequalities(LLIs), a quadratus lumborum (Q-L) syndrome and lack of depth in the investigation of the causes of the patient's complaints—how the injury occurred and what factors in the patient's lifestyle and work are aggravating the problem.

Where one begins treatment will depend on the physician's individual approach and the stage of the disease. Acute injury would benefit from rapid anti-inflammatory therapy, such as ice, protolytic enzymes, rest, calcium for spasm or other modalities, and procedures or supplements that are useful to one's individual practice. Manipulation should be judicious.

A chronic case would benefit from increased circulatory exchanges, such as ROM exercises, hot/cold applications, ultrasound, and most importantly, a manipulative program to restore joint function and stability (see Appendix B).

Proper control of the patient during treatment is essential, and at the same time difficult to achieve. Patients are likely to ignore instructions for home care. So make things as simple as possible. Be clear as to what you expect from patients and make sure that they understand the procedures and the consequences of not participating in their recovery.

INFLAMMATION AND CONNECTIVE TISSUE

The single, most common factor in dealing with neuromusculoskeletal pathology is the acute and chronic effects of the inflammatory process on the connective tissue. The low back, hip, and pelvis are more likely to break down and degenerate than articulations, such as the ankle mortise, which takes far more pounds per square inch force with rarely a complaint. The degree and frequency of inflammatory incidents in a patient's history and the degree of appropriate treatment for those injuries determine the thoroughness of recovery.

It seems to be the trend to consider inflammation as something to be stopped—an undesirable element that interferes with repair. A return to the basic texts on human physiology will remind one that inflammation is the healing process. To stop it could jeopardize healing. However, reducing the level of the reaction could be advantageous. Conservative management of inflammation is fast, direct, and has little likelihood of side effects.

Inflammation is the first stage—the acute stage—of healing. Swelling, redness, heat, and pain are the four aspects of inflammation. The problem with inflammation in aseptic strain/sprain injuries is the all-or-nothing response. It is not needed. If there is no threat by foreign invaders, there is no need for an all out response. Connective tissues are less likely to regenerate than are other tissues in the body. They are prone to scarring. The reparative effort produces a disorganized construction of fibers that are weaker and less elastic than the original fibers. If the swelling is encouraged, there is likely to be a more widespread involvement of connective tissue in this potential degenerative process.

Connective tissue, which includes the ligaments, tendons, and fascia, holds things together. The muscles and skin are specialized types of connective tissue. The fibrous tissues like the ligaments, tendons, and muscles tend to repair strains and tears with collagenous scar tissue. The membranous tissues, such as the fascia, also mend in this way and tend to form adhesions that bind tissues down, preventing movement. Skin, more often than not, will regenerate unless the damage is great or the healing is slow or interrupted. Then scars are likely.

The Acute Phase

When the cellular integrity is damaged, neurochemical reactions trigger the inflammatory response, which is an all-or-nothing reaction. It is designed to rapidly protect the body from infection by walling off the injured area, and preparing the tissue for repair. As a part of this mechanism, the serous exudate in the injured tissue begins coagulating, forming collagen fibers that blend to form fibrous barriers. Those barriers become the scars and adhesions that can degrade connective tissue.

The Subacute Phase

The reparative process begins in the subacute phase. The remains of the damaged tissue are on the way out and fresh blood with oxygen and nutrients is flowing in. Inflammation is less intense. Collagen fibers are being formed to mend the torn fibers.

The Chronic Phase

Resolution of the tissue to a patched up version of its former self takes place in the chronic phase. The chronic phase can be short, with complete repair and near 100% return of strength and function. Or, it can be a long, and sometimes, incomplete process leading to chronic dysfunction and degenerative changes.

In my opinion, the repair of injured connective tissue is a regenerative process, with a generic, lower-grade repair tissue. It is less elastic and is often so disorganized in its construction, that it causes contractions and shrinkage in the tissue. Adhesions in the fascial sheaths contribute to reducing the pliability and ease of movement of one tissue on another, one part on another.

This repair process does a miraculous job of patching up and restoring function. With our better understanding of human physiology and the use of simple therapeutics, it is possible to control and maximize the repair process. It is possible to come far closer to regeneration of tissue with the proper combination of conservative treatment and rehabilitation.

The conservative approach in the acute phase, using ice and rest, is far superior in the long run. By properly icing, a significant slowing of swelling will be accomplished. A reduced flow of blood through the capillaries over the first 8 to 36 hours coupled with rest can markedly reduce the area of involved tissue (see Appendix B).

In the subacute and chronic phases, with reduced swelling, a graduated introduction of heat, range of motion exercise, and ice (to control swelling), then progressing into toning exercises, will create the best environment for maximum repair. It has been shown that movement exercise, introduced early in the subacute phase, can create a better organized scar. The collagen fibers will tend to align themselves with the dynamics of movement. They become more like the tissue they are patching. This will greatly improve the strength and resilience of the repair.

Many patients are seen for the first time with chronic low back problems, some of them having suffered for years. A poorly healed injury, or degenerative changes and the long-term tissue changes that ensue, can challenge the practitioner. With proper care and patience, many cases of serious, chronic arthritic and myofascial inflammation can be controlled and the structure stabilized.

Connective tissue diseases are becoming more widely understood and accepted as a valid condition. The lumbosacral articulations, the dorsolumbar fascia, the sacroiliac, and iliolumbar ligaments are often found to be chronically inflamed, degenerated, and often slide into chronic fibrositis, myofascitis, or fibromyalgia-like syndromes. I have found this to be much more common in women, beginning in the early 40s after childbearing. These diseases are linked, according to some researchers, to chronic fatigue and Epstein-Barr virus (EBV) syndromes, and rheumatoid diseases. They are often clinically linked to strain/sprain or repetitive stress injuries. It makes the reduction of inflammation and the thorough resolution of such injuries important to the long-term health of the patient.

There is a growing body of literature on the subject of chronic connective tissue pathology. It is becoming clear that we have much to learn about the fascia and the interrelatedness of a variety of pain mechanisms that can be created by fascial irritation.[1,2] These conditions are benefited greatly by chiropractic intervention. Manipulation, especially spinal manipulation, is a powerful tool, affecting what is a combination of highly integrated tissues, neurologically and biomechanically. Manipulation coupled with soft tissue work (myofascial and ligamentous) can afford pain control and tissue stabilization. By maintaining that stability over a long enough time, what is known as degenerative joint disease (DJD) may actually show signs of regeneration.

STRAIN/SPRAIN INJURIES

Trauma to the musculoskeletal system is classified by the degree of injury and signs and symptoms. The tissues involved also need to be delineated. A strain is generally considered to be a degree of trauma, due to overstretching that causes incomplete tearing or rupturing of the connective tissues. A sprain injury will cause more severe tearing and disruption of tissue. We generally think of straining muscles and spraining joints.

Classifying strain/sprain injuries is based on an assessment of the severity of the injury. Consider the history and the clinical findings. We generally define an injury as acute, subacute, or chronic, depending on the time of injury and time elapsed before treatment. The first 36 hours is the acute stage. The subacute stage lasts from 3 to 14 days, and the chronic phase can last for 2 to 8 weeks, or as its name implies, it may never resolve.

The severity of the injury is categorized as mild, if it is a straining injury with minimal evidence of tissue damage or reaction. A moderate strain will involve a larger area of connective tissue, with mild swelling, and have some tissue close to the breaking point. A sprain would be diagnosed as mild if evaluation finds only the likelihood of a small tear with increased pain and evidence of swelling. I use the term strain/sprain as most injuries beyond this level are combinations of both types of damage. A moderate strain/sprain injury would find significant disruption of tissue and evidence of increased joint instability. A severe sprain is a major disruption of ligament or tendinous structure with serious joint instability that, in the extremities, can lead to the need for major orthopaedic intervention.

In dealing with strain injuries, after the inflammation is under control, the muscles involved can be evaluated for weakness. When found weak, goading the origin and insertion of the muscle will often bring the muscle up to near normal function.

Goading is a rapid, oscillating movement, deep enough to affect the underlying muscle/tendon tissue, without the examiner's contact being allowed to slide over the skin. This technique can be done on repeated treatments to help the body maintain as normal a function as possible during recovery.

The acute low back injury is commonly brought on by some type of injury, such as a fall or twisting while bending or lifting. A sudden onset usually suggests muscle strain and spasm. A more gradual onset, overnight, is more likely to be a sprain. However, there is no set rule that it cannot be any combination of factors. The patient will most often be aware of what brought on the episode. In some cases of spontaneous low back pain, it was not bending over the sink, but the ski trip two weeks earlier that set up a delayed reaction. Recall that an injury while bending down will involve the gluteus maximus more often than not (Fig. 6–1). Raising up or lifting will most often affect the psoas and especially the L4–5 segments (Fig. 6–2).

An examination should rule out pathology, such as kidney infection, vascular, or serious neurological problems. The age and any history of previous low back episodes will help determine the likelihood of degenerative changes.

Patients with acute low back strain/sprain can usually make it to your office and onto your table; however, sometimes it may take awhile. They may be antalgic, complain of low back

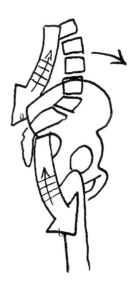

Fig. 6–1 Erector spinae and gluteus maximus contract eccentrically when bending over. The gluteus maximus can be strained. a. erector spinae, b. gluteus maximus.

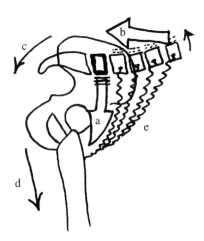

Fig 6–2 The lower psoas slips can be injured in the initial stage of arising from a bent position. a. L5 psoas slip contracts hard, b. erector spinae contracts, c. gluteus maximus contracts, d. hamstrings contract, e. relaxed upper psoas fibers.

pain, indicating the lumbosacral area, and often have pain in the buttock or thigh, but do not often complain of pain or numbness below the knee or into the foot. Their range of motion is limited, and although neurological testing is negative, some of the orthopaedic tests can give conflicting results. Even when it appears that there may be nerve root irritation, the early management would still be aimed at reduction of swelling, rest, and judicious correction of musculoskeletal imbalances. All lumbar strain/sprain injuries should, at first, include a possible discopathy in the working diagnosis. In many cases, early neurological symptoms will subside as inflammation is controlled.

Palpation will show areas of hypertonic muscles, hypomobile joints, and a good indication of the level of pain tolerance of the patient. That level will help determine how aggressive initial treatment should be. If a moderate-to-severe sprain is suspected, all manipulation during the acute phase should be light, with respect to the already damaged ligaments and the patient's comfort.

In the initial treatment, reducing muscle spasm, due either to strain or protective, antalgic hypertonicity, will often provide noticeable relief. The most common hypertonic muscles in low back/pelvic injuries will be one or more of the psoas, gluteus maximus, piriformis, iliacus, and paravertebral muscles. A patient with spasm or hypertonicity of the gluteus and erector muscles usually presents with a flat back. Psoas hypertonicity will cause an increased lordosis and anterior pelvis. Stretching can be accomplished in the acute stage with relative comfort and safety.

The acute phase blends into the subacute phase, as pain subsides and ROM is increased, even slightly. With inflammation down, a clearer idea of actual damage is easier to assess. Ma-

nipulation can become more aggressive. The use of combinations of heat, ROM exercise, and ice, along with any physical therapy modalities can be initiated. As a general rule, each treatment should include correcting any muscle imbalances by stretching or goading as needed. Dysfunction of the injured tissue and the adaptive changes needed to protect the area and support the body cause repeated neurological "imprinting" of aberrant function. That function can become habitual causing long-term damage and incomplete healing. Repeated correction of these dysfunctions "reminds" the body of normal function.

The chronic phase is the time of final resolution. Inflammation should be occasional and minimal at most, with steady improvement, noted subjectively by the patient, reporting less pain and increased function. This should be confirmed by objective signs, such as decreased pain, increased joint mobility, and improved findings upon orthopaedic testing. Patients are seen less frequently and should be educated as to proper lifting techniques and preventive lifestyle changes. They should also be progressed into an exercise program, specific to their particular weaknesses, but containing a generalized low back strengthening program (see Appendix B).

No two patients respond to their injuries in the same way. As a general rule, most simple strain/sprain injuries should be resolved in four to six weeks. Many differing attitudes and opinions exist about how much treatment is proper and how long the treatment should take. These are individual decisions based on the physician's understanding of the patient's condition, the technique being used, and the individual healing processes of the patient. Recent attempts to define the protocols for treatment are leading, in my opinion, to placing medically acceptable limitations on chiropractic treatment concepts.

In general, the Mercy guidelines, an intraprofessional attempt to standardize clinical chiropractic protocols acceptable to both chiropractors and managed care institutions, are reasonable but lack any consideration for corrective manipulative programs, or preventive checkups. The emphasis, like that in traditional medicine, is on the fast elimination of symptoms, which to some is equivalent to a cure. In my opinion, the chiropractic protocol should provide for longer term manipulative treatment programs to correct chronic subluxation patterns and express the benefits of preventive care. It is my experience that a series of adjustments can make significant improvements in joint function. The judicious use of specific, repetitive adjustments can break down fibrous adhesions and contractures restoring the functional integrity of the joints in question. This reduces nervous interference from aberrant sensory input and direct irritation of the spinal nerves and may contribute to regeneration of tissue.

LORDOTIC LUMBAR SYNDROME

The lordotic lumbar syndrome (LLS) is a common finding in patients with low back complaints (Fig. 6–3). If chronic, it

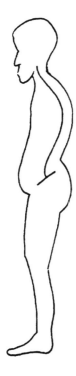

Fig. 6–3 Chronic LLS.

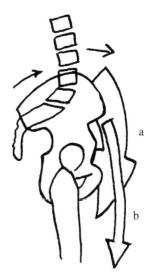

Fig. 6–4 Muscles that produce an anterior pelvi. a. psoas, iliacus, b. TFL, rectus femoris, sartorius.

is accompanied by long-term changes in function and intrinsic tissue changes. An acute injury with an underlying LLS may have complications in recovery due to a breakdown in the adaptive process. This can be a good time to initiate corrective intervention because the injured area is open to improvement. Old adhesions and contractures are likely to be disrupted, which can be an advantage.

The LLS is a persistent anterior tilt of the pelvis involving combinations of increased lordosis, anterior ilia, hypertonic psoas, and iliacus, and possibly, the sartorius, tensor fascia lata (TFL), and rectus femoris (Fig. 6–4). The gluteus maximus or abdominals or both will be weak or underfunctioning (Fig. 6–5). Weight is felt anteriorly, on the balls of the feet. The patient will describe the inability to stand still without pain. Patients may complain of pain and restricted ability to straighten up upon arising from a seated position. Both psoas often, in LLS, contract while a person is sitting and will not relax quickly enough due to irritation and hypertonicity. Patients may have pain when lying supine, and the gap between the table and the low back will be wide (Fig. 6–6). The spine remains arched by the tight musculature. Patients with LLS will commonly have medially rotated femurs with irritated piriformis muscles, compensating for the weak gluteus maximus, as well as laterally rotated tibias and changes in the feet as part of the compensatory mechanisms.[3]

LLS–type posture is encouraged by the fashion industry that requires models to pose in severe swayback positions,

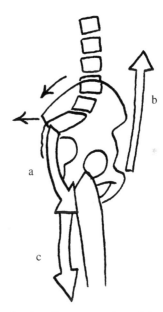

Fig. 6–5 Muscles that allow an anterior pelvis. a. gluteus maximus, b. abdominals, c. hamstrings.

which seem to be emulated by many young women. Such posture is also common in those who have been gymnasts. It is also caused by negligence, evident in the declining male physique, with a large pendulous abdomen hanging over a badly, anteriorly tipped pelvis (Fig. 6–7). LLS, however, affects more women than men. Women lose, and often never regain, abdominal strength after pregnancy. They are encouraged to conform to the fashionable styles that demand high heel shoes. Both of these factors will encourage LLS.

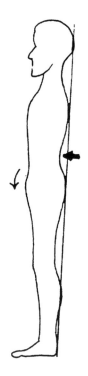

Fig. 6–6 Lordotic lumbar syndrome (LLS).

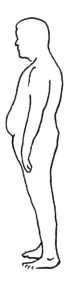

Fig. 6–7 Anterior pelvic tilt with weak abdominals and anterior head displacement.

In both the declining male physique and loss of abdominal strength after pregnancy, one will find the psoas or the iliacus or both in a state of hypertonicity with marked pain to palpation of the belly or origin/insertion. The abdominals are weak or stretched and the lower posterior fibers often are not work-

ing at all. The gluteus maximus will be weak and stretched. The piriformis may be hypertonic, or inflamed and weak. The piriformis will be attempting to compensate for the weak gluteus maximus.

Some patients with LLS are stomach sleepers. Prone sleeping habits will stress the lumbar spine anteriorly, irritating the psoas that becomes contracted increasing the lordosis. Stomach sleepers often throw one or the other leg out, which precipitates a lateral rotation subluxation of the femur (Fig. 6–8). This produces a long leg which will, itself, be the subject of adaptation and further complications.

The initial treatment must emphasize the reduction of inflammation. The hypertonic muscles, the psoas, and iliacus and, less likely, the sartorius, TFL, and rectus femoris, should be stretched, and the patient should be instructed about how to perform home stretches to reduce chronic muscle contracture. The stomach sleeper will need some aid in altering the sleep posture.

One method is to use a belt to hold the knees together. In sleep, it will be impossible to sleep prone. Another method that can be successful is to tape two marbles to each side of the umbilicus. Like the fable of the princess and the pea, most patients will not stay prone for long. It takes about 30 days to break the prone sleeping habit. The use of a body pillow that the patient can sleep over is helpful with difficult cases.

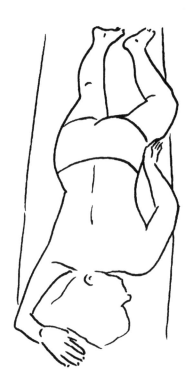

Fig. 6–8 Stomach sleeping.

Stretching Techniques

There are numerous methods of stretching muscles, from reflex methods that use the spindle cells and Golgi tendon organs to reset the neurological components of the muscle, to various combinations of contract/relax-and-stretch methods. The nature of the contracted muscle will determine the best method. An acutely strained muscle may be more comfortably relaxed by working the sensory organs and avoiding further damage by overstretching.

Proprioceptive Adjustment

Chaitow[1] describes spindle cell and Golgi tendon work as proprioceptive adjusting, but acknowledges its more common description: applied kinesiology. I agree with his statement that the tight hypertonic muscles should be dealt with first. Applied kinesiology stresses the weak muscles. The concept is to apply light thumb pressure (two pounds) toward the center of the muscle in the area of the spindle cells, or away from the center in the area of the Golgi tendon organs.

The spindle cells are located in the belly of the muscle, and the Golgi tendon organs are located near the origin and insertion. Spindle cells feed back contraction forces. Pushing toward the center of the muscle stimulates the spindle to signal the muscle to reduce its tone. The Golgi tendon sensors monitor forces at the tendinous origin and insertion. By stimulating the areas of the muscle near the origin and insertion, pushing away from the center, the Golgi tendon organs feed back the need to relax the muscle (Fig. 6–9). By working the spindle cells and Golgi tendon organs in the opposite manner, it is possible to activate a lax muscle to increase its tone. I have used these methods with inconsistent results.

I have found the method of stretching recommended by Robert Anderson[4] to be effective. He recommends a two-phase stretch. The first is the "easy stretch" at the tension point of the muscle for 10 to 30 seconds. Then a second "developmental stretch" at a mild tension for another 10 to 30 seconds. There should be no bouncing, and each stretch should be in a comfortable range. Overstretching activates the stretch reflex, which contracts the muscle, and the muscle ends up tighter.

Another effective method, postisometric relaxation (PIR),[5] uses muscular facilitation and inhibition to reduce muscle tone. The muscle that is being stretched is brought to its maximal length without stretching. The patient is asked to contract the muscle (with minimal force) against the examiner's resistance, for 10 seconds. The patient is then instructed to completely relax, and when the physician is certain of complete relaxation, the muscle is elongated further, beyond the original tension point for 10 seconds. If this is not successful, the phases can be increased to 30 seconds, or the isometric phase shortened and repeated three to five times.

Stretching the psoas can be achieved by adding tension to the Thomas test for hypertonicity (Fig. 6–10). By having the

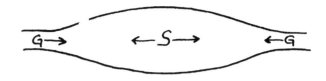

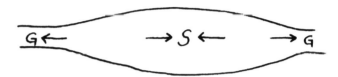

Fig. 6–9 Spindle cell (S) and Golgi tendon (G) procedure. Top: direction to strengthen tone, Bottom: direction to weaken tone.

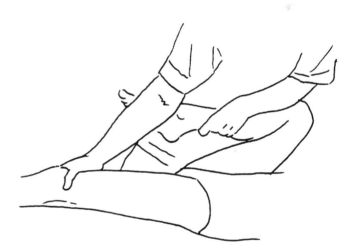

Fig. 6–10 Psoas stretch.

patient drop the extended leg off the table, into extension, holding the opposite knee flexed tight to the abdomen, the physician can apply extension pressure against the extended thigh. The patient can use this method to stretch at home.

The iliacus can be stretched by holding the supine patient's insertion area on the inner femur and applying posterior pressure on the ilium. This is a sensitive area, and the skin is often easily overstretched. Be sure to have plenty of slack.

The sartorius can be reached in the supine patient at its belly and origin or insertion. A direct stretch is best with a palm contact over the anterior superior iliac spine (ASIS) and an index contact at the medial aspect of the knee, where the sartorius passes on its way to the pes anserinus. Pressing down on the ASIS, rotating the ilium posterior, and pushing toward the insertion at the medial knee, the muscle is comfortably stretched.

The TFL can be stretched by placing the thigh (patient supine) into flexion, slight abduction, and slight internal rotation, leg extended. Support the leg by holding it at the ankle. The cephalad thumb is used to stretch the muscle fibers toward their origin on the iliac crest, as the thigh is lowered into extension and adduction.

The rectus femoris can be worked with the patient in the supine position by pushing inferiorly on the patella and superiorly on the anterior inferior iliac spine. The piriformis, if hypertonic, can be stretched by applying pressure toward the sacral origin while the patient is in the side posture (Fig. 6–11).

In LLS, the weak muscles, the gluteus maximus and piriformis and, most importantly, the abdominals, will need to be strengthened (see Chapter 7 on Exercises).

It is more common to find an inability to activate the abdominals in women. They are often unable to perform a pelvic rocking action, and it becomes necessary to train these patients to activate the pelvic rhythm. This is often a result of the inaction of the abdominals during pregnancy. With the patient in the supine position, ask them to rock the pelvis anteriorly to posteriorly. If they cannot, assist them by placing one hand over the lower abdomen and the other under the sacrum and actively rock the pelvis back and forth until the patient becomes aware of the necessary action. This is an exercise they should do several times a day to reestablish proper tone and function of the abdominals. Sit-ups may be necessary to completely strengthen the muscles.

Manipulation in LLS is directed at correcting any habitual subluxation patterns. Anterior fixations of the ilia are common. Along with correcting the muscles that allow and pro-

duce LLS, passive motion palpation (PMP) should be used to check for AS fixation (Fig. 6–12). The condition may require repeated adjustments due to habitual changes in the proprioceptive mechanisms adapting to the imbalance, and contractual changes in the connective tissue (Fig. 6–13).

Anterior fixation subluxations will be common in the lower lumbars. The hypertonic psoas slips to L4 and L5 can maintain vertebral anteriorities (Fig. 6–14). The knees and feet should be checked for subluxation patterns.

Exercises should be started as soon as the patient can do them without pain. Educate the patient on better postural habits. Stomach sleepers need to change their habits, or use a sup-

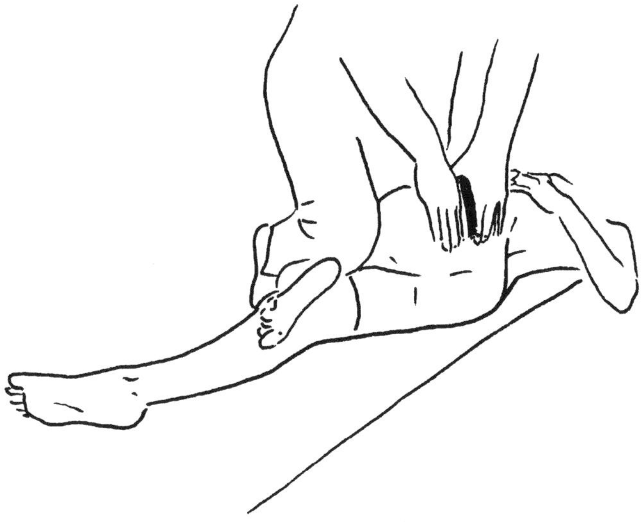

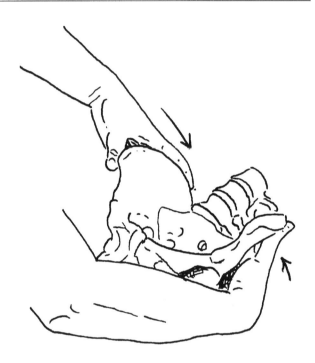

Fig. 6–12 Passive motion palpation for AS ilium fixation.

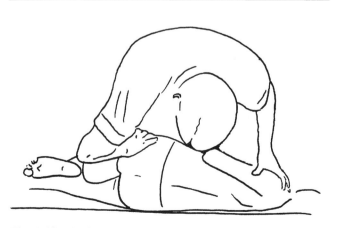

Fig. 6–13 AS ilium adjustment.

Fig. 6–11 Piriformis stretch.

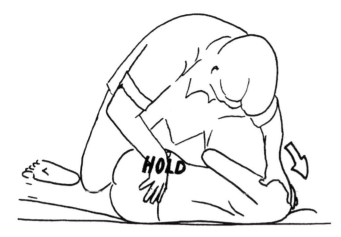

Fig. 6–14 Anterior lumbar adjustment.

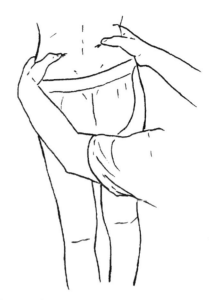

Fig. 6–15 Palpation of iliac crests and posterior superior iliac spine.

port pillow under the stomach, or sleep over a body pillow. The patient's work and play habits should be considered for any factors that are contributing to the LLS pattern.

LEG LENGTH INEQUALITY (LLI)

The exam finding of unequal leg length is very common. I would estimate that 80% of patients will show uneven legs. However, only 8% to 10% are anatomical. The functional short leg is controversial. A number of authors, writing on the subject of LLI, seem neither to reject nor accept the idea that lumbar and pelvic dynamics are capable of altering leg length. They will admit to the need for further study.[6] Most techniques in use consider the functional short leg.

Dr. Logan defined a clear set of functional factors that will cause a functional leg length inequality (LLIfn). He found in his preliminary clinical studies that he could consistently diagnose, by physical examination, an anatomical LLI and be within two to three mm of the most accepted radiological methods.

In the examination, a number of findings will lead to an investigation of LLI, such as unlevel iliac crests in the standing exam (Fig. 6–15) and gluteal folds and knee folds (Fig. 6–16). Look for signs of pronation (Fig. 6–17). Check for a history of leg fracture or hip dysplasia.

A patient with LLI will often stand with the short leg rotated outward (Fig. 6–18). This is a compensatory mechanism; lateral rotation can increase the leg length, and often the hip is chronically subluxated laterally. Some patients with LLI will stand with a wide stance with the long leg rotated laterally, another attempt to compensate.

In the supine position, check crest and ASIS levels. Check the leg levels at the medial malleoli and medial femoral condyles (see Chapter 2 on Examination). The best way is to hook the thumbs up under the bones on both sides with equal

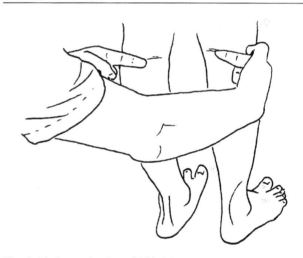

Fig. 6–16 Comparing knee fold heights.

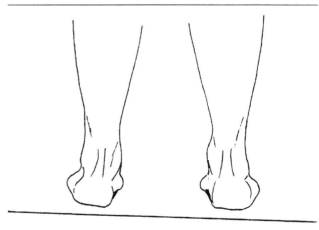

Fig. 6–17 Left Achilles tendon shows medial curve suggestive of pronation.

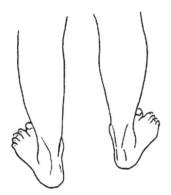

Fig. 6–18 Right leg rotated laterally to increase leg length.

pressure and sight down over them (Fig. 6–19). Check the heels for discrepancy.

A long leg can be functionally caused by: (1) laterally rotated femur, (2) an AS ilium, (3) an inferior ilium, (4) knee subluxation, and (5) high arch in the foot. A functional short leg can be caused by: (1) a PI ilium, (2) knee subluxation, and (3) pronation or dropped arch. The knee can subluxate laterally and rotate, more commonly laterally. It can simulate either a long or short leg depending on unique individual variations.[7]

By eliminating the functional causes listed above, the final outcome should be relatively equal leg lengths or a true anatomical difference. This method of evaluation will provide a

relatively accurate measurement of the difference. In my opinion, it is accurate enough for clinical purposes. The necessity of using a radiograph for the sole purpose of determining the inequality is not clinically necessary except in complicated cases.

A patient with true LLI will often create compensatory changes. Common among these are lateral rotation subluxation of the short side femur (Fig. 6–20), AS fixation on the short leg side, or PI on the long leg side. These are the same factors that cause a functional LLI (Fig. 6–21). The pronation of the long leg side foot or the high arch on the short leg side can be functional adaptations.[8] Another adaptation can cause the short side ilia to subluxate inferiorly with related Q-L stretching and weakness.

In true anatomical LLI, these imbalances are often chronic and will require corrective manipulation. The idea is to maintain function in the joints involved through manipulation and muscle balancing. They will remain healthier under the added stress of adapting to an imbalance. An LLIfn can also involve chronic adaptive changes that will require a program of correction. For instance, a chronic lateral rotation of the femur could cause a chronic PI ilium on that side. The patient with the persistent PI that is always corrected, but always there on the next appointment, may have a lateral femur that puts the ilium into PI as soon as the patient is on his or her feet.

Some patients have very stable adaptations. It would be unwise to attempt to alter anything in such a case. Use of a lift or attempts to stop adaptive functions may create pain and dysfunction where none existed. If dealing with a low back patient, be sure the LLI is actually a cause of the complaint before tampering with it.

The general consensus is that an inequality of more than ¼ inch is considered likely to cause problems. In practice, there

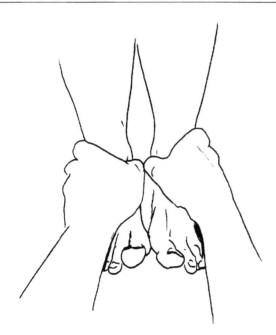

Fig. 6–19 Checking leg length at medial malleoli.

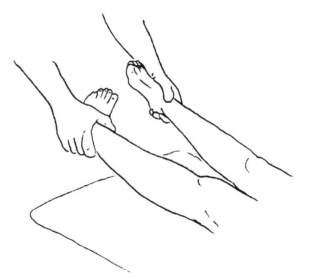

Fig. 6–20 Checking internal rotation of femurs. Note decreased rotation on right.

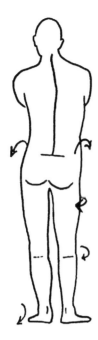

Fig. 6–21 LLI and compensations for a right leg deficiency: pelvic tilt and compensatory scoliosis, iliac rotations, knee and femur rotations, foot pronation.

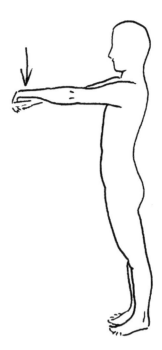

Fig. 6–22 Strength test for lift determination.

are some patients who have symptomatic dysfunction with less than ¼ inch and those who have stable adaptations with ½ inch or more. It would be unwise to introduce too much change into a stable adaptation. It is better to support the body's efforts by maintaining as normal a joint dynamic as possible and balancing and toning the muscles to accommodate the adaptation.

Lifts

When an LLI is determined, and all adaptive imbalances have been corrected, it is possible to determine the need for a lift. If the body is doing fine without support, it could be disastrous to add a lift automatically. Dr. Logan used a method presented by Dr. George Goodheart in the 1970s.[9] It is a direct challenge of the erect musculoskeletal support system. The patient stands barefoot with balanced posture and arms outstretched in front, hands together. The examiner contacts the hands and has the patient resist the effort to push the hands down (Fig. 6–22). Watch for an obvious weakness in the patient's efforts. The arms will not be able to resist, or the patient will make a noticeable effort to avoid falling forward. Look at the feet. If the heels lift off the floor or the toes grip with exaggerated effort, the need for a lift is indicated.

Start with a lift ½ the inequality. It is rare to need much more. Place it under the short heel and retest. If the patient's resistance is improved, it is dramatic proof of the need for a lift. Add or subtract from the height of the lift until the stron-

gest response is noted. By removing the lift, testing and replacing it, and testing it again, the patient is made well aware of the difference. This awareness can improve compliance. Periodic evaluation of the lift should be done to be sure it is still indicated, or the correct height. It is not uncommon to see changes over time.

Where pronation is a part of the adaptation to LLI, or is a factor in functional LLI, it is possible that correction of the other factors or support of the short leg with a lift may allow the foot to self-correct. When considering the use of orthotics, it is best to make sure the changes in the foot are permanent and not functional in nature.

Long-term adaptations to LLI may include degenerative changes in the hip, pelvis, and low back. The need for corrective manipulation will be likely. Changes need to be gradual in order to avoid reaction. All patients will need to exercise the muscles that are weak and stretch those that are hypertonic and contracted. The Q-L is often weak on the short leg side. The gluteus maximus will show weakness with an AS ilium. The abdominals are often involved. The psoas and iliacus may be hypertonic with an AS ilium.

THE UNSTABLE PELVIS

The unstable pelvis is the result of a laxity of the sacroiliac (SI) joints. The sacroiliac ligaments and the overlying lumbodorsal fascia are highly innervated with sensory nerves. The unstable pelvis is a common cause of severe acute low back episodes. This is the patient who presents with major pain, can-not sit or stand comfortably, but does not necessarily show antalgic leaning, as in a disk case. Motion palpation is not possible and muscle testing and orthopaedic testing are too painful, giving no useful information.

The history may be that of an underlying chronic condition with periodic exacerbations. Anatomical LLI can be a cause, as can a history of pregnancies, a prat fall, or other injury that damages the SI joints. This condition is more common in women because the female pelvis is subjected to the stresses of pregnancy and delivery. Also the laxity of the pelvic ligaments is enhanced by the hormonal changes of pregnancy. It seems that the pelvic structure never fully returns to its prepregnancy stability. Periodic strain/sprain injuries can lead to chronically unstable tissue.

I have found it very common in women approaching 50 to have exquisitely painful lumbosacral areas. Palpation is met with a major pain response and avoidance reaction. The connective tissue tends to become chronically involved with fibrositis. This tissue can be severely painful to the touch, but gives no indication to the patient except during exacerbations.

The supine position is best for evaluating this condition. Much can be discovered by palpating the SI joint and seeing how it responds to movements in all directions (see Chapter 2 on Examination). By pushing medially on the ischial tuberosity, a noticeable decrease in pain at the SI joint leads to the transversus peroneus as a causal factor. A lateral pull on the tuberosity that reduces pain indicates that the abdominals (transversus and posterior obliques) and the fourth segment of the Q-L are responsible. Relief with anterior pressure indicates the gluteus maximus, with superior pressure, the Q-L. If the pain is generated by muscle strain only, these maneuvers will noticeably reduce the pain. If it is an inflammatory condition, there will be little change.

The pubic symphysis should be palpated. Chronic pelvic instability can irritate the pubis, and there may be signs of subluxation (Fig. 6–23). Compress the ilia and repalpate to see if there is any relief. If so, iliac compression with a trochanter belt could be helpful in recovery. Toning the adductors and transversus perineus is warranted.

The muscles that are involved are those that allow a PI (or produce an AS), primarily the iliacus, and of the muscles that produce a PI (or allow an AS), the gluteus maximus is primary (Fig. 6–24). The muscles involved in a medial ischilum (MI) are the transversus perinei and gluteus medius, which produce it, and the iliacus (anterior fibers), Q-L fourth segment, transverse and posterior abdominals, which allow it (Fig. 6–25).

The piriformis can also figure in an unstable pelvis. There are three muscles that affect the sacrum. The gluteus maximus, the medial fibers of the iliacus, and the piriformis. These muscles will be either in states of hypertonicity or weak. If the condition is chronic, some of the hypertonic muscles may have undergone contracture and can show signs of myositis.

If the patient is able, further information can be obtained by

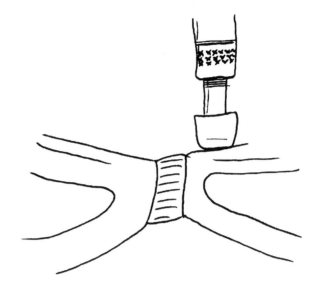

Fig. 6–23 Left superior pubis—adjusting with impactor.

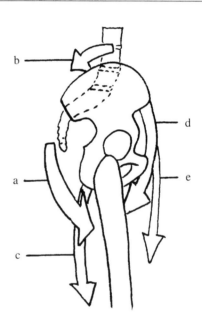

Fig. 6–24 Muscles producing a PI or allowing an AS ilium: a. gluteus maximus, b. quadratus lumborum and posterior abdominals, c. hamstrings. Muscles allowing a PI or producing an AS ilium: d. iliacus, e. TFL, sartorius, rectus femoris.

evaluating the function of these muscles in the act of arising and sitting (see Chapter 2 on Examination). Recall that the ischial tuberosities widen in the seated position, and pull together as we stand. Support the trochanters as the patient sits. This assists the piriformis and gluteus maximus. Support the ischial tuberosities. Such support helps the transversus peroneus and gluteus medius (Fig. 6–26). Reductions in pain or greater ease of movement can help pinpoint the problem.

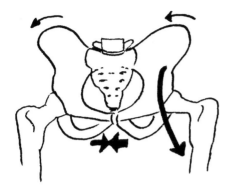

Fig. 6–25 Transversus perinei pulls ischium medially, causing a medial ischium. Anterior fibers of the iliacus pull iliac crest medially, reducing iliac flare and MI.

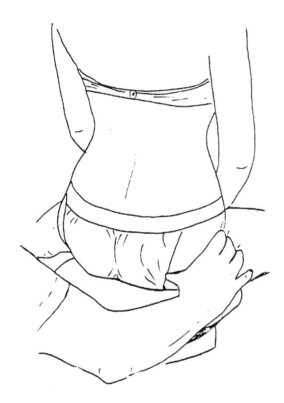

Fig. 6–26 Supporting ischial tuberosities as patient attempts to arise.

When observing the patient upon arising, note the knees. The patient keeping the knees close together may be indicative of a transverse peroneal strain or piriformis weakness. The piriformis acts as an abductor in the seated position and is active in the initial act of arising. It shifts to its lateral rotator role as the halfway point of standing is reached. A patient who stands with the knees far apart is usually protecting a bad lumbar spine and not an unstable pelvis.

Arising on one foot will be easier on the side of SI inflammation. When the weight is borne on the good side, the muscle actions, especially the Q-L, on the nonbearing, involved side will stress the inflamed SI joint.

A treatment program should start with the control of inflammation. The patient with an acute case should be ordered to bed, bearing no weight for two to three days. No adjusting of the SI should be done. Adjusting the T9–10–11 areas helps normalize the innervation of critical muscles (recall the actual origin of nerve roots on the spinal cord).

Adjusting of the SI should be judicious, for these joints are unstable. Too much adjusting could increase the instability. The best approach is to correct the pelvic imbalances, such as AS, PI, and MI. Use blocks in the severe stage if other approaches seem unwise. It is important in the treatment plan to emphasize strengthening exercises for the weak pelvic muscles. The ligaments may never regain their original tightness, elasticity, and ability to completely support the SI joints. The muscles become important secondary support. Chronic cases may take a long time to stabilize. There is usually enough steady improvement to keep the patient motivated.

SCIATICA

Radiating pain into the buttock, thigh, or leg is a common presenting symptom of sciatica. The examination will focus on differentiating between the various causes of sciatica.

Inflammation is often a factor in producing radicular symptoms. In the initial treatment, reducing swelling can often result in rapidly diminished symptoms of sciatica. When neurological findings are slight or inconclusive, often an initial period of rest, ice, and careful manipulation can eliminate a concern over a discogenic sciatica. Nervous tissue is slower to recover than other tissues. It is important to understand that to jump too soon to conclusions can lead to unnecessary invasive procedures. Depending on the severity of the neurological deficit, the patient should be informed as to available options. Usually the medical approach is to wait and provide pain, anti-inflammatory and muscle relaxant medications, which do not always relieve much of the discomfort.

Peripheral entrapment of the sciatic nerve can occur in the buttock. Piriformis syndrome is the irritation of the sciatic nerve by a dysfunction of the piriformis. This dysfunction can be due to spasm, or overstretching and laxity. Check the piriformis for strength and hypertonicity. The patient will have no signs or symptoms of spinal involvement. There is usually significant palpable pain in the sciatic notch. A lateral rotation subluxation of the femur can be a precipitating factor, causing irritation in the lateral rotatores.

Treatment should be directed at reducing the femoral subluxation (Fig. 6–27) and either stretching or toning exercises to normalize muscle function. Proceed with caution until the severity of the neuritis has subsided.

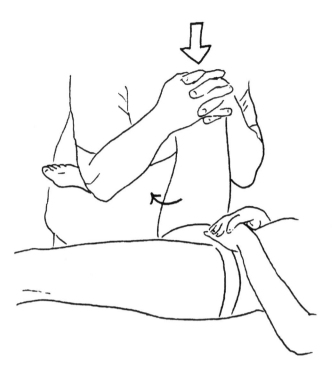

Fig. 6–27 Adjustment for lateral rotation subluxation of femur.

Another area where the nerves can be irritated is in the psoas muscle. The spinal nerves that make up the lumbar plexus pass through the psoas near its origins on the vertebrae. When the psoas is hypertonic or irritated and inflamed, the nerves passing through are in danger of being irritated as well. This could cause radiating pain into the anterolateral thigh. Stretching and correction of the factors involved in creating the hypertonicity are indicated.

The lateral femoral cutaneous nerve can become inflamed by compression or trauma over the anterior hip and ASIS area. Meralgia paresthetica, as it is known, can mimic arthritis of the hip joint and is a factor to consider in differential diagnosis.

There are several referred pain mechanisms that can cause radiating pain into the buttock, posterior thigh, and rarely the calf. The spinal ligaments like the ligamentum flavum and the facetal capsular ligaments can refer pain when irritated. The gluteus medius can, when inflamed, mimic sciatica (personal communication from R. Klein). It should be examined for weakness or inflammation or both.

Stenosis

Degenerative spondylosis and hypertrophy of the ligamentum flavum, in particular, added to degenerative changes in the disks can make the passage for the nerve root quite narrow. Patients with stenosis will suffer radicular symptoms that can

be managed with rest, ice for pain and inflammation, and careful manipulation. It is likely that too aggressive an approach will worsen the symptoms.

Intermittent claudication can mimic sciatica. It is more suspect in older men and is clearly related to activity, coming on with walking, and often quickly relieved with rest.

Discopathy

The increased use of computed tomography (C-T) scans and magnetic resonance imaging (MRI) have shown many protrusions that are incidental, causing no symptoms. When a discogenic radiculopathy is suspected, it is important to recognize when to refer for surgical consultation. If the neurological signs are significant, with severe weakness of muscles and signs of atrophy, the patient should be referred for possible surgery. Signs of bladder or bowel disturbances are also serious signs. If initial treatment shows no improvement, it is best to seek another opinion.

In treating patients with acute disk problems, the first two weeks should show some positive improvement. If the neurological signs are severe, the longer one hesitates, the more likely there will be permanent damage. Some patients should be referred right away. They may not always take the advice of the surgeon and prefer to avoid surgery by toughing it out with conservative management. Many discopathies can be satisfactorily resolved with time, rest, and conservative treatment, including rehabilitation.

Manipulation should be judicious. In my opinion, it is not necessary to avoid adjusting, but care should be used to be as specific as possible and use less force. I have found the flexion/traction technique, pioneered by the osteopathic profession and carried on in the chiropractic profession by James Cox, D.C.,[10] to be effective in many cases. It is specific and gentle. Improvement should be noted within the first 10 to 14 days. If improvement is not noted by this time the problem may be a more serious herniation that may require surgery. I have found that central protrusions or ruptures are less successfully treated by manipulation. The patients who have an antalgic lean into the side with sciatic symptoms or present with marked flexion antalgia or signs of multiple levels of involvement may also be surgical candidates.

QUADRATUS LUMBORUM

In his later research, Dr. Logan focused his attention on the quadratus lumborum (Q-L; Fig. 6–28) as an important muscle in the functional stability of the low back and pelvis. In Dr. Logan's clinical studies, he found Q-L involvement in 90% of unstable pelvis cases. As discussed earlier, the Q-L is a multifunctional muscle. Its main functions are lateral bending of the lumbar spine and depression of the twelfth ribs. Even though it is a thin muscle, it exerts significant influence on the balance

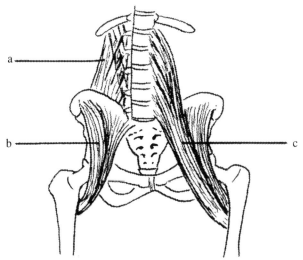

Fig. 6–28 Anterior view of deep muscles. a. quadratus lumborum, b. iliacus, c. psoas.

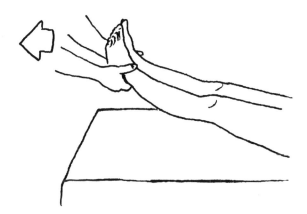

Fig. 6–29 Tug inferiorly for Q-L imbalance.

of the lumbars in lateral stability and iliac support. The fourth segment checks anterior iliac rotation and flare. The entire muscle supports the ilia, influencing it superiorly.

The Q-L is often found to be weak, often unilaterally, in such conditions as the unstable pelvis or functional and anatomical LLI. The pain when performing a Valsalva maneuver or when coughing may be caused by Q-L irritation. It must contract before the diaphragm. This should be considered in the differential diagnosis. This muscle is difficult to assess. Its tone can be determined by tractioning the legs inferiorly with a pull that rocks the pelvis (Fig. 6–29). Note if there is excessive pelvic rocking, as this is indicative of abdominal weakness. If one of the Q-L muscles is weak, it will show as an inferior ilia and longer leg with this traction. Q-L problems can cause palpable pain at the L1–2 level.

If a unilateral weakness is found, adjust T9–10–11 and recheck. Adjusting this level stimulates the nerve supply at the level on the spinal cord where the nerve roots originate.

If there is no improvement, the patient should be given a specific exercise (see Chapter 7 on Exercises) for the Q-L and instructed to do it unilaterally for two weeks. In most cases, the weakness will be corrected. The Q-L should be checked as a matter of routine and any weakness corrected. If this muscle is overlooked, it may be difficult or impossible to effect a complete cure.

ARTHRITIC LUMBOSACRAL SPINE

Many patients that present for treatment will have some degree of degenerative joint disease in the hips, sacroiliac joints, and lumbar spine. In my experience, there is no consistent correlation between the degree of degeneration and symptoms. Some of the worst degeneration, as evidenced on radiographs,

can be relatively stable and cause the patient little or no pain or disability.

In approaching the treatment of a patient with "arthritis," it is wise to use caution and light manipulation initially. If the patient has been told by another physician that they indeed have arthritis, they are often left with the impression that there is nothing that can be done, they will have to live with it, it will get worse, and it is dangerous to tamper with it as they are now very fragile.

In actuality, these patients can be treated successfully and with relative aggressiveness. Treatment directed at restoring joint mobility and reducing abnormal stress due to dysfunctioning muscles and related imbalances can afford relief from pain and improve performance. It is important to re-educate these patients to see their condition as controllable and not so delicate.

Using modalities, such as heat, ultrasound, and electrical muscle stimulation, can improve circulation in stagnant tissue. Manipulation should fit the condition of the patient. One with severe spondylosis and near ankylosis should be treated with gentle techniques designed to maintain as much movement and alignment as possible, and attention should be paid to the adaptations the patient has made to their particular situation. Keeping those adaptations balanced and free of problems is the key.

Many older patients with arthritis need to be encouraged to exercise. A lack of tone is often responsible for the failure of adaptation and keeps the degenerated areas inflamed. I have recommended yoga and t'ai chi (a gentle, slow-motion form of martial art) as excellent exercises that are gentle and safe.

HIP CONDITIONS

The most common hip problems seen clinically are related to straining injuries (not always associated with trauma, but related to chronic dysfunction in the lower back, pelvis, and lower extremities) and degenerative changes.

Pain in the hip can come from several sources. The bursae of the hip can be the source of pain and limitation of motion. The iliopectineal bursa (Fig. 6–30) can be irritated by a chronically laterally rotated femur. The trochanteric and the ischiogluteal bursae can be injured and inflamed. The joint capsule may be involved, and chronic capsulitis will cause contracture and reduced motion. Degeneration of the joint will cause local pain and referred pain down the anteromedial thigh, often to the knee.

Iliopectineal bursitis will show significant pain on direct palpation, and full flexion with adduction will be restricted. The hip flexors will test weak due to pain, and the pectineus may become hypertonic, reducing abduction. There is often an anterior ilia. If the femur is chronically subluxated, it is important to reduce it and keep it reduced. Besides adjusting and ice therapy, instruct the patient to avoid sitting cross-legged, and caution the patient against stomach sleeping.

In the examination of the hip, findings of reduced range of motion that increases after distraction is likely with degenerative changes. Treatment of degenerative hip conditions should be directed toward controlling inflammation and correcting all factors that will stress the hip. Any muscle imbalances, whether hypertonic or weak, will need to be addressed.

Edema of the hip can slightly lengthen the leg. Compression of the joint will temporarily reduce the length (Fig. 6–31). Pain can be elicited upon palpation behind the trochanter, superior to the piriformis and anterolateral to the ischial tuberosity. Rest and ice therapy are recommended.

Differential diagnosis is important. In children, the hip can be involved in pathological processes, such as Legg-Calve-Perth's disease or coxa plana, and a slipped capital femoral epiphysis. The early presentation may be of mild hip strain with signs of inflammation. Radiographs should be ordered.

In older patients, Paget's disease, meralgia paresthetica (an inflammation of the lateral femoral cutaneous nerve), osteoporotic fracture, intermittent claudication, and discopathy should be considered. As a rule, any nontraumatic hip pain should be thoroughly investigated. I have had an elderly patient actually walk into my office with a femoral neck fracture.

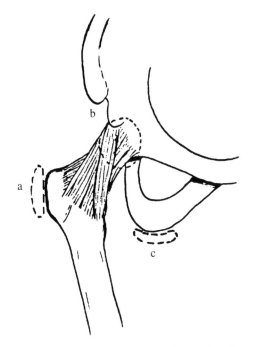

Fig. 6–30 a. trochanteric bursa, b. iliopectinea bursa, c. ischial bursa.

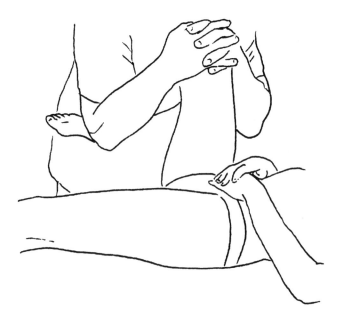

Fig. 6–31 Compress hip—checking for edema.

REFERENCES

1. Chaitow L. *Soft Tissue Manipulation.* Wellingborough: Thorsons Publishing Group; 1987.

2. Black J. Primary Fibromyalgia Syndrome. Ortho-Briefs: *American College of Chiropractic Orthopedists.* 1993;15:40–50.

3. Logan A. *Foot and Ankle: Clinical Aspects.* Gaithersburg, Md: Aspen; 1995.

4. Anderson R. *Stretching.* Bolinas: Shelter Publications, Inc.; 1980.

5. Hannon J, Scaringe J. New directions in the management of musculoskeletal conditions. Lecture notes presented at the Los Angeles College of Chiropractic License Renewal Program; Sacramento, Calif: April 23–24, 1994.

6. Manello D. Leg length inequality: A literature review. Presented at the Seventh Annual Conference of the Consortium for Chiropractic Research; California Chiropractic Association; Palm Springs, Calif: June 19–21, 1992.

7. Logan A. *The Knee: Clinical Aspects.* Gaithersburg, Md: Aspen; 1994.

8. Gillet H. *Belgian Chiropractic Research Notes, 1985.* Huntington Beach, Calif: Motion Palpation Institute; 1985.

9. Goodheart G. Applied Kinesiology Notes. Presented at Applied Kinesiology Seminars; 1972–1976.

10. Cox J. Low back pain: Recent statistics and data on its mechanism, diagnosis and treatment from chiropractic manipulation. *Journal of Chiropractic: American Chiropractic Association.* 1979;13:125–137.

Chapter 7

Exercises

A key factor in the successful outcome of treatment is the rehabilitative exercise necessary to restore normal muscle function. Getting patient compliance in this phase of treatment is likely to be difficult. Most patients are cooperative as long as they are in pain, but as pain subsides, their interest in rehabilitative processes diminishes.

In some cases, the best way to ensure compliance is to refer the patient to a rehab facility with a prescription. A rehab center will be staffed with trained therapists who can monitor the patient, ensuring proper compliance. There is a growing interest among many practitioners in establishing in-house rehab centers. This is an excellent way to control the patient's exercise program.

Some patients are already members of health clubs with adequately equipped gyms. They can be educated in the office and released on their own recognizance. Those patients who cannot afford rehab or gyms can be given training in the office and provided with inexpensive resistance exercise tubing and can work out at home. These patients are the most difficult to control, however. To ensure the exercises are performed and performed correctly, the following must be done:

1. Give a careful explanation in lay terms of exactly what the problem is.
2. Test the muscle and demonstrate to the patient how weak it is and stress the importance of strengthening it.
3. Demonstrate the exercise.
4. Have the patient perform the exercise, making sure that cheating (recruitment of other muscles) does not occur.
5. Provide, where possible, a diagram of the exercise as a reminder.
6. Make available exercise tubing if it is to be used. Do not rely on the patient to obtain it on his or her own.
7. If a spouse is available, he or she can be enlisted to ensure compliance.
8. Clearly explain the number of repetitions and number of sessions to be completed per day.
9. Review the exercise and check muscles for improvement on subsequent visits.

When relying on the cooperation of the patient, the simpler the exercise process, the easier its execution, the more likely it will be followed. Instead of describing the number of sets and repetitions per set, I have found it easier, in some cases, to give the patient a time line. For instance, I will instruct the patient to start with a one or two minute set, or until the muscle "burns," a few minutes of rest, then repeat again. The patient can gradually increase the time as the muscle responds. The extent of the program should be tailored to the patient's condition and ability.

The exercise concepts described in this chapter are those developed over many years of clinical experience. They have proved to be the most successful exercises when relying on the patient to comply. The muscles considered are the most commonly found to be weak or dysfunctional. There are numerous theories and methods of toning muscles. The exercise concepts described here can be modified to fit any program and should be an example of how to figure out creative ways to isolate and tone practically any muscle.

ABDOMINALS

There are countless "ab" exercise techniques. The evolution of the sit-up has progressed from the old straight legged full sit-up to the more correct current "cruncher." Dr. Logan devised his sit-up exercise to fully activate the total abdominal group. In many cases the rectus is the most emphasized, and the obliques and transverse groups get minimally worked, especially the lower pelvic fibers. The full sit-up will enlist the psoas muscles in the second half of the movement. In more cases than not, the psoas muscles are already too tight, and a full sit-up will exaggerate the imbalance between these two antagonistic muscles.

A "half" sit-up that isolates the abdominals and deactivates the psoas is advantageous. By putting the legs up over a chair with the hips at 90°, the psoas muscles are unable to assist with any strength. By limiting the sit-up to the first half (raising up only to elevate the shoulder blades from the floor), the abdominals are used fully. At the same time, flattening the low back to the floor, which tilts the pelvis posteriorly, works the lower abdominal fibers.

With the arms outstretched, rise up to touch an imaginary point to the extreme left (Fig. 7–1), hold for a count of two, and slowly return to the floor. This is position one. With each successive sit-up, move the imaginary point to the right passing the center point (over the knees) and ending with point six far to the right (Fig. 7–2). Then work back to the left. This six point radius of sit-ups works all the oblique and transverse fibers. The patient can be instructed to assess each position and add extra repetitions to those positions that seem weaker.

GLUTEUS MAXIMUS

Exercise 1

Instruct the patient to start on hands and knees. Raise one leg up and "push" the foot towards the ceiling (Fig. 7–3). Do not move the pelvis. The hip joint does not normally extend beyond neutral more than 10°. Further extension will be ac-

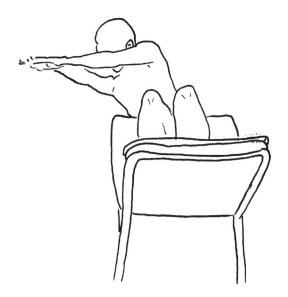

Fig. 7–2 Sit-up position 6.

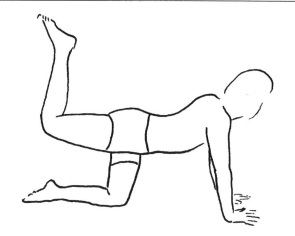

Fig. 7–3 Gluteus maximus exercise 1.

complished with pelvic rotation that defeats the purpose of the exercise. Start with 8 to 10 repetitions on each side and compare efforts. Add extra repetitions to the weaker side. As strength increases, ankle weights can be added as well as the number of repetitions increased.

Exercise 2

Using resistance tubing, a standing exercise can be done. Stand next to a desk or table and rest the weight-bearing hip against the edge of the table. Flex the hip and knee of the side to be worked and secure the tubing around the heel. Secure the other end against the desk with both hands. Push the foot back against the resistance no more than eight inches past the other leg (Fig. 7–4).

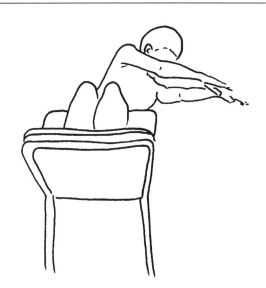

Fig. 7–1 Sit-up position 1.

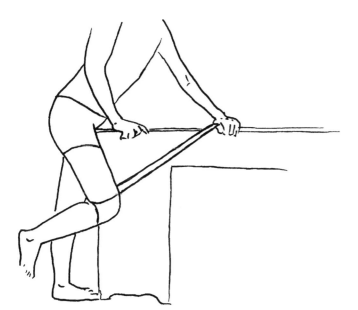

Fig. 7–4 Gluteus maximus exercise 2.

Repeat 6 to 8 times and reverse to work the other side. Compare the efforts and work the weaker side a little more.

Exercise 3

This is a non–weight-bearing position that is easier to do if the patient is unable to perform the first two methods. The patient lies supine with the hip and knee flexed to 90°. The resistance tubing is hooked around the heel, and the hip is extended to a 45° angle. This is actually the same as the standing exercise done supine. Repeat 6 to 8 times and switch to the opposite side. Compare and add repetitions to the weaker side.

GLUTEUS MEDIUS

Exercise 1

The most successful way to work the gluteus medius is to instruct the patient in side lifts (abduction with slight extension) in the same position as the test, lying on one side, then the other (Fig. 7–5). Increase repetitions or add ankle weights or both.

Exercise 2

A standing exercise can be achieved by supporting the body by holding on to a wall or chair back. The leg is abducted and slightly extended while the pelvis remains level. This resembles a ballet exercise.

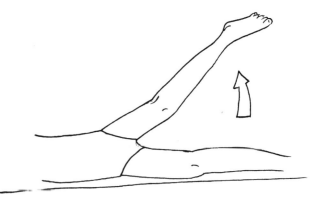

Fig. 7–5 Gluteus medius exercise.

LATERAL HIP ROTATORS

These exercises include the piriformis and gluteal muscles.

Exercise 1

Secure the resistance tubing to the leg of a heavy piece of furniture to the side being exercised. Sit in as reclined a position as possible, with the hip as extended toward neutral as is possible (about 30°—recall that the piriformis becomes an abductor as the hip is flexed toward 90°). Hook the tubing around the foot and pull across toward the opposite leg, which rotates the hip laterally (Fig. 7–6).

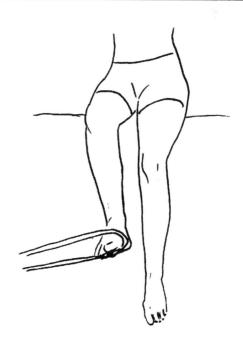

Fig. 7–6 Piriformis exercise 1.

Repeat 8 to 10 times. If both sides are to be worked, compare and add repetitions to the weaker side.

Exercise 2

Sitting up straight, hook the tubing around the thigh near the knee. Secure the other end around the opposite knee. Abduct the thigh to exercise the piriformis, which, in this position, acts as an abductor (Fig. 7–7).

QUADRATUS LUMBORUM

Secure the tubing at chest level. Closing a knotted end in a door jamb is a convenient method for home use.

Extend and "lock" the knees. They should not bend during the exercise. All movement should be from the waist up. Make sure the pelvis does not shift. Lean toward the door and take tension on the tubing holding the end to the chest with both hands (Fig. 7–8).

Pull against the resistance and do a side bend to the opposite side (Fig. 7–9). Be sure the shoulders remain in line and do not rotate to recruit other muscles and "cheat." Repeat 8 to 10 times.

Repeat the above exercise first with one foot 6 to 8 inches behind and then 6 to 8 inches in front of the other foot. Compare the effort and add 8 to 10 additional repetitions to the weaker foot position. This positional change emphasizes different portions of the muscles being worked.

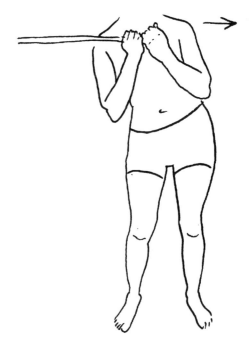

Fig. 7–8 Beginning position for Q-L exercise.

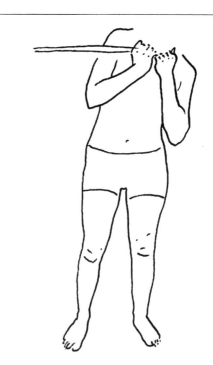

Fig. 7–9 Q-L exercise ending position.

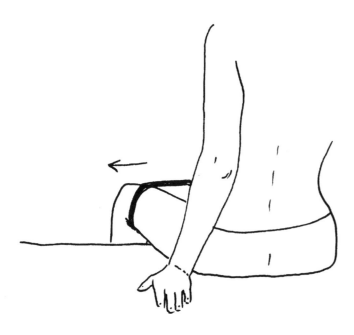

Fig. 7–7 Piriformis exercise 2.

TRANSVERSUS PERINEI

This muscle is activated to stabilize the ischial tuberosities prior to the activation of the adductors in returning the thigh from an abducted state.

The best way to perform this exercise is to sit slumped in a chair with the legs extended out and clamped against the legs of a facing chair, in slight abduction. An isometric contraction to bring the legs together will activate and work the transversus perinei (Fig. 7–10). Have the patient do a ten second isometric contraction 2 to 3 times a day.

A standing exercise can be done by standing with a wide stance and isometrically contract the adductors, which necessitates the initial action of the transversus perinei (Fig. 7–11).

LOWER Q-L AND COCCYGEAL FIBERS OF THE GLUTEUS MAXIMUS

Exercise 1

The fourth Q-L segment and posterior abdominals are part of the system that pulls the iliac crest medially, countering the transversus perinei. When weak, they will allow a medial ischium. The coccygeal fibers of the gluteus maximus are often weak with an anterior coccyx.

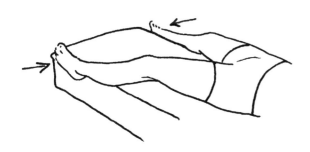

Fig. 7–10 Transversus perinei exercise.

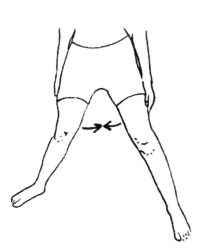

Fig. 7–11 Standing exercise for transversus perinei.

The patient is prone. Flex the knee to 90°. Abduct the hip as far as is comfortable. Then lift the foot toward the ceiling without rotating the leg (Fig. 7–12). Repeat 8 to 10 times.

Exercise 2

A sitting version can be done with tubing. The tubing is secured around the back of the neck and held tight on the opposite side. The other end is secured to the knee. Sit on the edge of the chair and abduct and flex the hip; take up all slack in the tubing and move the knee toward the floor, keeping the knee abducted (Fig. 7–13).

FIFTH SEGMENT OF THE PSOAS

The lower psoas and iliacus can be isolated when found weak. The fifth segment of the psoas is often weak from lifting injuries that occur upon rising up.

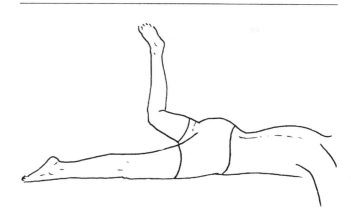

Fig. 7–12 Exercising the lower Q-L and coccygeal fibers of the gluteus maximus.

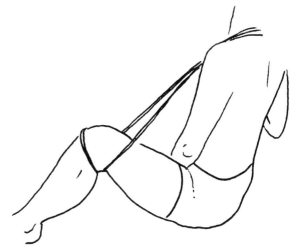

Fig. 7–13 Sitting exercise for lower Q-L and coccygeal fibers of the gluteus maximus.

In the sitting position, secure the tubing over the knee and the other end under the opposite foot. Take up all slack, and lift the knee toward the chest. This will work the whole psoas. By bending forward, further flexing the spine and hip, the lower psoas fibers and the iliacus can be isolated (Fig. 7–14).

These last three exercises are the most important in the rehabilitation of the unstable pelvis.

HIP AND WAIST EXERCISES

Adductors

The pull is to and beyond the opposite leg into adduction (Fig. 7–15). With each repetition, move the foot forward, and then reverse direction and move posteriorly, stepping over the tubing and progressing three or four increments into extension (Fig. 7–16).

Abductors

Stand with the tube secured at foot level and secure firmly around the ankle. With the knee straight, abduct the hip to a comfortable end point (Fig. 7–17). With each successive repetition, move the foot forward three or four increments and then back to a point three or four increments behind the opposite foot, stepping over the tubing as you pass neutral.

Repeat this sequence with the knee bent and the waist muscles more activated (Fig. 7–18).

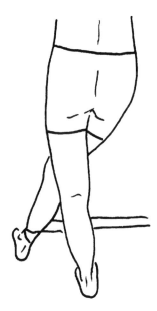

Fig. 7–15 Adduction exercise—anterior starting position.

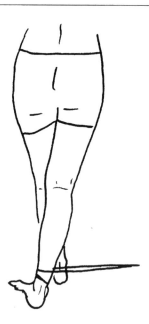

Fig. 7–16 Adduction exercise—posterior ending position.

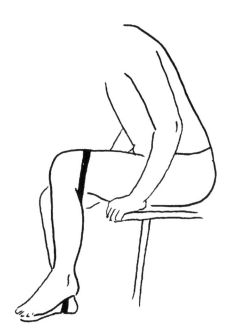

Fig. 7–14 Sitting exercise for lower psoas and iliacus.

These exercises should be done bilaterally. Any positions that seem weaker should be stressed with extra repetitions.

LORDOTIC LUMBAR EXERCISES

The lordotic lumbar syndrome (LLS) is a most common finding in chiropractic practice. The sedentary lifestyle of the modern age will weaken the support system of the erect body unless it is properly exercised.

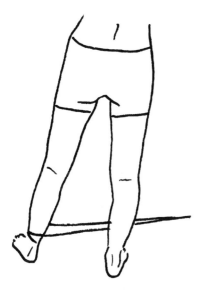

Fig. 7–17 Abduction exercise.

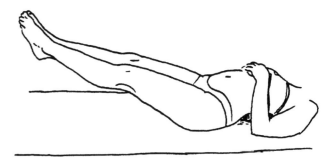

Fig. 7–19 Active bilateral SLR. Note increased lordosis and pubic symphysis lower than anterior superior iliac spine indicative of weak abdominals.

ors can go to work properly. They are likely weak, and in most cases will be dysfunctioning proprioceptively.

When this finding is positive, press on the lower abdomen and support the abdominals. Then have the patient attempt a bilateral SLR (Fig. 7–20). The difference should be significant, which can be a good example for compliance.

The following exercise can tone the gluteals and abdominals as well as reestablish normal proprioceptive function. Have the patient lie supine and place 5 to 10 lbs of weight on the abdomen below the umbilicus. Bend one knee, and place the foot on the floor. Raise the pelvis off the floor with that leg (Fig. 7–21). At the same time, rotate the pelvis posteriorly. Hold for 5 to 6 seconds. Repeat 6 to 8 times and reverse sides. Depending on the chronicity of the case, several sessions a day can be prescribed. This works both the gluteals and the abdominals.

When instructing the patient in this exercise, it may be necessary to consciously reeducate the patient to use the abdominals to posteriorly rotate the pelvis, rocking it back and

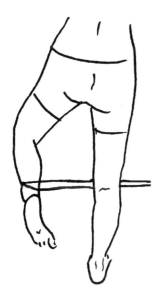

Fig. 7–18 Abduction exercise with knee bent.

The patient with LLS has a chronic anteriorly rotated pelvis with stretched and weakened abdominals, gluteus maximus, and possibly the piriformis muscles. The iliacus and psoas will be hypertonic and in need of stretching.

Test for abdominal function in LLS patients by having them attempt a bilateral straight leg raise (SLR). If the pelvis tilts anteriorly before the legs lift off, it is a sign that the abdominals are not participating properly (Fig. 7–19). They should be contracting and stabilizing the pelvis so the hip flex-

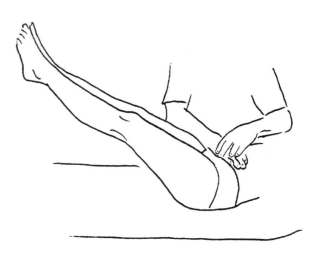

Fig. 7–20 Active bilateral SLR with abdominal support.

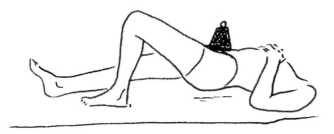

Fig. 7–21 LLS exercise with weight.

forth. Place a hand on the supine patient's abdomen and the other under the lumbar spine. Actively work the pelvis and have the patient flatten the lumbar spine while attempting to pull the pubis toward the chin. This pelvic rocking exercise will help the patient understand what is necessary to normalize function. This condition is most common in women who have had children. The muscles are weak and often have not reestablished normal proprioceptive integration after being stretched and nonfunctional during pregnancy.

Organic Problems and the Low Back

Organic problems may produce many signs and symptoms, which may include interference with the function of specific muscles. Muscle weakness in the low back and hip should warn the examiner of the possibility of organic problems. Questioning the patient as to other related symptoms will lead to further investigation to rule out organic pathology as a cause or contributor to the complaints of low back, pelvic, or hip problems.

The theories and application of reflex and organ-muscle techniques is controversial. Yet, there is a growing awarness that a common thread links the many applications of the viscerosomatic reflex. The ancient practice of yoga demonstrates a relationship between organs and muscles. The stretching techniques of theraputic yoga are designed to stimulate specific muscles that can affect specific organic functions. The muscles affected by stretching are strikingly similiar to the organ–muscle relationships introduced by Geroge Goodheart in the 1960s.

The work of Frank Chapman, DO,[1] Francis Pottenger, MD,[2] and Terrance Bennett, DC,[3] have introduced concepts of somatic signs and symptoms that can be detected and used to diagnose and influence the function of internal organs, via reflex techniques. Dr. Logan spent many years studying the various methods and became convinced of the validity of applying them clinically. There is little research in this area. The inclusion of these concepts in his teaching comes from his belief in their validity and his desire to perpetuate these helpful methods of treatment and perhaps encourage research to validate their inclusion in accepted treatment protocols in the future. It is up to each individual practitioner to apply these techniques and determine if they offer any consistent way to improve the health of their patients. I have used these techniques and found them effective.

FIXATION-ORGAN THEORY

From the begining, chiropractic has emphasized the relation of areas of fixation or subluxation and organic problems. In 1895, D.D. Palmer claimed to have restored the hearing of a patient by adjusting the dorsal spine of a patient—the first chiropractic patient.[4]

Many technique proponents have labeled various areas of the spine as organic places. In 1939, Biron, Wells, and Houser, in *Chiropractic Principles and Technique*,[5] refer to the organic places in use by many chiropractors at that time. The most prominent chiropractic system to propose organic places was the Meric System, which relates organs to specific spinal levels. The levels vary from author to author but are usually no more than one or two vertebral levels apart. It is likely that variations in patient anatomy and methods of palpation account for the differences.

MERIC SYSTEM

T1–2	Heart
T3	Lung
T4–5	Gallbladder
T6–8	Liver
T7–8	Pancreas
T7–11	Small Intestine
T9	Adrenals
T9–11	Kidneys
T12–L1	Ileocecal Valve, Appendix
L5	Uterus, Prostate

Even though there are overlapping areas in the list above, persistent fixations in the area should alert the practitioner to investigate the possibility of organic problems associated with that area. Further investigation may be necessary to differentiate between an undetected structural fault and an organic problem.

NEUROVASCULAR DYNAMICS (NVD)

Terrence Bennett, DC, established reflex areas that he believed related to each organ of the body. He claimed success in some organic problems by using the reflexes as treatment points.

The contact points on the ventral surface of the body (Fig. A–1) are either over the location of the organ, or, as Bennett described them, reflexes from the organ or sphincter valves. The contact points along the spine (Fig. A–2) are palpated as

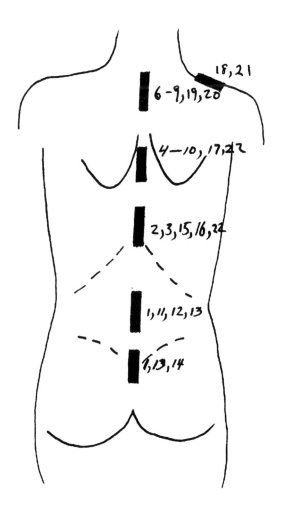

Fig. A–2 Neurovascular dynamics—posterior contact areas.

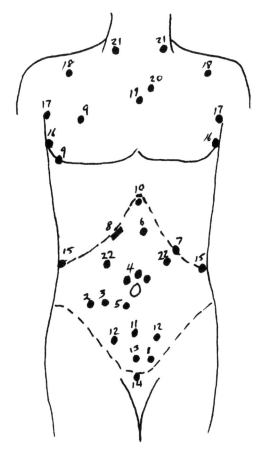

1. internal rectal sphincter	12. ovary/testicle
2. iliocecal valve	13. bladder/prostate
3. appendix	14. urethra
4. small intestine	15. adrenals
5. pyloric valve	16. spleen
6. pancreas head	17. bronchi/lungs
7. pancreas tail	18. bronchi
8. gall bladder	19. cortic sinus
9. liver	20. heart tone
10. cardiac sphincter	21. thyroid
11. uterus	22. kidney

Fig. A–1 Neurovascular dynamics—anterior reflex points.

areas of muscle tension or sensitivity or both. Some of these spinal contacts coincide with the fixation places.

Treatment using NVD consists of passive holding of contacts at the appropriate dorsal and ventral points specific to the organ or system being treated. The physician should stand to the right side of the patient. The right hand should contact the ventral point while the left contacts the dorsal, along the paravertebral tissues. Pressure is light. According to Bennett, the point should be held until a pulsation is felt under the ventral contact hand, signifying a completion of stimulation and a normalization of the viscerosomatic pathways. This pulsation is not always easy to detect. In some cases, it may take several treatments to restore normality. The points should be held for at least 45 seconds to 1 minute. I have had results without feeling the pulsation. If there is no pulsation or no evident results, try reversing position and contacts; the physician on the patient's left side, left hand on ventral points, right hand on dorsal contacts. This may alter polarity between physician and patient.

NVD is a heplful tool in decongesting organs or relaxing visceral muscles and sphincters. It is highly effective in calming down an overactive gastrointestinal (GI) tract in cases of spasm or diarrhea. It is an amazing tool in the treatment of infant colic. Tracing the digestive tract from the internal rectal sphincter to the cardiac sphincter, can quickly relax and normalize function. The same pattern of reflex treatment can activate a sluggish organ as well. The treatment by reflexes seems to normalize the function of the target organ whether it is over- or underactive. The charts for NVD (Figures A–1 and A–2) are expanded to include points for the lungs, heart, and thyroid as Bennett described them. In my experience with NVD, I have had more consistent results with the points for abdominal viscera.

ORGAN–MUSCLE RELATIONSHIPS

Chapman, an osteopath, found that patients with organic problems usually had related areas of sensitivity. Like Bennett, he found related dorsal and ventral areas of sensitivity, although they are not similiar in location. Chapman claimed sucess in treating these areas by goading.

George Goodheart, DC, introduced to the profession the importance of muscle balance and function as part of diagnosis and treatment.[6] He found that patients with known organic problems had specific muscles that tested weak (Table A–1). He discovered that goading of the Chapman reflex points related to the organ resulted in an increased response in the muscle's strength.

With further testing, Goodheart found that in the presence of organic problems the reflexes would be present and the muscle would be inhibited. If the muscle was injured, however, there was no reciprocal organ dysfunction. Goodheart

theorized that the relation was via common lymphatic drainage channels that are affected by goading. He coined the term neurolymphatic (NL) reflexes to describe his findings.

CLINICAL PROOF—METHODOLOGY

The foregoing description of NVD and NL is an interpretation of the work of Chapman, Goodheart, and Bennett and does not necessarily reflect the theories as originally presented. Further study is the prerogative of the reader. The following is Dr. Logan's account of his attempt to prove clinically, at the Anglo-European College of Chiropractic, the theories of NVD, muscle weakness, fixations, and NVD.

To prove or disprove the organ-muscle relationship, it was necessary to prove or disprove the fixation and NVD theories. Several things had to be considered:

- If a patient with organic symptoms presented with a muscle weakness, would the fixation be present? Would the NVD reflex be present?
- If a fixation is persistent, returning time after time, and other postural and functional faults have been corrected, would the muscle related to the organ that is related to the fixation be weak?
- If distortions in the posture can be related to one muscle or muscle group, would investigation find that the fixation is present? With further investigation, would the patient have clinical or subclinical symptoms of organic problems?
- If a muscle is inhibited from functioning as a result of an organ dysfunction, would the muscle respond if the NVD reflexes were used?

Table A–1 Organ/Muscle/Fixation Relationship

Symptoms	Organ	Muscle	Fixation
1. Inverted foot	Bladder	Peroneus tertius	L4–5
2. Low back	Bladder	Piriformis	L4–5
3. Everted foot	Urethra	Anterior tibialis	L5–S1
4. Knee problems	Gall bladder	Popliteus	T4–5
	Small intestine	Quad. femoris	T7–11
5. Low Back	Uterus	Glut. max and med	L5
6. Bowel	Colon	Tensor fascia lata, iliotibial tract	L4–5
7. Menopause	Adrenal	Sartorius	T9
8. Appendicitis	Appendix	Quadratus lumborum	L1
9. Bowel	Ileocecal valve	Quadratus lumborum	L1
10. Urinary	Kidney	Psoas	T9–11
11. Digestion	Stomach	Pectoralis major—clavicular division	T6–7
12. Digestion	Pancreas	Latissimus dorsi	T7–8
13. Digestion	Gall bladder	Popliteus	T4–5
		Pectoralis major—sternal division	T4–5
14. Respiration	Lung	Deltoids	T3
15. Shoulder-heart	Heart	Subscapularis	T1–2
16. Shoulder-thyroid	Thyroid	Infraspinatous teres minor	C7–T1
17. Endonasal	Endonasal	Upper trapezius	C1

- If a muscle is inhibited from functioning as a result of an organ dysfunction, would the muscle respond to adjustment of the fixation?

I used several methods to find the answers. Students in several postgraduate classes were instructed to dine on spicy Mexican or Italian food for lunch. Upon their return to class, all the muscles related to digestion were tested and retested during the remaining three hours after the meal. This was not a scientific study because both the students and examiners were aware of the test. Nevertheless, each time this method was used, the majority of the muscles that presented weak corresponded with the organ required to function at that time during digestion. As the three hours passed and the food passed, the muscles associated with the stomach returned to normal, and those associated with the pancreas, small intestine, and so forth weakened and then returned to normal. It would seem reasonable that, if the muscle is inhibited when the organ is overworked, it should be affected during any dysfunction.

All patients with known (or at least diagnosed) organic symptoms were checked for fixation, NVD reflexes, and muscle weakness. Fixations were found in the majority of the cases with proven organ problems (on ultrasound, radiography, computed tomagraphy, etc.). In several cases where fixations were not present, investigation proved the original diagnosis to be incorrect, with the new diagnosis later being confirmed on surgery. The NVD reflexes were present in most proven organic cases. One exception was the presence of stones in the gallbladder. The reflex was not always present without symptoms. A reasonable explanation is that, where stones are present and are not blocking the duct, the reflex would not be triggered. Gallstones are present in many individuals who have never experienced symptoms and are an incidental finding on another investigation or surgery. The muscles were affected in almost all the proven organic problems. In the majority of the proven organic cases, fixation, NVD reflex, and muscle inhibition were all present.

Patients who presented with persistent fixations in an area related to an organ were investigated as thoroughly as possible for other structural faults. If the fixations were still persistent, the patients were investigated for organic problems. The number of clinical and subclinical problems was great enough to justify the use of persistent fixation as a major sign of organic disease. Some patients without obvious signs and symptoms limited this investigation. The patients could not ethically be referred for investigation without justification. Of course, some persistent fixations could have been, and probably were, compensatory for problems not found on the examination.

One procedure used on several occasions with classes of both students and doctors of chiropractic in a workshop setting involved the reflex relationship between the popliteus muscle,

T4–5, and gallbladder. Without explanation, the students were instructed to examine each other in the erect posture for flexion-hyperextension of the knees and to examine in the supine posture with the legs suspended by the heels (for those hyperextended without weight-bearing). Those with bilateral hyperextension were eliminated from the test. Using only those cases with unilateral hyperextended knees, the students were instructed to test the popliteus muscles bilaterally. Ninety-six percent of the hyperextended knees (mostly left knees) tested weak compared with the opposite knee. Careful palpation in the supine position found fixation at T4–5 in all cases. In two groups, I adjusted each student in the supine position, and in two other groups, the students were adjusted by the examiners, both with similiar results. Seventy-seven percent of those adjusted revealed upon reexamination that both the weakness and the hyperextension were eliminated. Of the remainder, six responded when NVD was used. One failed to respond; he reported that he had recently had an injury to the knee.

One can only conclude that, if the gallbladder is under stress,

- a fixation will be present at T4–5
- the popliteus muscle will test weak
- the affected knee will be hyperextended
- the NVD reflexes will be present
- by adjusting the T4–5 fixation, a response may be expected by the weak popliteus muscle (with no direct neurologic explanation) most of the time
- use of the NVD reflex (passive) after all else fails may produce improved function of the popliteus muscle (with no neurological explanation) and possibly will help gallbladder function

The value of the above testing is proved often. When an examination reveals a hyperextended knee, a tight, sensitive area is usually present under the right rib cage, and a persistent T4–5 fixation is present. Inquiry into symptoms of gallbladder dysfunction many times surprises patients because they usually do not believe that a relationship exists between the gallbladder symptoms and their structural problems. With the use of organ–muscle relationships and subsequent investigation into the organ problems, the treatment program must be improved.

OPINION

Nothing is absolute. Each reflex, fixation, and muscle test requires judgement on the examiner's part to determine the reflex, the degree of fixation, or the loss of normal strength or both. Accuracy again depends on the degree of experience and ability of the examiner. To cloud the issue further, patient reaction varies from individual to individual.

Most signs and symptoms accepted by the medical community also require the judgement of the examiner and patient reaction. One study in Australia (where, with socialized medicine, one would expect fewer needless surgeries) showed that only 57% of the appendicies removed from female patients were pathologic. Other studies in California, showed even a lower percentage of accuracy.[7] The accepted signs of nausea, elevated temperature, rebound tenderness over McBurney's point, and elevated white cell count were the criteria used to determine the necessity for surgery.

If the area of fixation (T12–L1) had been palpated and found sensitive, and if the quadratus lumborum muscle had been tested and found lacking in its normal strength, could needless surgery have been prevented? Would the percentage of pathological appendicies be higher? No one can answer those questions after the fact. If the examiner has the advantage of the additional signs and symptoms provided by the fixation, NVD and organ–muscle relationships, however, the diagnosis must certainly be more accurate.

There definitely is validity to the existence of an organic place, and this should be taught in palpation and examination and as a part of diagnosis together with accepted diagnostic signs and symptoms. NVD reflexes are valuable in the diagnosis and treatment of organic problems and should be taught as a part of diagnosis as well as technique. The organ–muscle relationship is sufficiently correct to include it as one of the signs and symptoms of organic disease and as part of structural analysis.

Using the three theories as a cross-check, some of the muscles proposed by applied kinesiologists proved clinically incorrect, but the majority proved correct. Only those proved correct are discussed here. Most of the NVD points coincided with the affected muscles and fixations. The fixations were found to be consistently correct in known, proven organic problems. None of the above is intended to endorse or discredit applied kinesiology. The neurolymphatic reflexes were not used as a part of the tests because my intention was to cross-check NVD. Therefore, the validity of treatment through the use of the neurolymphatic reflexes was not a consideration.

A knowledge of normal muscle function is necessary to enable the examiner to detect malfunction or dysfunction or both. Determining the cause requires investigation and should include orthopaedic testing, neurologic testing, palpation for fixations, muscle testing, and testing of all the reflexes known to be helpful in arriving at a correct diagnosis. The use of organ–muscle relationships, fixations, and NVD reflexes helps in determining that an organ problem exists, pinpointing the organ involved, and adding to existing accepted medical diagnostic signs and symptoms. Their use can only enhance the diagnostic ability of our profession.

The examples used above are related to muscles affecting the knee. They may also relate to muscles affecting the low back, hip and pelvis. For instance, persistent weakness of the gluteus maximus should lead to an investigation of the reproductive system. Kidney problems can affect the psoas.

REFERENCES

1. Owens C. *An Endocrine Interpretation of Chapman's Reflexes.* Colorado Springs, Colo: American Academy of Osteopathy; 1937.

2. Pottenger F. *Symptoms of Visceral Disease.* St. Louis, Mo: Mosby; 1953.

3. Bennett T. *A New Clinical Basis for the Correction of Abnormal Physiology.* Des Moines, Iowa: Foundation for Chiropractic Education and Research; 1967.

4. Palmer DD. *The Science, Art and Philosophy of Chiropractic.* Portland, Oreg: Portland Printing House Co; 1910.

5. Biron W, Welles B, Houser R. *Chiropractic Principles and Technique.* Chicago, Ill: National College of Chiropractic; 1939.

6. Goodheart G. Applied Kinesiology Notes. Presented at Applied Kinesiology Seminars; 1972–1976.

7. Chang A. An Analysis of the Pathology of 3003 Appendices. *Aust NZ J Surg.* 1981;151:169–178.

Physical Therapeutics

Depending on the approach of the individual practitioner, the use of therapeutic modalities can be employed to enhance the healing process. Below, I have listed the modalities that Dr. Logan and I have found consistently effective in controlling the inflammatory and repair processes. This is not intended to be a complete list or to discount other modalities that are in wide use.

CRYOTHERAPY

The use of ice to control pain and inflammation is recognized as an efficient method in the acute stage of injury. Unfortunately, many medical practitioners continue to advise patients to put heat on a fresh strain/sprain injury, which will, more often than not, cause an increase in swelling.

I recommend my patients use ice on any injury they are unsure of unless there is obvious muscle spasm. Less harm will be done. Most people want to use heat because it feels better. Ice will reduce circulation and control pain more effectively with fewer side effects than medication.

Ice is best used in the acute stage of inflammation—the first 8 to 72 hours. The most efficient and effective method is a 30 minute interrupted session (10 minutes on, 10 off, and 10 on again). It is my understanding that this interrupted method will maximize the decrease in temperature for the longest time (over 60 minutes). The frequency should vary with the severity of the injury. The most frequent application would allow 1 hour between sessions. Patients with less severe injuries should apply ice three to six times per day.

HEAT

The use of heat is best in subacute and chronic conditions. It aids in the relaxation of tight muscles and increases circulation. The use of heat in too acute a case will likely increase swelling.

There is some controversy over the use of wet or dry heat. I believe that wet heat will affect deeper tissues, but the difference is probably insignificant. The use of moist heat is often awkward for home therapy and an electrical heating pad is usually sufficient. An easy way to do moist heat therapy at home is to microwave a damp towel. It will hold heat for about 15 minutes.

I recommend heating for no more than 20 minutes. If multiple sessions are recommended, there should be an hour break between sessions to minimize the possibility of a recurrence of swelling.

HOT/COLD

The alternating of heat and ice is a very effective way to create a tissue flushing effect in the subacute or chronic stages. The alternate dilation and constriction of blood vessels in the injured tissue seems to aid in the exchange of waste products and fresh oxygen and repair materials. It is effective in controlling muscle spasm while also reducing the propensity for swelling in some tricky acute strain/sprain injuries where the muscles are prone to spasm.

The method I have used most successfully is to alternate for 10 minutes each, heat, then cold, then heat again. I have the patient do four 10-minute heat sessions with a 10-minute ice session in between. In other words, four heat sessions with three ice sessions interspersed, so that the patient starts and ends with heat. If you are concerned about inflammation, have the patient end the session with ice. This is a lengthy process taking about 90 minutes. I will have the patient do this one to two times a day for two to five days.

HEAT/RANGE OF MOTION

When the patient is approaching the end of the subacute stage and is beginning rehab exercises, the use of heat for 10 minutes prior to a range of motion exercise can be effective in increasing circulation and relaxing tight muscles. If the patient notices any increased pain after such a workout, have them ice down afterward.

ELECTRICAL STIMULATION—SINE WAVE

There are a number of sophisticated electrical stimulation instruments available, from sine wave generators to interferential and microcurrent instruments. I have found the use of simple sine wave to be helpful in reducing muscle tension. In some cases of severe spasm, I have used tetanizing sine to fatigue muscles that would not relax with manual techniques. The use of intermittent sine with heat is an excellent way to work muscles in injured areas without irritating damaged joints.

ULTRASOUND

Ultrasound can be helpful in the subacute and chronic stages when the need to break up congestion and reduce the tendency for serous exudate to coagulate and begin the formation of collagenous scar tissue.

Index

Notes

Notes

Notes

Notes

Notes

Notes

23494704R00118

Printed in Great Britain
by Amazon